D1323562

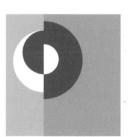

Macleod's
Clinical OSCEs

For Elsevier:
Content Strategist: *Laurence Hunter*
Content Development Specialist: *Fiona Conn*
Project Manager: *Andrew Riley*
Designer: *Miles Hitchen*
Illustration Manager: *Karen Giacomucci*
Illustrator: *Robert Britton*

Macleod's

Clinical OSCEs

Paul O'Neill
BSc(Hons), MBChB, FRCP (Lon), MD, FAcadMed, FHEA
Professor of Medical Education, University of Manchester;
Honorary Consultant Physician, University Hospital of South
Manchester NHS Foundation Trust, Manchester, UK

Alexandra Evans
MBChB, MRCGP, DRCOG, DFRSH
General Practitioner, Brooklands Medical Practice,
Manchester, UK

Tim Pattison
BSc, MBChB, MRCP, MSc, PGCert (Med Ed)
Consultant, Department of Ageing and Complex Medicine,
Salford Royal NHS Foundation Trust, Manchester, UK;
Honorary Lecturer, University of Manchester, Manchester, UK

Meriel Tolhurst-Cleaver
MA (Cantab), MB BChir, MRCPCH
Paediatric Specialist Trainee, North Western Deanery, UK

Serena Tolhurst-Cleaver
MBChB, MRCP(Lon), FFICM, PGCert(MMC)
Consultant in Intensive Care Medicine, Salford Royal NHS
Foundation Trust, Manchester, UK

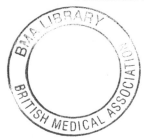

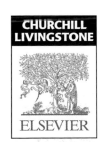

CHURCHILL
LIVINGSTONE

ELSEVIER

Edinburgh London New York Oxford Philadelphia St Louis Sydney Toronto 2016

CHURCHILL
LIVINGSTONE
ELSEVIER

ISBN   978-0-7020-5481-5

British Library Cataloguing in Publication Data
A catalogue record for this book is available from the British Library

Library of Congress Cataloging in Publication Data
A catalog record for this book is available from the Library of Congress

Printed in China
Last digit is the print number: 9 8 7 6 5 4 3 2 1

Contents

Preface

Objective Structured Clinical Examinations (OSCEs) or their variants are now almost universal formats in either postgraduate or undergraduate assessments. This is why there have been increasing references to these in successive editions of *Macleods Clinical Examination* and, in the latest edition, a chapter focused on OSCEs.

This new book takes the chapter in the *Macleods Clinical Examination* and expands and builds on it so that *Macleod's Clinical OSCEs* is a self-contained guide to the likely structure, domains and content of an OSCE with an easy-to-understand framework for revision. The two books are inter-connected and complementary, but *Macleod's Clinical OSCEs* focuses entirely on passing and doing well in a clinical examination.

We have provided a complete set of mark sheets online (http://coursewareobjects.elsevier. com/objects/elr/ExpertConsult/Oneill/macleod1e/PDFs/) which, together with access to *Macleod's Clinical Examination* video material (http://coursewareobjects.elsevier.com/ objects/elr/ExpertConsult/Oneill/macleod1e/videos/), mean that you can work with your friends and colleagues in preparation for the OSCE. We strongly recommend this collaborative approach to OSCEs as this will reinforce everybody's learning and will bring out all the detail, tips and approaches we have included in *Macleod's Clinical OSCEs*.

Acknowledgement

Peter Yeates was instrumental in planning this book and drafting some chapters. We are very grateful for his input and creativity. We all benefit from very supportive partners and loving families and want to dedicate this book to them.

Introduction to the OSCE

Introduction to the book

This book is designed to give you an approach to each type of OSCE station that you are likely to encounter but does not contain every possible OSCE scenario. It is not just a collection of facts or lists but is a workbook to help you prepare effectively. Often the approach to a station is as important as the underlying knowledge.

Use this book later on in your revision so you can have it as a guide to practice in conditions as close to your examination as possible. We suggest not using this book in the initial revision stages or simply reading it cover to cover, as it does not contain all of the required knowledge. Other books in the *Macleod's Clinical Examination* series will be more useful in the early revision stages, such as *Macleod's Clinical Examination* or *Macleod's Clinical Diagnosis*.

This introduction gives you some hints and tips for the OSCE as well as how to use the book within a revision programme. You should use it to practise real-time stations in groups so you can learn from each other under examination conditions. For ease, we have divided station types into six chapters,

- Chapter 2: History taking
- Chapter 3: Examination skills
- Chapter 4: Practical skills
- Chapter 5: Communication, ethics and explanation
- Chapter 6: Prescribing and handover
- Chapter 7: Acutely unwell patients

Each chapter contains a broad range of scenarios that could be tested in OSCEs. Each scenario follows the same template that highlights important points. Some of these are about how to approach the station; some relate to clinical knowledge and expertise. We have included hazard warnings for key points in the station and also a guide on how to excel or common mistakes that are made. We have included online mark-sheets and other material to structure and guide your learning.

Each station is graded as below, but many have station extensions that make the station more (or less) complex. You can also think of your own variations to each station. Obviously the OSCE that you take will depend on your level of experience, with more complex stations coming later in your career.

Basic stations — These are designed for candidates who are taking their first OSCE, usually at the start of clinical practice. They are often based on one particular skill, such as performing an examination or a practical procedure.

Intermediate stations — These are designed for candidates who are further on in their training and may combine some diagnostic and clinical reasoning skills or data interpretation and explanation.

Advanced stations — These are likely to come at the end of medical school or in postgraduate exams. They include focused examinations, often combining a number of skills to be close to a real clinical experience. Candidates who have spent extensive time with patients are more likely to perform well. Timing is always crucial in these complex situations.

We realise that exams can be very stressful, but would encourage you to use this book with friends to help each other. The best way to pass the OCSE is to practise the OSCE. In the words of Arnold Palmer, 'The more I practice, the luckier I get.'

What is an OSCE?

1.1

An OSCE is an Objective Structured Clinical Examination, which has been in common use for over twenty years. OSCEs are becoming increasingly sophisticated and more like real clinical situations, rather than a test of a particular skill (Fig. 1.1.1). They often contain an element of different skills, such as taking a history, interpreting a relevant result and then explaining to the patient.

OSCEs were developed to reduce the variability in marking candidates. In an ideal assessment, the variability in scores should all come from the difference in the competence of the students. Unfortunately, in clinical examinations much of the variability can come from other factors.

The OSCE reduces the variability by decreasing some of these factors. Usually, the OSCE takes the form of a 'circus' with a number of 'stations'. Each station lasts a fixed time and then the student rotates. In this way, all students perform the same task and are asked the same questions by the same examiner(s) at each station. The exam often has between 10 and 20 stations, with each lasting between 5 and 15 minutes and the exam usually taking 1–2 hours.

Each medical school or postgraduate body will design their OSCE differently and you should make sure that you know the following:
• What disciplines are being tested?
• How many stations are there?
• How long is each station?
• What are the different types of station?
• Is this a formative OSCE (designed to improve your performance) or a summative OSCE (i.e., counts towards your overall result – pass/fail)?

We have included some example OSCEs in Section 1.4 that you can use for a complete practice examination cycle.

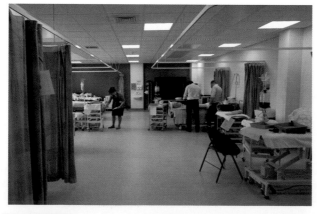

Figure 1.1.1 Clinical skills lab

How to get the most from this book

1.2

You should work through stations with your peers under conditions as close to the examination as possible. We suggest that you practise in groups of two or three (Fig. 1.2.1) and the more realistic you make the session, the more you are going to benefit. You may want to complete one station at a time or use a template (see Appendix) to set up a practice OSCE. You could run a mock OSCE or mini-OSCE with the use of a clinical skills lab and enough volunteers to play all the roles.

Once you have worked through one of the example stations, then we suggest altering it to have a different diagnosis, clinical condition or explanation of a procedure. This way you will be able to practise the same skills, but use different clinical information. In this way you will get the most use out of this book. We have summarised this below in Fig. 1.2.2.

ROLES

The candidate should read only the candidate information. One of you should be the examiner and use the mark-sheets that are provided (on the website). Ideally a third person should be present to assume the role of the patient where this is required. While some stations do not need this (for example, in Chapter 6) you will gain most benefit from the combined feedback of two individuals and your own self-assessment. It is also useful when playing the examiner to watch the candidate and note what is a good performance and what could be improved. Remember you all learn from each other.

TIMING

Run through the station in real time. The examiner should have a stopwatch as it is essential to time the stations as this is a common problem in OSCEs. If your OSCE has standard timings then use these for every station.

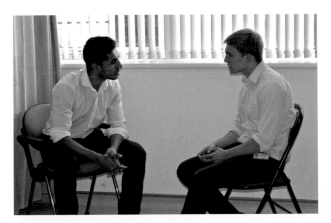

Figure 1.2.1 Reflection and feedback on performance

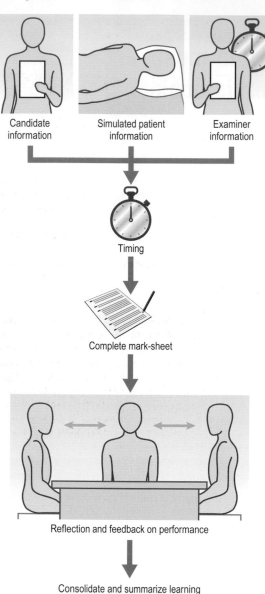

Figure 1.2.2 How to get the most out of the book

Candidate information

Simulated patient information

Examiner information

Timing

Complete mark-sheet

Reflection and feedback on performance

Consolidate and summarize learning

MARK-SHEET COMPLETION

The person playing the examiner should complete the mark-sheet, which is then used for reflection and feedback. The mark-sheets allow you to record specific feedback to review later. An example mark-sheet is included at the end of this chapter with all others available online at http://coursewareobjects.elsevier.com/objects/elr/ExpertConsult/Oneill/macleod1e/PDFs/.

The mark-sheet for your examination may be different, but ours will serve as a guide. When playing the examiner, try to learn from this—what makes you think that a candidate is doing well or badly? What do candidates do to make this easier or more difficult to judge? Share these points as they provide insight into examination technique.

REFLECTION ON FEEDBACK AND PERFORMANCE

To get the most from the book, you must reflect and get feedback on your performance. There are several models of feedback, but the important principle is that the individual thinks about their performance rather than just being told what they have done right or wrong. This encourages deeper learning and will help with performance in examinations and beyond.

The best feedback is as specific as possible. Write down actual quotes of what the candidate said or did. For example, 'I thought it was really good how you asked about allergies and then went on to ask about the specific reaction to each of the drugs' or 'when you tested the reflexes you missed the left biceps reflex.'

Pendleton's feedback rules are simple and provide a structure to enhance learning:
1. Ask the candidate to comment on what went well.
2. The observers (examiner and/or simulated patient) comment on what went well.
3. Ask the candidate what could be improved.
4. The observers comment on what could be improved.
5. Develop an action plan for improvement.

The last point is crucial—the mark-sheets have been designed to help with this. As a group you should discuss the stations including the extensions and record specific points for revision. You should use each station as a platform for learning from each other. Ask probing questions to help you understand why your colleagues have approached a scenario in a particular way—for example, 'You said that you thought the most likely cause of this man's chest pain was cardiac. What made you think this?'

After you have finished your session we suggest using a summary sheet to record what you have learned and what else you need to focus on. We have included an example of a summary sheet with the mark-sheets online and have reproduced it in the Appendix. Keep a collection of these as a useful revision resource.

General tips for OSCE candidates

1.3

ON THE DAY OF THE EXAMINATION

- Try and get a good night's sleep before — don't stay up cramming.
- Dress smartly and appropriately.
- Bring a pen (even better, bring two).
- Bring a stethoscope (but not around your neck).
- Come on time (plan your journey). Remember the hospital might be far away with lots of traffic so leave plenty of time (less stressful).

IN THE OSCE

General tips
- Be as calm as possible.
- Be nice to simulated patients and to examiners — be polite and considerate.
- Watch your time in a station — it is a very common mistake to run out of time — see below for tips on what to do if this happens.
- Be structured in your approaches and presentations.

Whilst preparing for a station
- Move on from the previous station in good time — you need time to prepare.
- *Carefully* read the instructions — these are often specific in what you must do or not do.
- Plan your approach — make a mental tick-list of things to do.

Starting the station (Fig. 1.3.1)
The first 30 seconds are very important. It is important to get this part right as it will help you to relax and focus. It is also a chance to pick up some easy marks. A generic introduction should include:
- Introduce yourself.
- Check the patient's name and identifiers (date of birth/ wristband).
- Explain what you are going to do.
- Get permission.
- Clean your hands.
- Put on gloves if required.

If you are running out of time
- Unless you are very nearly finished, do not carry on as before.
- Think about any important points you have not covered.
- Cover as many broad areas as you can before the finish.
- Don't keep talking after the final buzzer, leave to prepare for the next station.

At the end of the station
- Make a differential diagnosis if required.
- Give the most likely diagnosis and your rationale.

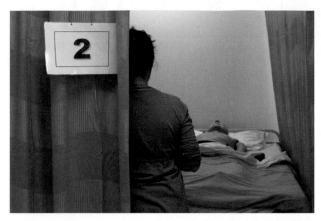

Figure 1.3.1 Starting the station

- Do not worry about getting it wrong as long as you have a sensible explanation.
- Ask (simulated) patients 'Is there anything you would like to ask me or is there anything you are not sure about?' This is a good way of making sure you have not missed anything.
- If it is a test you are performing on the patient, explain how and when they will get the result.
- If you are suggesting any follow-up, say when this might be.
- Thank the examiner and simulated patient.

If you think you are not doing well in a station
- Do not panic.
- Try not to let a poor performance on one station affect your performance on the rest.
- You may not have done as badly as you thought.
- Even if you have failed, this is only a small proportion of the exam and there will be more stations to come.

On examiners
- Examiners will normally be doing the same station many times.
- They will be swayed towards giving you better marks if you get the introduction right and are confident in your approach.
- They expect you to be nice and interact with and respond to the patient.
- They are generally sympathetic and want you to pass the exam if possible.
- They may write both positive and negative comments on mark-sheets — do not second-guess your mark, focus on the task.
- Do not make things up!

On simulated patients
- They are acting a role.
- They will not tell you all the information straight away.
- They will often give you hints or cues — don't miss these.
- Avoid using medical jargon with them.
- Summarise regularly.
- Check the understanding of the patient.
- Interact with them — respond to what they say rather than going through a checklist of answers.

Specimen OSCEs

1.4

We have included some examples of potential OSCE examinations which you can use as a 'complete' examination.

Basic — short 'mini OSCE' — could be completed in about an hour.
- Station 2.1 Pains in the chest
- Station 6.4 Prescribing insulin
- Station 3.13 Knee examination
- Station 2.4 Abdominal pain
- Station 4.4 Capillary blood glucose measurement
- Section 5.2 Consent for gastroscopy (basic station extension)

Advanced OSCE — could be used at finals level and designed to test the competency of a newly qualified doctor. We have included 15 stations as this reflects usual practice.
- Station 7.2 Acute management of breathlessness 1
- Station 3.10 The patient with a tremor
- Station 4.5 Urinary catheter insertion
- Station 2.8 A child with fits
- Station 6.7 Referring a patient
- Station 5.9 Discuss a 'do not resuscitate' order
- Station 4.7 Suturing a wound
- Station 7.7 Acute management of postpartum bleeding
- Station 6.3 Prescribing postoperative fluids
- Station 5.11 A dissatisfied relative
- Station 3.5 Chronic liver disease
- Station 2.5 Collapse
- Station 5.4 Explaining a new diagnosis of type 2 diabetes
- Station 6.6 Prescribing antibiotics
- Station 3.3 The breathless patient

Sample mark-sheet and summary of learning sheet

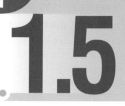

1.5

This sheet is for station 3.1 Examination of the cardiovascular system. (The full set of mark-sheets for all 65 stations can be found at http://coursewareobjects.elsevier.com/objects/elr/ExpertConsult/Oneill/macleod1e/PDFs/.)

1. Introduction and approach to the patient

No elements   All elements

| 1 | 2 | 3 | 4 | 5 |
| ☐ | ☐ | ☐ | ☐ | ☐ |

2. Communication with patient

No elements   All elements

| 1 | 2 | 3 | 4 | 5 |
| ☐ | ☐ | ☐ | ☐ | ☐ |

3. Inspection of patient and palpation of pulses

No elements   All elements

| 1 | 2 | 3 | 4 | 5 |
| ☐ | ☐ | ☐ | ☐ | ☐ |

4. Auscultation and augmentation of murmurs/heart sounds

No elements   All elements

| 1 | 2 | 3 | 4 | 5 |
| ☐ | ☐ | ☐ | ☐ | ☐ |

5. Differential diagnosis

No elements   All elements

| 1 | 2 | 3 | 4 | 5 |
| ☐ | ☐ | ☐ | ☐ | ☐ |

6. Discussion of further tests

No elements   All elements

| 1 | 2 | 3 | 4 | 5 |
| ☐ | ☐ | ☐ | ☐ | ☐ |

Overall impression

Clear fail	Borderline fail	Pass	Good	Excellent
1	2	3	4	5
☐	☐	☐	☐	☐

Please record specific feedback below for discussion:

1

SPECIFIC CHECKLIST FOR THIS STATION

1. Introduction and approach to the patient
- Introduces themselves to patient
- Ensures privacy and comfort of patient
- Optimises examination environment (patient positioning and exposure)
- Hand hygiene prior to examination

2. Communication with patient
- Obtains consent for examination
- Polite and courteous throughout
- Sets patient at ease
- Explains actions throughout, appropriate pace of examination

3. Inspection of patient and palpation of pulses
- Inspects in a systematic fashion
- Comments on any positive findings
- Tests for radio-radial delay and collapsing pulse, and palpates a central pulse
- Measures pulse rate
- Examines the JVP
- Palpates for apex beat and ventricular heave

4. Auscultation and augmentation of murmurs/heart sounds
- Auscultates in systematic fashion over correct areas
- Takes the pulse during auscultation
- Listens with bell and diaphragm
- Performs appropriate manoeuvres to improve quality of any murmurs
- Listens for radiation of murmurs in appropriate positions
- Listens at lung bases (or states they would do this)

5. Differential diagnosis
- Gives a logical differential diagnosis
- Gives most likely diagnosis
- Explains positive and negative features suggesting most likely diagnosis

6. Discussion of further tests
- Discusses following investigations with reasons why they are required
- Explains what they would be looking for in each investigation
- Tests may include ECG, full blood count, U&Es, CXR, echocardiography, cardiac angiography

SUMMARY OF LEARNING SHEET

This summary of learning sheet can also be found at http://coursewareobjects. elsevier.com/objects/elr/ExpertConsult/Oneill/macleod1e/PDFs/.

Summarising learning

Date of session

Stations completed

What went well today?

What could be improved on?

What new information did we learn?

What do we need to follow up on?

1

History taking

Introduction to history taking in OSCEs

History taking is a core skill that forms the basis of diagnosis. All OSCEs include history taking stations, often several. In most OSCEs time is limited, and so you will have to be focused in your history taking. Many candidates assume that history taking is easy, and that it is physical examination which requires practice. You will not appear fluent by just reading; it is important to practise ways of phrasing questions and using non-verbal communication.

Usually these stations involve a brief description of the presenting complaint with 1–2 min preparation time. The station then consists of a simulated patient with the examiner observing. Very occasionally, 'real' patients are still used, but this is becoming rare as it is more difficult to standardise these stations. At the end of the station you will usually be asked to summarise, and will often be asked to discuss differential diagnoses and initial management.

➡ KEY SKILLS

Some core knowledge is required to take a tailored history, as well as experience in recognising the patterns of symptoms in different conditions. It is impossible to cover all the possible conditions that could appear in OSCEs. However, this chapter covers some of the more frequently encountered history taking stations and also gives you an approach to improve your general technique so that you can better adapt to different situations. For these stations it is important to:

1. Introduce yourself, begin the interview and establish a rapport.
2. Obtain a clear account of the relevant symptoms and allow the patient to express their problem fully and in their words.
3. Address their symptoms and their ideas about their condition, and explore their concerns and expectations.
4. Summarise and check the accuracy of what you have understood.
5. Suggest likely diagnoses and discuss further investigations and management.

GENERAL HINTS AND TIPS

- Do not write extensively as it can interfere with establishing a rapport. One approach is to use the (1 min) preparation time to note headings and key symptoms that you want to cover.
- Note key statements by the patient to enable accurate summarising.
- Do not ask questions too quickly or interrogate the patient.
- Do not be afraid of brief thinking time. Better to pause than to repeat, mumble or miss out something important. Avoid long awkward silences.
- Do not be so focused on obtaining information that you miss what the patient is saying. Listen for cues. Decide whether to follow at the time, or to acknowledge a cue, and say that you will return to it.
- Allow space when expressing empathy—pause and acknowledge.
- Think about how you use language, particularly technical terms.

2

GENERAL FORMAT

Even in a short station, you can use many parts of the structure set out below. For a longer station, try to include all elements.

Introduction
- Introduce yourself/use appropriate clinical title.
- Obtain permission to speak with the patient.
- Check their details — name/date of birth or age.
- Assure them about confidentiality.

Presenting problem
- Start with an open question: 'I understand you've been breathless. Could you tell me about that please?'
- Listen attentively to response. Avoid interrupting.

History of presenting complaint
- Use further open questions to encourage description of symptoms.
- Focus history with specific closed questions.
- Verbally and non-verbally encourage patient's responses.
- Clarify issues that are uncertain or require expansion.
- Summarise — check accuracy of your understanding.
- Notice and pick up on cues — verbal or non-verbal.
- Acknowledge, legitimise and respond to patient cues.
- Different symptoms are clarified in different ways, but usually include:
  - Characteristics/severity/onset/duration/timing/aggravating/relieving factors/associated symptoms — relevant symptom clusters.
- For common symptoms, have in mind a list of related symptoms which characterise patterns of disease.
- Ask about important *negative symptoms* (i.e., absence).

Important risk factors or red flags
- Depending on the condition, check for important specific risk factors or 'red flags' for the condition.

Past medical history (PMH)
- Ask about both current or active medical conditions and past conditions.
- Use open questions.
- Note dates where possible.
- May need focused questions to exclude some conditions.

Drug history (DH)
- Ask about current medication (or recent — depending on history).
- Ask about over-the-counter or non-prescription medication.

Allergy history
- Enquire about allergies or intolerance to medication.

Family history (FH)
- Ask whether any of their family suffer or suffered from particular problems.

Social history (SH)
- Relevance varies depending on situation.
  - Smoking, alcohol, recreational drug use
  - Diet and exercise
  - Employment

- Home circumstances, relationship status, children, pets
- Functional status/level of help required with activities of daily living (ADLs)
- Recent travel
- There may be issues that are very personal; enquire sensitively into areas that are relevant.

Systems enquiry
- It may not be necessary in an OSCE focused history.
- Be systematic, avoid repetition and phrase questions clearly.

Patient perspective
- Three distinct parts:
  - Ideas (I): what the patient knows, or thinks. What they think might be wrong; what they have heard about this condition.
  - Concerns (C): worries or fears that arise in response to either their ideas or the information that you may give.
  - Expectations (E): what they think will happen if symptoms are treated or untreated. What they hope will happen next, or what you should do.
- ICE do not need to be kept to the end. They are often best addressed as they arise, by noticing and responding to cues.

Giving information
- You may repeat your summary, depending on time.
- Check whether they want to know your provisional diagnosis(es).
- Explain this or these in plain language—check their understanding.

Develop plan
- Discuss the plan and next steps—investigations or treatment.
- Often examiners will discuss diagnosis/investigations or management.

Conclude
- Address any outstanding questions the patient may have.
- Thank them.

The best way to practise these stations is with a colleague, with one of you taking the role of candidate, and the other the role of the simulated patient. All of the stations include a script for the simulated patient. If there are a group of you, then another person can act as the examiner using the mark-sheets provided, with any others being additional observers.

2

Chest pain

2.1

CANDIDATE INFORMATION

Background: You are the junior doctor in a general practice and are seeing Mr Keith Jones (58 years old), who is complaining of chest pain.

Task: Please take a history from Mr Jones and discuss the diagnosis with the patient.

APPROACH TO THE STATION

This type of station is common in OSCEs and, as with all history stations, you must plan your time and decide how long you are going to allocate to each section. Remember the marks will be allocated between the history and discussion, so even if you take a perfect history, but take 10 minutes, you will only get a portion of the marks.

Given that the patient is a middle-aged male, the most likely diagnosis is cardiac chest pain and atypical features should not necessarily put you off (high 'pre-test probability'). You should consider the differential diagnosis of chest pain before you start and listen for cues in the story that point towards the diagnosis.

A general approach when someone complains of pain is to listen for the features captured by the mnemonic **SOCRATES** — **S**ite, **O**nset, **C**haracter, **R**adiation, **A**ssociated features, **T**iming and **S**everity.

PATIENT INFORMATION

Name: Mr Keith Jones   **Age:** 58 years   **Sex:** Male

Occupation: Labourer on building site

Presenting symptom: Chest pain

You have been having pains in your chest on and off for the past month. Prior to this you have never had any chest pain. Initially you thought that it was indigestion and took some antacids but they did not help.

The pain feels like tightness in the middle of your chest. It came on when you were walking to work. When it comes on, you stop and the pain goes away within a few minutes. The first time it happened, you kept walking and the pain got worse and went into your jaw. You have had the pain about once a week for the past 4 weeks. It has never lasted for more than 5 minutes.

Other symptoms (if asked): No breathlessness, cough (including blood), leg swelling or pain. You do a lot of lifting at work but don't remember injuring yourself.

Other medical problems: You have had high blood pressure for 5 years and you take Ramipril 5 mg.

You work as a bricklayer and have done all your life. You have smoked 20 cigarettes a day since you were 16 years old. You have not drunk alcohol for over 10 years.

In your family, your father had angina from his 40s. He died at the age of 60 from a heart attack.

If asked:

Ideas: You thought it was indigestion at first but now you're worried that it may be your heart. You understand what angina is as your dad had it from the age of 40.

Concerns: You are worried as your father died of a heart attack at 60. You also don't want to give up work.

Expectations: You hope the doctor will take your pain seriously and tell you what's wrong.

2

CLINICAL KNOWLEDGE AND EXPERTISE

Cues that point towards the diagnosis are known as **positive diagnostic factors**. Those that suggest an alternative diagnosis are known as negative diagnostic factors.

Positive diagnostic factors in chest pain
- Ischaemic/cardiac pain
  - Onset with exercise, relieved by rest
  - Central dull/tight pain, radiates to arm/jaw
  - More concerning if pain is worsening or occurring at rest
  - Presence of cardiac risk factors
- Pulmonary embolism
  - Associated with shortness of breath
  - Pleuritic pain
  - Sudden onset
  - Risk factors for thromboembolism
- Oesophageal spasm
  - Associated with indigestion
  - Usually described as a burning pain
  - Related to eating
  - Relieved by antacids.
  - Can be very similar to cardiac pain
- Muscular pain
  - History of chest wall or muscular injury
  - Pain on movement (and possibly tenderness over chest wall)
- Aortic dissection (rare)
  - 'Tearing' interscapular pain
  - Neurological features (branches of aortic arch)
  - Differential blood pressure, absent pulses
  - Shock

2

Box 2.1.1	Main risk factors for cardiac disease

- Increasing age and male
- Hypertension
- Hypercholesterolaemia
- Smoking and obesity
- Other vascular disease—stroke, peripheral vascular disease
- Diabetes
- Family history of cardiac disease

The main **negative diagnostic factors** for angina are if the chest pain is:
- Continuous or very prolonged
- Unrelated to activity
- Brought on by breathing and association with symptoms such as dizziness, palpitations, tingling or difficulty swallowing.

Main risk factors for cardiac disease
See Box 2.1.1.

 WARNING

If the history suggests an acute coronary syndrome this needs urgent assessment in hospital. If appropriate, at the end of the station, you should inform the patient to attend hospital immediately if they develop:
- Cardiac pain lasting more than 15 min at a time
- Associated symptoms of sweating, breathlessness
- Pain occurring on minimal exertion or at increasing frequency and severity.

✓	How to excel in this station	
Action	**Reason**	**How**
Ask about risk factors.	Show the examiner that you know what the risk factors for cardiac disease are by asking the patient directly if not mentioned.	In this case, if they do not mention any risk factors other than hypertension, then ask 'Can I ask specifically ask if you have diabetes or...'
Explore the patient's personal perspective.	Can impact on acceptance of diagnosis, investigations and treatment.	What do they think is causing the pain? How is it affecting them? Is there anything they are particularly worried about and what do they want from the consultation? If you elicit any concerns, be sure to respond to them.
Explain in everyday language and avoid jargon.	Patients often are confused by medical terms, but may not ask for clarification.	Explain to the patient the likely diagnosis is cardiac chest pain or angina. Ask them if they know what angina means. Give a simple explanation: 'lack of blood flow to the heart due to fatty deposits in the arteries'. Check that the patient understands what you mean.
Counsel the patient about what they can do.	Important to have a focus on patient-centred care and empowerment.	How to minimise risk factors—for example, losing weight, stopping smoking, better control of hypertension (if present). Explain about any drug treatment and advise on the use of a glycerol trinitrate spray. You should offer an information leaflet (http://www.patient.co.uk).

Common error	Remedy	Reason
Use of a 'shopping list'.	Aim to have a 'conversation' with the patient to draw out the information, even allowing for the pressure of an OSCE.	Poor candidates will take a tick box approach (shopping list)—asking a long list of closed questions.
Reliance on closed questions.	Ask the patient to describe the pain in their own words and listen carefully. People will usually mention most of the features of the pain—follow up with a few closed ones.	Easy to put words into the patient's mouth (e.g., a poor candidate may say 'Was the pain stabbing?', whereas a good candidate would say 'Tell me about this pain in as much detail as possible'). Closed questions descend into an interrogation of Yes/No answers.

Common errors in this station

STATION VARIATIONS

○ Advanced

Can be extended to a focused examination of the patient, then explaining a management plan to the patient including a resting ECG and screening for risk factors. You may need to explain referral for further tests—may include an exercise tolerance test or an angiogram. See Chapter 7.1 for more details.

Further reading

Douglas, G., Nicol, F., Robertson, C., 2013. Macleod's Clinical Examination, 14th ed. Chapter 6: Cardiovascular System, Churchill Livingstone.

NICE clinical guideline 95: chest pain of recent onset http://www.nice.org.uk.

NICE clinical guideline 126: management of stable angina http://www.nice.org.uk.

2

A breathless young woman

2.2

CANDIDATE INFORMATION

Background: You are a final year medical student on an attachment in general practice. Kerry is a 22-year-old woman who is short of breath.

Task: Please take a history; near the end of the station, you will be asked to discuss the diagnosis, investigations and initial management with the examiner.

APPROACH TO THE STATION

You've been asked to take a history from a young breathless woman, so what conditions would be common? Although there are a number of possibilities, most likely is asthma followed by infection, pneumonia, pneumothorax or pulmonary emboli. Functional breathing disorders are also common, but as these are complex they are unlikely to included as an intermediate level station. An advanced station could focus on a more complex condition like pulmonary arterial hypertension.

Think about the onset, duration and severity of the breathlessness (rapidity of onset, whether it is constant or episodic) and associated symptoms: fever and sputum, variable wheeze, sharp pain with haemoptysis. Next consider risk factors, lifestyle and their linked medical conditions.

Remember that you must make a diagnosis and be able to justify it. You might want to take a moment before starting to consider investigations and management of each of the differential diagnoses, so that you can be 'smooth' when the examiner questions you at the end.

PATIENT INFORMATION

Name: Ms Kerry Woodloft   **Age:** 22 years   **Sex:** Female

Opening statement: Over the past few months when you go running you feel more breathless, and your chest feels tight. You find this troubling and would like it treated. Recently it has happened once or twice when you've just been walking.

If asked: As well as shortness of breath and chest tightness, you have noticed a dry cough during these episodes. All of these symptoms are worse if it is damp or cold. Also, you have started to wake up a few nights per week coughing and feeling tightchested. Over the past few months these symptoms have gradually increased, although varying each day. You feel moderately breathless, but never had a frightening episode where your breathing was so bad. After running, your symptoms ease gradually. You've noted that using hair spray can make your chest feel tight. You are not really sure of anything else that makes them better or worse. You can't think of anything that started it all.

Previous medical history: Childhood asthma, but it went away in your early teens. You were never hospitalised.

Mild eczema.

No recent colds or infections.

Family history: Nil.

2

Drugs history: Hydrocortisone cream, oral contraceptive pill.

Drug allergies: Nil.

Social history: You recently moved in with your boyfriend, who has a cat and two dogs, and enjoy helping to wash and brush the dogs. You work as a hair stylist. Your boyfriend smokes, and although you know you shouldn't, you've started smoking about five cigarettes/day over the past 6 months.

Ideas: You wonder if this is asthma — it feels a bit like what you had as a child — and whether cigarettes could be responsible, but feel fairly sure that five/day are too few to do any harm. You have not thought of pets or your job as contributing.

Concerns: You're not particularly concerned, but feel annoyed as you were told you would grow out of asthma and it feels unfair.

Expectations: You expect the doctor to prescribe a treatment that will make your symptoms go away. You remember taking an inhaler when you were younger and wouldn't mind taking one again for a bit.

CLINICAL KNOWLEDGE AND EXPERTISE

Often, a diagnosis of asthma can be made just from the history — the likelihood is increased with two or more of the following features:
• Shortness of breath, cough or wheeze, especially if:
  • Worse at night/early morning
  • Worse with exercise/cold air/exposure to allergens
  • Symptoms after taking aspirin or beta blockers
• Presence of atopy (eczema/hay fever)
• Family history of asthma or atopy

Adding a measure of airflow obstruction — ideally spirometry, but possibly peak expiratory flow rate (PEFR) — helps to confirm the diagnosis. These tests should show *variable* airway *obstruction*. Clinical examination which identifies *wheeze* helps, and *eosinophilia* also supports asthma. In less clear-cut cases, or with poor treatment response, further investigations are needed.

You must ask about other situations that might worsen the condition — particularly exposure to allergens or irritants. These might be at home, at work (occupational asthma) or leisure. Ask about whether it is better when away from work for a few days. Always ask about smoking!

2

Try to determine the degree of *control* — use of the '3 questions': In the last week (or month)

1. Have you had difficulty sleeping because of your asthma symptoms (including cough)?
2. Have you had your usual asthma symptoms during the day (cough, wheeze, chest tightness or breathlessness)?
3. Has your asthma interfered with your usual activities (e.g., housework, work/school, etc.)?

Also ask about rescue medication (short acting beta agonists), changes in PEFR, steroid courses (number and date), hospital admissions and whether the patient ever needed ventilatory support. In a new presentation, these will not be relevant.

Non-pharmacological management involves avoiding allergens and stopping smoking. Pharmacological management should use the *lowest* step on the ladder that achieves control (see Fig. 2.2.1). However, you can start higher if the symptoms seem to warrant more intensive treatment. All patients should have an action plan, detailing what to do in an emergency.

This patient has a classical history: *variable* chest tightness (or wheeze), cough and shortness of breath. She has a history of childhood asthma, and is atopic (eczema).

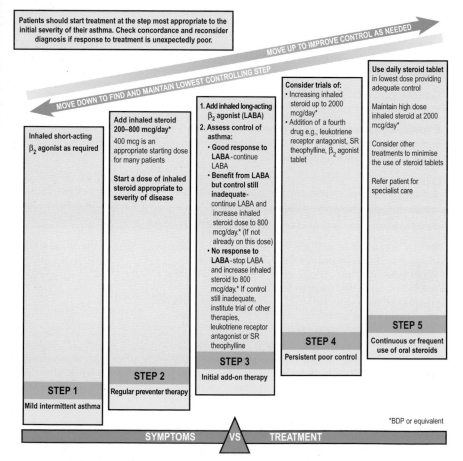

Figure 2.2.1 Stepped management of asthma (From British Thoracic Society asthma guidelines 2012 update, with permission.)

Her symptoms are worsened by cold and damp. More specifically, she is getting frequent exertional symptoms and night-time symptoms—both indicate 'poor control'. Exposure to:

- cigarette smoke
- cats and dogs
- occupational triggers

are all likely to have worsened her condition—through either sensitisation or irritation.

In addition to the history, investigations should show airflow obstruction. With frequent symptoms, she should start treatment at step 2, as well as non-pharmacological measures—stop smoking and consider other exposures (pets/possibly occupation). Response to treatment must be reviewed and increased or decreased appropriately.

2

⚠ WARNING

- Haemoptysis would suggest pulmonary emboli.
- A severe attack might require admission.

How to excel in this station		
Action	**Reason**	**How**
Get a clear description.	Diagnosis, severity and control	Cover the specific symptoms and changes with time. Ask about severity and episodicity. Enquire about night/early morning variation, effect of exercise and whether symptoms interfere with normal activities.
Take a thorough social history.	Linked triggers, impacts on quality of life	Leisure or social activities that make symptoms worse. Ask about pets, smoking and occupation. Ask whether aero-allergens—dust, diesel fumes, air fresheners, etc.—cause or worsen symptoms.
Listen and respond.	Her acceptance of the diagnosis and taking responsibility for its management are crucial	Explore ideas, provide information and then use this to have a dialogue around lifestyle issues. Discuss medication. Explain that she may need long-term treatment, but (with her efforts) symptom control can be very good.

Common errors in this station		
Common error	**Remedy**	**Reason**
Rapid-fire questions.	Not—'symptoms worse at night, early morning, work' but 'tell me about how your symptoms vary'.	Let the story come out in her own words—build relationships, and avoid false tracks and inappropriate weightings.
Use of a checklist approach to symptoms.	Listen first, then clarify or ask.	Don't simply ask about the presence or absence of symptoms in a checklist fashion; characterise each symptom—when/how/how often/how much/what it is like.
Critical of lifestyle—e.g., smoking.	Consider non-verbal as well as verbal communication. Do not judge. Explore, discuss and involve.	Will upset her, break trust in the doctor–patient relationship and reduce her self-efficacy. As with all chronic disease management, asthma relies on patient involvement.

2 STATION VARIATIONS

○ Basic: Patient with known asthma

- You will be asked a basic question about a patient with known asthma such as 'clarify her treatment and also what affects her asthma'. This gives you the structure you require.
- Treatment:
  - Consider the treatment step ladder shown in Fig. 2.2.1.
  - Ask about side effects and compliance.
  - Ask what works for her.
  - Any change recently.
- Consider smoking, lifestyle, occupation, animals and other potential allergens.
- Present your findings in a logical structure and be able to explain your questioning.
- There will be a strong emphasis in the mark-sheet about communication skills.

○ Advanced: Patient with unusual respiratory cause of breathlessness

This would include pulmonary fibrosis, pulmonary hypertension, pulmonary apsergillosis complicating asthma. Consider what would be the pointers towards each of these in the history. For example in bronchiectasis, you need to look for:

- Productive cough with infective exacerbations (green sputum) — quantify amount.
- Frequent courses of antibiotics.
- Use of postural drainage.
- Previous history of lung damage — e.g., tuberculosis.
- Patients with cystic fibrosis — this could form an advanced station on its own.
- If asked — on examination, look for clubbing (chronic pulmonary sepsis), localised crackles.
- Chest radiograph might show focal changes (CT thorax best).

Further reading

2011 revision of the British Thoracic Society/Scottish Intercollegiate Guidelines Network (BTS/SIGN) Asthma Guideline. Full guideline or quick reference guide. Available at: https://www.brit-thoracic.org.uk/guidelines-and-quality-standards/asthma-guideline/.

Persistent diarrhoea

2.3

CANDIDATE INFORMATION

Background: You are a junior doctor in the gastroenterology outpatients and are seeing Justine Olowu (32 years old), who has been referred complaining of persistent diarrhoea.

Task: Please take a history from her, and address any issues that you believe may be important. Towards the end, the examiner will ask you about your differential diagnosis.

APPROACH TO THE STATION

Diarrhoea has a large number of potential causes, and obtaining a clear history—although not always diagnostic—is a key starting point. The background states that the diarrhoea is 'persistent', without making the duration clear—there are many potential causes for chronic diarrhoea. You also need to get a description of the nature of the bowel disturbance, and the presence or absence of related symptoms. Next, specifically consider causes of diarrhoea with any pointers in the history.

Based on the briefing, consider what are the important areas to focus on before starting and then listen for cues as you proceed. Make sure you address the patient's perspective.

PATIENT INFORMATION

Name: Justine Olowu   **Age:** 32 years   **Sex:** Female

Occupation: Temporary work as cleaner in a residential home

Presenting symptom: Diarrhoea and abdominal pain

Opening statement: You've been having diarrhoea most days for just over a month. It has fluctuated, and you kept thinking that it would stop, but it has persisted. The diarrhoea is watery, and has occurred 3–4/day on most days. Your stomach has felt bloated and uncomfortable although not painful. You're a bit embarrassed that you have been passing a lot of wind, which has been offensive. You have been off your food, and you think that you have lost a few pounds. You have generally felt tired.

If asked: You returned from Vietnam 2 weeks before this started—you have assumed that this is not connected. You only drank bottled water, but you did buy a bottle on the way to the airport, and noticed that the seal was already broken. Most of your food was from restaurants, although conditions were often rustic.

(Continued)

2

You've travelled extensively in the developing world in the past and never had stomach problems. On this occasion you stayed for 6 weeks, mostly taking photographs in rural areas.

Although you have been off your food, you have kept drinking plenty of fluids, and you don't feel dehydrated.

There has been no blood in your stools, although there has been some slime and mucus, and occasionally they are difficult to flush away. You haven't noticed any change in the colour of your skin, and your urine has not darkened. You have had no heartburn, and no trouble swallowing. You do not have a rash, and you have had no problems with your joints.

Otherwise well.

Previous medical history: Hay fever. No surgery. No episodes of pancreatitis.

Drugs history: Malaria prophylaxis — you started taking this a week before travelling and haven't missed any doses, despite being ill. You do not use the oral contraceptive pill or any other medication.

Social history: You smoke 20 cigarettes per day, and drink two or three beers a few times/week.

You've tended to work casually in the care industry for the past several years, whilst you try to develop as a professional photographer. You haven't been at work since the diarrhoea started.

You've never noticed problems in relation to particular types of food.

Family history: No significant family history.

Ideas: You're not sure what this is. You think that you might have developed a chronic bowel disorder. You've read about coeliac disease in a magazine and wondered if that might be the cause.

Concerns: Your main concern is getting back to work soon, as you're almost out of money. As you are a temp, if you do not work, you do not get paid.

Expectations: You're hoping to be given something that will stop all of this and get you back to work.

CLINICAL KNOWLEDGE AND EXPERTISE

Diarrhoea can be defined as the passage of greater than three stools per day and it becomes chronic after 4 weeks.

Acute diarrhoea is almost always due to infection and establishing the causal agent and the source can be very important for public health. By contrast, chronic diarrhoea has a long list of causes. History alone will not distinguish between all of these — further investigations will be needed — but getting a clear history helps narrow down the list. Important things to cover are:

- **Family history** — any history of coeliac disease, inflammatory bowel disease or GI cancer.
- **Social history** — other family members or friends affected. Employment.
- **Surgery** — resections of the GI tract — including gastrectomies, gastric bypass surgery or resections of parts of the small bowel.
- **Previous pancreatic disease** — the exocrine function may be impaired, causing malabsorption.

- **Systemic disease** — e.g., hyperthyroidism or diabetes (autonomic dysfunction).
- **Excess alcohol consumption** — pancreatic damage.
- **Medication** — magnesium containing drugs, NSAIDs; some antihypertensives, antiarrhythmics and theophylline.
- **Recent antibiotics** — risk of antibiotic-associated diarrhoea or *C. difficile* infection.
- **Travel** — particularly to areas where parasitic cystic disease is endemic.
- **Lactase deficiency** — problems after consuming milk or cheese.

If cues pointing to any of these arise in the history, then relevant information, including any relationship to the current symptoms, should be explored.

In the station, when asked about next steps, you should include:

- Clinical examination.
- Basic investigations:
  - FBC (anaemia, macro- or microcytosis)
  - Liver function tests (alcohol)
  - U&Es (dehydration)
  - Plasma viscosity & CRP (general inflammation — cancer or IBD)
  - B_{12}, folate, iron (malabsorption)
  - thyroid-function tests (hyperthyroidism).

Additionally, it is important to request anti-endomysial antibodies because coeliac disease is an important cause of chronic diarrhoea. Stool samples should be sent for microbiology for common bacteria — *E. coli*, *Salmonella* sp., *Campylobacter*, *C. difficile* and toxin, and examination for 'ova, cysts and parasites' (giardia or amoeba).

The history is typical of chronic diarrhoea and could be due to a range of diagnoses. In the UK, in this age group, the most likely are:

- Coeliac disease
- Functional bowel disorders (irritable bowel syndrome)
- Inflammatory bowel disease.

Whilst infective causes of chronic diarrhoea are rare in the UK, the recent travel — with possible consumption of contaminated water or food — makes this more probable. In particular, giardia can present up to 2 weeks after ingestion of contaminated food and can persist for much longer than other infective causes (as can *Entamoeba histolytica* infection).

Working in a care home with a potentially infective diarrhoea would pose an important risk to the residents. If proven, she will not be able to return to work until stool samples are clear.

⚠ WARNING

- Ensure you ask about weight loss and PR bleeding. The presence of these symptoms should prompt urgent investigations (regardless of age) as they may indicate bowel cancer or active inflammatory bowel disease.

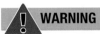

How to excel in this station

Action	Reason	How
Get a clear description of diarrhoea.	Provides the basis for a differential diagnosis to be confirmed on examination and investigations.	Ask specifically about duration, time course, frequency, characteristics of stools including any blood or mucus. Are there any associated symptoms: pain, bloating, flatus, nausea, weight loss, sweats or fevers, skin rashes (coeliac disease) or any joint problems?

(Continued)   31

2

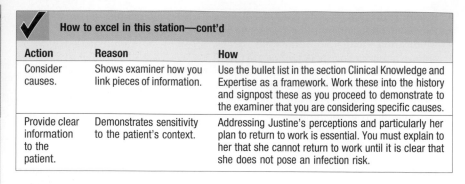

How to excel in this station—cont'd

Action	Reason	How
Consider causes.	Shows examiner how you link pieces of information.	Use the bullet list in the section Clinical Knowledge and Expertise as a framework. Work these into the history and signpost these as you proceed to demonstrate to the examiner that you are considering specific causes.
Provide clear information to the patient.	Demonstrates sensitivity to the patient's context.	Addressing Justine's perceptions and particularly her plan to return to work is essential. You must explain to her that she cannot return to work until it is clear that she does not pose an infection risk.

Common errors in this station

Common error	Remedy	Reason
Assuming too early that the diagnosis is IBS.	Look and listen for clues that point elsewhere.	Although IBS is common, other possibilities must be excluded. Equally, avoid assuming that the cause is infective. Despite the travel history, this requires confirmation.
Giving false reassurance.	Do not simply try to 'please the patient'.	Hopefully she will be able to return to work soon—either treated adequately or because it is non-infective. However, until she's had more investigations, it is difficult to give accurate predictions.

STATION VARIATIONS

○ Advanced

The station may ask you, with justification, about an investigation plan. The examiner may then provide some results and ask you to discuss your interpretation, next steps and management.

Further reading

Chronic Diarrhoea in Adults: PatientPlus web resource. http://www.patient.co.uk/doctor/Chronic-Diarrhoea-in-Adults (accessed 29.11.11.).

Thomas, P.D., et al., 2003. Guidelines for the investigation of chronic diarrhoea, 2nd edition. Gut 52 (Suppl. V), v1–v15. Available at, http://www.bsg.org.uk/clinical-guidelines/small-bowel-nutrition/index.html.

Abdominal pain

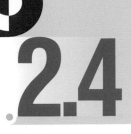

CANDIDATE INFORMATION

Background: You are a junior doctor in general practice assessing Amy Adams (36 years old), who is complaining of severe abdominal pain which started this morning.

Task: Please take a history and then discuss the likely diagnosis with the examiner.

APPROACH TO THE STATION

Abdominal pain in a 36-year-old woman could be due to any number of causes—surgical, gynaecological, urological and possibly obstetric. You will need to rely on the history to reach the likely diagnosis. Remember the mnemonic for pain: **SOCRATES**

- Site
- Onset
- Character
- Radiation
- Associated features
- Timing
- Severity.

An abdominal pain history in a female should include questions about menstruation, and a sexual history should be taken in both sexes (see *Macleod's Clinical Examination*, Chapter 10, The reproductive system).

PATIENT INFORMATION

You should practise taking a history from a colleague using this simulated patient script.

Name: Amy Adams   **Age:** 36 years   **Sex:** Female

Presenting symptom: Abdominal pain

Opening statement: You have intermittent abdominal pain. It is in your right side towards the back (loin). It started suddenly this morning. It lasts a few minutes and feels sharp and very severe and then it fades a little and comes back a few moments later. It never goes completely and there are waves of extremely severe pain.

(Continued)

2

The pain radiates into your groin at times, especially when you pass urine. It is the worst pain you have ever experienced.

If asked: Your menstrual periods are regular, your last period was one week ago. You have had a normal cervical smear one year ago. You have no children. You are not currently in a sexual relationship after breaking up with your long-term boyfriend 6 months ago.

Other symptoms (if asked): No diarrhoea or vomiting. You opened your bowels normally yesterday. You have not had a fever or flu-like symptoms. It does not sting or burn when you pass urine, but the pain radiates into your groin. You are not passing urine more frequently than normal. You have not seen blood in the urine.

Previous medical history: You had your appendix removed when you were 10 years old. You have had a urinary tract infection before, but it did not feel like this, although you had some pain in the same place on your back.

Drugs history: You have been told that you had a reaction to penicillin when you were a child, but are unsure about the details. You take an over-the-counter multivitamin tablet. You do not take any regular prescribed medications. You do not use recreational drugs.

Social history: You gave up smoking one year ago. You drink a glass of wine most evenings and have two or three glasses if you go out at the weekend. You work as a legal secretary and you live with a friend.

Family history: Your parents are in reasonable health, although you think your father has urinary problems — he may have stones but you are not sure. You have a younger sister who has no health problems. As far as you know no diseases run in the family.

If asked:

Ideas: You are frightened and upset about the pain.

Concerns: You are worried that it could be something serious and you might need an operation to fix it, which worries you.

Expectations: You want to know what the problem is and whether you will need an operation.

CLINICAL KNOWLEDGE AND EXPERTISE

A number of differentials are excluded from taking a careful history — you should have found out that the patient has had an appendectomy and a normal menstrual period one week ago, and is not currently in a sexual relationship. This effectively excludes appendicitis and obstetric causes, as well as making sexually transmitted infections much less likely. Despite renal or ureteric colic being less common in women, this is a classical history for ureteric colic. The main differential would be a complicated urinary tract infection (which can coexist with ureteric colic), but this is unlikely as the patient does not have a fever or flu-like symptoms, and although the pain radiates into the groin, she does not have any urinary frequency.

Ureteric colic is often relieved when the patient passes the stone, which can result in immediate relief. Taking oral fluids can help to pass the stone. Even if the stone is passed, the patient should still have investigations as there may be multiple stones at the pelvi-ureteric junction. Patients who suffer with recurrent episodes or have any obstruction may require lithotripsy or surgery. Staying well hydrated and reducing alcohol intake can reduce the risk of having future episodes.

Another possibility is an ovarian cyst. Although this could potentially cause colicky pain, it should not cause loin pain. This pain would normally be located in the right or left iliac fossae and could radiate into the anterior thighs.

After taking a history, the second part of the station is to discuss the likely diagnosis with the examiner. Remember that, most likely, the examiner will ask how you would manage the patient.

 WARNING

- You should exclude a pregnancy in any female presenting with abdominal pain who could be potentially fertile (consider from ages 11 to 55) — this needs to be done sensitively particularly in younger and older women. Early pregnancy complications (such as an ectopic pregnancy) can cause death if not recognised.
- An acute abdomen can worsen over a period of hours — if there is any doubt, arrange to re-assess or re-contact the patient later, or give clear instructions for them to return if worsening.

2

✓ How to excel in this station

Action	Reason	How
Listen and respond.	The history should evolve based on what the patient is telling you—then ask a few clarifying questions.	Even when faced with a raft of possible diagnoses, a careful history should mean you are able to whittle it right down to one likely diagnosis.
Ask about menstrual and sexual history.	Filters the differential diagnosis—without this it is impossible to exclude potential causes.	First listen then ask specifically about these areas. You must be clear as to the date of the patient's last menstrual period—influences management—a menstrual period one week ago in a woman with regular periods means you could safely perform an abdominal radiograph.
Provide information.	Useful for avoiding future episodes.	Suggest to the examiner that you might give the patient a patient information leaflet (see http://www.patient.co.uk).

✗ Common errors in this station

Common error	Remedy	Reason
Ignoring the patient's distress	Acknowledge this and state that you will arrange for some analgesia after a brief discussion.	Ureteric colic is usually described as 'excruciating' pain. Be sensitive to this when taking the history; pain is very distracting. Most general practices have analgesia available, sometimes in IM form.
Simply saying that the patient should be referred.	State that you would examine the urine (dip–infection) and suggest urinary tract imaging.	It is correct to refer for urgent assessment, but the examiner will want to assess your knowledge of ongoing management. Microscopic haematuria supports ureteric colic. If there are leucocytes and/or nitrites as well, the urine should be sent for culture and sensitivity. You should suggest urinary tract imaging: • KUB (kidneys, ureters, bladder) radiographs show around 70% of stones—but require a large dose of ionising radiation. • An ultrasound scan will reveal any stones greater than 0.5 cm as well as any obstruction or hydronephrosis.

2 **STATION VARIATIONS**

○ Intermediate

The examiner may show you the results of the urine dip and ask for your interpretation. Similarly, they may ask you to interpret a KUB radiograph.

○ Advanced

The patient may have a complicated sexual and gynaecological history with possible infection including chlamydia.

Further reading

A Clinical Knowledge Summary (CKS) is available from the National Institute for Clinical Excellence (NICE) on the management of acute renal colic. Available online at: http://cks.nice.org.uk/renal-colic-acute.

Collapse

.2.5

CANDIDATE INFORMATION

Background: You are in the Emergency Department and Mrs Lisa Roberts is a 45-year-old woman who has been brought in by her husband after collapsing in a restaurant.

Task: Please take a history then explain the likely diagnosis and a management plan to her.

APPROACH TO THE STATION

In a patient who has collapsed, the history is the key, so you need as much detail as possible (including witnesses) so that you can visualise exactly what happened. Listen to the patient's story and be sure to determine whether there was any loss of consciousness. Then get the patient to 'walk you through' what happened before, during and after the episode. Listening then clarifying/expanding on some points will often provide this information. Mirroring information back to the patient is an effective technique to use to check your understanding. The key structure is the following:

Before

Where were they? What were they doing? What position were they in? Did they get any prior symptoms such as nausea or palpitations? Have they been unwell recently (e.g., flu, change in tablets)? Patients often describe 'dizziness' — clarify what they mean. For example, was there true vertigo (room spinning, indicating possible vestibular disease), light-headedness or feeling faint (pointing towards syncope) or just a general feeling of being unbalanced (non-specific, often related to gait abnormalities)?

During

Did they lose consciousness? Did anyone witness the collapse? (If so, indicate you would like to speak to them.) Did the person fall straight to the ground? (They may have sustained facial/head injuries.) Did their colour change? Were there any abnormal movements? Did they bite their tongue or have any incontinence?

After

How long did it take to regain consciousness? Were they confused or drowsy? Were they injured? Was there any nausea? Patients with vasovagal syncope feel sick because of the excessive vagal tone.

2

Then look for clues in the past medical history. Specifically,

- Previous episodes of collapse/loss of consciousness
- History of cardiac disease
- History of diabetes (What was their blood sugar? Do they have an autonomic neuropathy?)
- Drug history—especially recent changes (anti-hypertensives or other drugs—postural hypotension)
- Previous stroke, head injury or family history of epilepsy or family history of sudden cardiac death.

PATIENT INFORMATION

Name: Mrs Lisa Roberts   **Age:** 45 years   **Sex:** Female

Occupation: Taxi driver

Presenting symptom: Collapse

Opening statement: You were out for a meal with your husband and the restaurant was warm and made you feel uncomfortable. After 30 min you got up to go to the toilet. You felt unwell when you stood up, hot, sick and sweaty. Then you couldn't see properly and everything went black. The next thing you remember is your husband asking if you were ok and looking worried. You looked around and realised you were in the restaurant. You tried to get up but had to wait a few minutes, as you felt drained. Your husband said he was going to bring you to hospital because you looked pale and had jerked briefly. Now you feel fine.

If asked: You fainted a few times when you were a teenager, but never since. You did not bite your tongue, sustain any injuries or become incontinent. Your husband has gone to pick up the children but will be back soon. He has told you that you jerked once when on the floor for a second. He also says that you went very pale and were sweating. He thinks you were unconscious for about 10 s before you started mumbling. You were back talking normally within 1 min. You had not been drinking alcohol as you start work early.

Previous medical history: None.

Drugs history: Nil. No allergies.

Social history: You do not smoke. You do not drink alcohol because of your job as a taxi driver.

Family history: Your cousin has epilepsy.

If asked:

Ideas: You think that you have fainted as it felt the same as when you were a teenager.

Concerns: You are worried the doctor will say it is epilepsy because of your job.

Expectations: You want the doctor to say everything is fine and let you go home.

CLINICAL KNOWLEDGE AND EXPERTISE

The first step is to decide whether there was loss of consciousness, in which the differential diagnosis is mainly between cardiovascular causes (syncope) and epilepsy (Table 2.5.1). The history here is consistent with a vasovagal syncope. There is brief jerking, but this can occur in syncope and does not point to a seizure. The appropriate investigations would be a 12-lead ECG and lying and standing blood pressure. If these are normal, the diagnosis of vasovagal syncope should be explained and she should be reassured. If there are uncertainties, her care should be discussed with a senior doctor to decide about further investigations. As this is a vasovagal syncope, there is no restriction on driving; however, given her occupation, she should consult with the local taxi licensing authority.

The cardiovascular causes include all forms of syncope, detailed in Table 2.5.2.

2

 WARNINGS

The following 'red flag' features require urgent further investigation:
- ECG abnormalities (see NICE guidance)
- History or signs of heart failure
- Transient loss of consciousness during exercise (structural heart disease/arrhythmia
- Family history of sudden cardiac death
- New shortness of breath.

Table 2.5.1 Differences between epilepsy and syncope

	Diagnostic features	Syncope	Epilepsy
Before	PMH	Cardiac disease/drugs	Epilepsy, stroke, head injury
	Prodrome	Sweating, light-headed	Déjà vu/jamais vu
	Provocation	Postural, situational	Flashing lights
During	Duration LoC	Usually brief	Prolonged
	Limb jerking	Brief	Prolonged. Tonic-clonic phases
	Tongue biting	Less common	Common
	Faecal incontinence	Rare	More common
	Head turning	Rare	Common
After	Confusion	Less common	More common
	Amnesia	Less common	Very common

Table 2.5.2 Causes of syncope

Type of syncope	Features
Vasovagal syncope	Provoked by standing/pain, strong emotion, typical prodrome
Situational syncope	E.g., when coughing, micturition
Syncope secondary to arrhythmias	Usually bradyarrhythmias
Carotid sinus syncope	Symptoms on looking up or to the side
Postural hypotension	Worse on standing up from sitting

2

✓ How to excel in this station		
Action	**Reason**	**How**
Ask about driving.	Some causes will mean counselling not to drive and informing the licensing authority.	Ask directly. If you are unsure about the guidance, state you would ask for senior advice.
Ask about witnesses.	This is often key to obtaining crucial information.	Tell the patient you would like to speak to anyone who saw the event.
Find out about occupation.	This is often a major concern for the patient and must be addressed.	If patient does not mention their work, enquire directly.
Offer reassurance.	Even a faint can be frightening and lead to ongoing worries—driving, occupation.	Explain that it is a simple faint, and no further investigations are required if her ECG is normal.

✗ Common errors in this station		
Common error	**Remedy**	**Reason**
Poor timing.	Focus on relevance to the differential diagnosis and then on concerns.	There is a lot to do in 10 min. It is important to get a detailed history about the collapse and the relevant past history and social circumstances.
Too many closed questions.	Listen more than speaking, use clarification and 'mirroring'. Only ask essential closed questions.	Will reduce your rapport with the patient, can miss important clues and come across like an interrogation.
Fixing on one diagnosis.	Do not close off your thinking too early—ask why it cannot be this (ruling out) rather than always asking confirmatory (ruling in) questions.	Some candidates will quickly class this as a seizure as there was brief jerking. However, this is the only symptom that *may* suggest a seizure, everything else points towards vasovagal syncope. Weigh up the number of positive diagnostic features for each condition and avoid jumping to a conclusion based on one piece of information.

STATION VARIATIONS

⭕ Advanced

Please assess this (elderly) person with falls:
- Falls in older people are more complicated than simple collapses, although there are obviously overlaps between the two. The style of history taking is the same—discovering what happens before, during and after the fall. A fall in an older person may be a sign of a new acute illness and a marker for underlying frailty.
- Remember, not all fallers will lose consciousness; the key aspect is that falls are often multifactorial, so you must widen your history (and examination if this is required).
- Use the mnemonic **DAME** to consider the multifactorial causes of falls in older people:
  - **D**rugs (hypnotics, anti-hypertensives, antipsychotics, etc.)
  - **A**geing processes (decreasing postural stability, slowing of reflexes)
  - **M**edical causes (syncope and epilepsy as above, plus neurological disorders and sensory impairment)
  - **E**nvironmental causes—lighting, stairs, rugs, steps, footwear.

Further reading

NICE transient loss of consciousness guidance. http://guidance.nice.org.uk/CG109.
DVLA medical information. http://www.dft.gov.uk/dvla/medical.aspx.

Back pain

2.6

CANDIDATE INFORMATION

Background: You are a junior doctor in a general practice surgery. Mrs Jean Smith (70 years old) has made an appointment due to back pain.

Task: Please take a history from Mrs Smith and explain the likely diagnosis to her.

You do NOT need to discuss investigations or a management plan with the patient or the examiner.

APPROACH TO THE STATION

It is important to take note of the tasks that the candidate information specifically says you do NOT have to do; it wastes time and you will potentially miss out on marks. Some examiners may stop you if you go outside the remit, but others will not!

Back pain is a very common reason for people to consult their general practitioner. There will not usually be a serious underlying pathological condition but it is important not to miss these. Finding out about 'red flag' symptoms is therefore crucial. Back pain also has a huge impact on people's lives and ability to live, work and exercise. You should ask yourself the following:
1. Is there serious pathology? Are there any 'red flags'? (Table 2.6.1)
2. What impact does the back pain have on this person's life?

Lower back pain commonly radiates down the back of the leg—this is sometimes referred to as 'sciatica'. This is not specific of any particular cause of back pain but suggests involvement of nerve roots. If it is persistent/disabling for more than 6 weeks, then further assessment is indicated.

Table 2.6.1 Red flags for back pain	
Disease	**Red flags**
Cauda equina syndrome	'Saddle area' paraesthesia (perineal sensation) New onset bladder dysfunction (retention/ continence) New onset faecal incontinence Difficulty walking
Spinal cancer	Previous history of cancer New onset in > 50 years old Weight loss Symptoms of specific cancers

(Continued)

2

Table 2.6.1 Red flags for back pain—cont'd	
Disease	**Red flags**
Spinal fracture	History of osteoporosis/other fragility fractures Sudden onset severe central back pain Major trauma Minor trauma in osteoporotic people
Spinal infection (Infective discitis)	Symptoms of infection—fever, rigors, weight loss Recent bacterial infection Intravenous drug use
Inflammatory arthropathy	Young age Early morning stiffness Joint swelling Systemic features—rash, iritis, bowel symptoms

PATIENT INFORMATION

Name: Mrs Jean Smith   **Age:** 70 years   **Sex:** Female

Occupation: Retired

Presenting symptom: Back pain

Opening statement: You have had pains in your lower back for about 6 weeks. The pain is in the middle of your back and came on when you were lifting some shopping out of the car. You have been taking some painkillers but they have not helped and you are struggling as the pain is so bad.

When asked about the pain: The pain is low down in the middle of your back. It is present as a constant dull ache, but made worse by movement and especially with lifting. Mention that you have not been able to do the shopping recently. The pain has not improved much over the past 6 weeks. You took some ibuprofen as you thought it was a muscle sprain but it has not helped.

If asked: The pain does not go anywhere else.

Other symptoms (if asked): No weight loss, no fevers. Bladder and bowel function is normal. No numbness around your bottom. You have otherwise been feeling well.

Previous medical history: Left wrist fracture last year after a fall on the ice (you had an operation to fix this). If asked, you have never been tested for osteoporosis.

Drugs history: No allergies. You take Ramipril 5 mg for your blood pressure. You do not take any other medications.

Social history: You have smoked 10 cigarettes per day since the age of 20. You do not drink alcohol. You live alone (your husband has died of lung cancer). You are finding it hard to get out because of the back pain. Your daughter is doing your shopping and helping round the house.

Family history: Your mother died after she fell and broke her hip at 80 years old. Father died of a heart attack.

If asked:

Ideas: You thought it was a muscle sprain but it has not got better and now wonder whether it is something more serious.

Concerns: You are worried it could be cancer, as your husband died of cancer 5 years ago.

Expectations: You want to be reassured that it is not cancer and are expecting to have an X-ray. You know a little about osteoporosis (weak bones) as you read about it in the newspaper.

CLINICAL KNOWLEDGE AND EXPERTISE

Pre-station clues. The patient is a 70-year-old woman, so this should alert you to any 'red flags'. In post-menopausal women you should consider whether they have osteoporosis (previous fractures, smoking and family history). It is also important to exclude malignancy. The patient's age makes it very unlikely to be an inflammatory arthropathy such as ankylosing spondylitis (usually less than 30 years old).

Positive diagnostic features for a vertebral fracture in this case include:
- The pain is 'mechanical' — this means that it is worse on movement.
- There is a history of smoking, a previous wrist fracture and maternal hip fracture, suggesting underlying osteoporosis.
- The pain came on suddenly whilst lifting.
- The pain has been present for 6 weeks, making muscular pain unlikely.

 WARNINGS

Table 2.6.1 lists the red flags that you should consider for back pain.

✓	How to excel in this station	
Action	**Reason**	**How**
Listen and respond.	Builds a rapport with the patient.	Respond to cues with empathy, for example when patient is discussing their struggles: 'That must be difficult for you. How else does the pain affect you?'
Think about associated conditions.	Demonstrates wider knowledge about risk factors for illness.	Ask specifically about history of and risk factors for osteoporosis—time of menopause, family history, smoking and alcohol use.
Reassure	Patient is concerned about cancer; from the history you can reassure her that other diagnoses are more likely.	Explore Mrs Smith's ideas, concerns and expectations. Say, 'I know that you are worried that this may be cancer but from what you have told me I think this is unlikely. We can do some further tests to check.'
Give information.	It is good practice to point patients in the direction of good quality information sources so they can learn more about their condition.	There may be a condition-specific leaflet that you can offer the patient, or point them to a condition-specific website (in this case, the National Osteoporosis Society, http://www.nos.org.uk) or a reliable general website such as http://www.patient.co.uk.

2

Common errors in this station		
Common error	Remedy	Reason
Too general review of symptoms.	Get focused systems review specific to the case—here concentrate on the red flag symptoms.	You may run out of time and also it suggests that you do not know which specific questions to ask.
Missing effects on patient.	Ask specifically about how the pain affects the patient—how does it restrict them? How is their mood? Does it affect their ability to work?	Chronic lower back pain is often associated with depression, psychosocial factors and disability claims ('yellow flag' symptoms). You should consider whether these factors are relevant here.

STATION VARIATIONS

O Advanced

A similar patient, but with a red flag and the task would include: *How would you investigate lower back pain?*

Current guidance suggests that further investigations are required only if red flag symptoms are present.

- Prescribe analgesia—see Chapter 6.5, Prescribing analgesia.
- In this case, where vertebral fracture is suspected, then the patient should be referred for imaging of the spine, either a spinal radiograph or magnetic resonance imaging (MRI) scan.
- If Cauda equina syndrome or infective discitis is suspected, the patient should be referred to hospital for an urgent spinal MRI scan.
- If a spinal tumour is suspected, imaging should be arranged and the patient should be screened for a primary cause for the malignancy (as most spinal tumours will be metastatic in nature).
- To investigate a patient for osteoporosis, the national osteoporosis guidelines group suggest the following as first-line tests:
  - Full blood count (to exclude infection, anaemia suggesting chronic disease or infection);
  - Erythrocyte sedimentation rate (ESR) or CRP to look for inflammatory conditions;
  - Creatinine to look for osteoporosis secondary to renal failure;
  - Calcium, albumin, phosphate and alkaline phosphatase to look for problems with calcium homeostasis and thyroid function tests; and
  - A bone densitometry (DXA) scan should be requested.

Further reading

NICE clinical guideline 88: lower back pain. http://www.nice.org.uk.

National Osteoporosis Guidelines Group, Guideline for the Diagnosis and Management of Osteoporosis. http://www.shef.ac.uk/NOGG/downloads.html.

Vaginal bleeding

2.7

CANDIDATE INFORMATION

Background: You are a junior doctor in a general practice surgery and your next patient is Miss Katherine O'Brien (32 years old) who is complaining of heavy periods.

Task: Please take a history from this patient; find out more about her menorrhagia.

APPROACH TO THE STATION

Heavy menstrual loss, or menorrhagia, is common in primary care, with one-third of women experiencing it at some point and one in 20 women aged between 30 and 49 consulting their GP each year. Where severe, it can have a significant effect on a patient's life. A patient's perception of what constitutes heavy menstrual loss differs in terms of amount of blood lost and duration and it is important to quantify these. Although the definition of menorrhagia is a monthly menstrual loss greater than 80 ml, it is more relevant for management to focus on the effect on the patient's quality of life, not just physically, but also psychologically and socially.

Around 40–60% of heavy loss has no identifiable cause and is classified as dysfunctional uterine bleeding. It is important, however, to exclude possible reversible underlying causes, which may be systemic, such as a clotting disorder, or local, such as fibroids. The history can be as useful as a clinical examination or further investigations. NICE guidelines on heavy menstrual bleeding state that, in cases of menorrhagia where no structural or histological abnormality is suspected, a full blood count (FBC) and detailed history is all that is required prior to commencing pharmacological treatment.

You are not required to formulate a management plan (though this could be offered as an advanced station), but your history must include the patient's ideas, concerns and expectations, especially with regards to treatment options, as the patient may have fixed views and management plans vary, depending upon the patient's need for contraception and whether the patient and her partner have completed their family.

PATIENT INFORMATION

Name: Katherine O'Brien   **Age:** 32 years   **Sex:** Female

Occupation: Nursery nurse

Opening statement: You're fed up with your heavy periods, which have been getting worse over the past 6 months. You have had to take time off work twice in the past 2 months and you ended up leaving work early last week due to an embarrassing episode where the blood leaked through your clothing. Your manager has advised you to get it sorted out, and you have been warned about further time off work.

If asked: You have to wear a super-absorbency tampon and sanitary towel for the first 5 days of your period, which you change roughly every 2 h during the day. Your normal menstrual cycle is 30 days with your period lasting 8 days. You often pass large clots at the beginning and have had a few episodes of 'flooding' over the past few months where blood leaks onto your clothing or bedding, which has caused you distress and embarrassment. You do not suffer from bleeding between periods or after sex. You've been with your current partner for 4 years and do not think that you are at risk of sexually transmitted infection. You currently use condoms for contraception, but are considering pregnancy in the next year or two. You used to be on the (combined) oral contraceptive pill 10 years ago but stopped it because of mood swings and weight gain. You have never had any treatment for heavy periods. You sometimes feel dizzy if you stand too quickly and are generally tired but otherwise feel well and have no other symptoms **if asked** (e.g., no excess bruising, bleeding, hair loss or skin changes). You are up-to-date with your cervical smear tests and they have always been normal.

Past medical history: Childhood asthma but have not needed inhalers for several years.

Family history: Mother had a hysterectomy at 44 for heavy periods due to fibroids.

Drug history: You take over-the-counter antihistamines as required for hay fever.

Social history: Live with partner who has two children from a previous relationship who stay at the weekends. You smoke 10 cigarettes per day and drink approximately 12 units of wine per week. You work as a nursery nurse and enjoy your job but struggle to cope when your periods are very heavy, as you need to rush to the toilet regularly.

If asked:

Ideas: You wonder what can be done for your heavy periods and whether you could be anaemic because your mum mentioned that you looked pale and you've been feeling tired.

Concerns: You are worried about the effect on your work and that you need to take regular time off and may be disciplined in future.

Expectations: You hope that you will be given something to stop or ease the bleeding. You don't want a hysterectomy like your mum as you are thinking of having children in the next couple of years but you're not sure about going on the pill again given the problems that you had in the past with weight gain and mood swings.

CLINICAL KNOWLEDGE AND EXPERTISE

Causes of heavy menstrual loss

It is important to ask questions to exclude possible underlying causes that may require further investigation. When considering causes, they can be considered in three different areas although several factors may coexist and contribute to the heavy menstrual loss. A few examples are listed here. These are not exhaustive, and remember that the majority of cases in general practice will not have an identifiable cause.

Systemic: Obesity
Hypothyroidism
Coagulation disorder, e.g., Von Willebrand's disease
Diabetes

Local: Fibroids
Endometrial/cervical polyps
Adenomyosis or endometriosis
Endometrial carcinoma

Iatrogenic: Anti-coagulants/anti-platelet medications
Use of the copper IUD (contraceptive intrauterine device)

2

Any menstrual history should be taken with sensitivity as heavy loss may cause distress and embarrassment for the patient, and may be difficult to discuss. Listed below are examples of useful questions to qualify and quantify the extent of the problem although a good candidate would allow the questions to flow together rather than rely on a 'tick box' approach to history taking. Using open questions may allow the patient to volunteer the information needed, whilst explaining in their own words the effect that heavy menstrual loss has on their daily life and therefore what management plan is likely to be the most appropriate.

Key questions in a menstrual history

- Age of menarche
- Length and variability of cycle
- Duration of menses and how many days within that are heavy
- Amount of tampons/pads used daily and whether requires double protection
- Any episodes of clots or flooding?
- Any recent change in menstrual flow or pattern?
- Duration of menorrhagia (how many cycles) and previous menstrual pattern
- Any intermenstrual or post-coital bleeding?
- Associated symptoms, e.g., dysmenorrhoea, pelvic pain, dyspareunia, pressure symptoms
- Impact of bleeding on quality of life
- Family history of menstrual disorders.

Additional questions to ask

- Sexual health screening
- Cervical smears
- Features of systemic disease, e.g., hair loss and weight gain (hypothyroidism) or excess bruising (clotting disorders)
- Features of anaemia, e.g., pallor, tiredness
- Current/future contraceptive plans
- Any plans for conception now or in the future?
- Drug history (especially anti-coagulants/anti-platelet medications).

Management of heavy menstrual loss

Although you do not need to discuss management with the patient, it is important to have a good understanding of the initial management of menorrhagia, and which

2

patients might be referred early for further gynaecological assessment as it is possible that the patient may raise concerns and expectations that may warrant further consideration.

In the absence of any red flags within the history or background of the patient, initial drug treatment may include:

- Mefenamic acid: a non-steroidal anti-inflammatory drug
- Tranexamic acid: an anti-fibrinolytic drug
- The combined oral contraceptive pill
- The progesterone-containing intrauterine system (Mirena coil)
- Other continuous forms of progesterone-only contraception that can lead to amenorrhoea, e.g., the depo injection or progesterone-only contraceptive pill.

Factors that may suggest a referral is indicated include:

- Any red flags within the history that may suggest endometrial carcinoma (see below);
- Failure to respond to treatment given; and
- Features suggestive of a secondary cause of menorrhagia that may require surgical intervention, e.g., significant fibroids.

It is worth noting that a hysterectomy is now regarded as very much the 'last resort' in gynaecological management of heavy menstrual loss, with many other less invasive options available, and women should be counselled that a gynaecological referral does not automatically mean that surgical intervention is necessary or appropriate.

⚠ WARNINGS

- Do not forget endometrial carcinoma as a cause of menorrhagia — strongly consider if the patient is over 45, overweight or obese, has intermenstrual bleeding and treatments for menorrhagia have failed.
- Other symptoms suggesting the need for further investigation include post-coital bleeding, dyspareunia, pelvic pain and sudden change in pattern of blood loss.

✓ How to excel in this station

Action	Reason	How
Listening to the patient.	The patient has often had to cope with heavy menstrual loss for some time and can often provide useful information without a long list of questions.	Ensure that open questions are used early followed by pauses to allow the patient time to respond fully. Examples of this could be: 'Tell me about your heavy periods' or 'Describe to me a typical period'. Reserve closed questions for finer clarification or if the history risks going off topic.
Remember ICE.	The patient's agenda for the consultation can be very different from what you assume; for example, the patient may be more concerned about something serious underlying their heavy bleeding than the bleeding itself.	Explore early in the consultation what the patient's ideas, concerns and expectations are so that any management plan can be tailored to address their needs and allow a patient-centred approach. Make sure that the patient does not feel that their concerns are dismissed or regarded as unimportant.

Common error	Remedy	Reason
Not considering the impact of symptoms on the patient's quality of life.	Although it is important to review the pattern of menorrhagia and elicit whether the patient has definite heavy menstrual loss, allow time to discuss the consequences of their menstrual loss and the physical, emotional and social effects.	Often it is possible to become so focused on quantifying the significance and amount of menstrual loss that the impact on the patient's life may be overlooked and there is not always a correlation between the amount of blood loss and the distress.
Assuming there must be an underlying cause.	Taking a thorough detailed history, looking for unusual features or possible symptoms of systemic disease, will mostly differentiate between menorrhagia that is likely to have an organic cause and that more likely to be dysfunctional uterine bleeding.	The temptation can often be to arrange investigations instantly rather than consider the most likely differential diagnosis, which can be costly and unnecessary as well as being invasive and distressing for the patient.

Common errors in this station

2

STATION VARIATIONS

○ Intermediate

The station could be increased in complexity by asking you to formulate a management plan based on your diagnosis (dysfunctional uterine bleeding) and the patient context (e.g., completed their family). The examiner would observe you negotiating this with the patient.

○ Advanced

The patient may be older with risk factors for uterine cancer. You would be required to set out your plan for investigations and the utility of each of these.

Further reading

Clinical Knowledge Summaries, National Institute for Clinical Excellence. Available at: http://cks.nice.org.uk/menorrhagia.
NICE clinical guideline CG44. Available at: http://www.nice.org.uk/guidance/cg44.

An unwell child

.2.8

Background: You are a junior doctor in paediatrics and Sumit Chandra (18-month-old boy) has been brought into hospital after a short period of unresponsiveness and shaking, during which time he had a temperature. He has now recovered and is being observed on the ward.

Task: Please take a history from the baby's mother, Rashmi Chandra, and answer her questions.

APPROACH TO THE STATION

As you read the information, a likely diagnosis of febrile convulsion may stand out to you. Bearing this in mind, think about how you will approach the task. You would be expected to be sensitive to the distress that witnessing such an event would cause to the child's parents.

As well as a history of the event itself, you need to remember to cover the following areas:

- Obtain information about the child's delivery and immediate post-partum progress. Was the child born at term, following a normal delivery? Were there any complications and did the baby require admission to the Special Care Baby Unit (SCBU)?
- Is the child generally well? Are they thriving and developing normally?

You can refer to *Macleod's Clinical Examination*, Chapter 15, 'Babies and Children', if you need a reminder on how to go about taking a birth history or developmental assessment.

PATIENT INFORMATION

Name: Sumit Chandra, history from mother, Rashmi Chandra   **Age:** 18 months
Sex: Male

Presenting symptom: Shaking episode

Opening: Sumit has been unwell for a day or so with a high fever. His GP had diagnosed an ear infection today and started treatment. This evening Sumit had a temperature again of 38.9 °C. Before you had a chance to give him paracetamol, he went suddenly rigid and unresponsive then started shaking with a clenched jaw. This probably lasted 2–3 min, during which time your husband called an ambulance. When the shaking stopped, Sumit was sleepy at first but started to wake in the ambulance. He is now awake and seems much better. Nothing like this has ever happened before.

Other symptoms (if asked): No diarrhoea or vomiting. No rash. He had a fever at the time of the shaking. He is not drowsy or floppy any more, and was not before the shaking.

Previous medical history: Sumit has been well up till now. He was born at term by vaginal delivery. He was healthy at birth. He has had his vaccinations and has developed normally and is gaining weight. Specifically — he is walking, climbs stairs and says several single words. He was weighed in A&E and was 14 kg (charted close to the 50th centile).

Drugs history: No known allergies. Sumit has been given paracetamol whilst unwell and was started on amoxicillin suspension today by his GP, though he has only had one dose so far.

Social history: Sumit is your second child; he has a 4-year-old older sister. Neither you nor your husband smoke. You have no pets. No one else lives at home. Sumit's father is a secondary school teacher and you are a stay-at-home mum.

Family history: You and the baby's father are both well. The only family history is of type II diabetes (your mother, Sumit's maternal grandmother), and ischaemic heart disease (Sumit's paternal grandfather).

If asked:

Ideas: You are extremely frightened and distressed by what you witnessed.

Concerns: You are worried about Sumit having another episode of shaking and what it means.

Expectations: You want to be reassured that Sumit is OK. You are worried this means he has epilepsy or some other serious illness.

CLINICAL KNOWLEDGE AND EXPERTISE

This history is classical of a febrile convulsion, as short-lived generalised (tonic-clonic) seizures are quite common in previously well children associated with a fever. A febrile convulsion is largely a clinical diagnosis and the history is key.

Please see Table 2.8.1 for information on the features of a typical febrile convulsion. You should confirm these features to diagnose a febrile convulsion.

The birth and developmental history is very important, as seizures in this age group can be associated with cerebral palsy and several clinical syndromes, though these often present as afebrile seizures.

It may be useful to give the parents information about general first-aid measures. However, you need to be pragmatic about how to deal with further febrile illnesses — there is no good evidence that further convulsions can be avoided in susceptible children so advise the parents that they should take the usual steps to treat a febrile illness, e.g., paracetamol, offering fluids, but no special measures need to be taken, and that the child may have further seizures in any case. Try to avoid instilling 'fever fear' in the parents — remember that febrile convulsions are basically benign and if this is explained at the first event it can have a beneficial impact on how parents deal with any future seizures.

2

Table 2.8.1 Typical features of a febrile convulsion	
Essential elements	**Description**
Child's age	6 months to 6 years
Fever	Must be present
	Must precede or be found during convulsion (not develop afterwards)
Convulsion	Generalised not focal
	Usually lasting less than 5 minutes
	Usually self-terminating Recovery usually within about an hour
Also common	
Family history	One of the child's parents may have had febrile convulsions

 WARNING

- Afebrile seizures are much more likely to be pathological, and although treatment is rarely commenced after a first episode, a child would normally be investigated to identify a cause. Therefore, the history of a fever being present is very important.
- It is mandatory to assess whether the child has any risk factors for brain damage (such as meningitis as an infant, or hypoxia requiring resuscitation and admission to SCBU at birth), and whether they are developing normally, when taking a history regarding a seizure. You must, therefore, be aware of the most common developmental milestones.

How to excel in this station

Action	Reason	How
Listen and respond.	The child's parent/s should be able to give a description of the event with minimal or no prompting by you.	A strong candidate will be empathetic and sensitive, offering reassurance from an early stage. The mainstay of the history is to confirm points regarding the convulsion, and to ask about the child's birth and developmental history before moving on to answer the parents' questions.
Associated conditions.	The parent/s may ask about whether this is epilepsy, or whether this episode heralds a tendency towards epilepsy.	Demonstrate your knowledge that <1% of children with febrile convulsions will go on to develop epilepsy.
Reassure.	Mrs Chandra will be understandably extremely frightened at having seen her child having a seizure.	Reassurance is a major requirement and as febrile convulsions are benign you must explain this to the parents. If there is time, it may be helpful to counsel the parents on the likelihood of further seizures in the future.
General advice.	Offer first-aid advice if time.	The child may have a further febrile convulsion so it is useful to offer general first-aid tips—place the child on their side, move objects away that they could injure themselves on, avoid restraining when they are fitting and call an ambulance if it lasts over 5 minutes.
Provide information.	Reassure parents further.	Knowledge is power, and an advice leaflet lets the parents digest the information when they are less distressed and they can keep it for further reference.

Common errors in this station

Common error	Remedy	Reason
Interrupting the history.	Good listening skills.	The parent is likely to offer most of the key information so listen to the story and keep interruptions to a minimum. The parents will not respond to empathy or reassurance if they do not feel you are listening and understanding their concerns. The birth and developmental history are key areas and you will not score well without covering these.
Using jargon.	Make sure parents are happy with the terms you are using, e.g., 'fit' or 'convulsion', and say fever rather than febrile.	Avoid jargon in history taking, but remember that lay people may refer to seizures using a variety of terms—it may be helpful to use whatever term the parent/s use.
Dismissing the parents fears.	Empathetic body language and approach to parents.	Avoid being dismissive. Although febrile convulsions are common, the experience is nevertheless frightening for the parents who may worry that their child was going to die. Avoid offering false reassurance—although febrile convulsions are relatively benign, this does not mean the child will not have a further one. It may be helpful to explain the rule of thirds—roughly a third of children will have no further episodes, another third will only have one further episode, and the final third may have recurrent convulsions with fevers over the next few years.

2

STATION VARIATIONS

O Advanced

Discuss with parents after a child has had a second afebrile seizure

- Epilepsy is very rarely diagnosed after only one seizure; however, after a second seizure the diagnosis of epilepsy would need to be discussed.
- Explain that further investigations are necessary, including basic blood tests, brain imaging (often an MRI—more detailed imaging and avoids radiation) and an EEG.
- The child may need admission if the parents are very distressed or there are other worrying features, but otherwise, further assessment and follow-up can take place with the child as an outpatient.
- Tell parents that once investigations have been performed, the child is likely to be started on anti-epileptic medication; however, avoid talking about specific drugs at this time. Explain that medication depends on the epilepsy type and using the information from investigations.
- Remember to give first-aid and safety advice such as never to let the child bathe or swim alone and that the child should always wear a helmet when on a scooter or bike, etc.

Further reading

Clinical Guideline 47—Feverish illness in children. Available at http://www.nice.org.uk.

2

Clinical Guidance 137—The epilepsies: diagnosis and management of the epilepsies in adults and children in primary and secondary care. Available at http://guidance.nice.org.uk/CG137.

Douglas G., et al., Macleod's Clinical Examination, 13th edn (Churchill Livingstone, 2013), Ch. 15.

First Aid Advice for parents. http://www.nct.org.uk.

http://www.patient.co.uk/health/febrile-seizure-febrile-convulsion.

http://www.nhs.uk/conditions/Febrile-convulsions.

A child with breathing problems

2.9

CANDIDATE INFORMATION

Background: It is November and you are a junior doctor in Paediatrics. Sam Roberts is a 10-month-old baby brought in with breathing difficulties.

Task: Please take a history and answer any questions from Sam's mother, Mrs Sarah Roberts.

APPROACH TO STATION

The background information should give you a clear nudge as to the likely diagnosis; i.e., it is November – within the seasonal peak for respiratory viruses. Viral illnesses are extremely common in babies in winter, particularly in the age group 6–18 months, so this is also a strong indicator. Some will require admission for oxygen and support with feeding, but many can be safely discharged, provided the baby's caregivers are provided with appropriate information.

When taking a history from parents of a small child it is imperative to ask about the birth and delivery, vaccination history and health up till now. You should always include some questions about the developmental history and whether the child is 'thriving', i.e., gaining weight, growing and developing normally. In a respiratory history, the social and family histories are also key areas (parental smoking and damp living conditions). See *Macleod's Clinical Examination*, Chapter 15, 'Babies and Children', for more information on paediatric history taking.

A history taking for acute illness in an infant must also include questions about feeding and current hydration, as well as excluding serious infections, such as pneumonia or meningitis.

PATIENT INFORMATION

Name: Sam Roberts, history from mother, Sarah Roberts   **Age:** 10 months
Sex: Male

Presenting symptom: Breathing difficulty

Opening statement: Sam has been unwell for a day or so with a dry cough and breathing more quickly than usual. He is not sleeping well and seems to have gone off food. The cough is not noisy or barking and he is not making much noise breathing but sometimes sounds a little wheezy.

(Continued)

2

When asked about feeding: Sam is refusing solids but has taken some milk and some water. (**If asked:** Sam is fully weaned on solids but still has follow-on formula milk normally. He was formula-fed prior to weaning.)

If asked: Sam is producing wet nappies. Although he is refusing solids, he has had half a bottle of milk about an hour ago. He has also had some water earlier (about 100 ml) and his full bottle this morning.

Other symptoms (if asked): No diarrhoea or vomiting. No rash. He had a fever of 37.9°C at home, but this responded to paracetamol. Sam is fully alert but a little miserable. He is not drowsy or floppy. He has a runny nose with lots of secretions.

Previous medical history: Sam has been well up till now. He was born at term but was delivered by Caesarean section for failure to progress in second stage of labour. He was healthy at birth. He is up-to-date with his vaccinations. He has reached his developmental milestones at the usual time and is gaining weight normally. Specifically, he is able to sit unsupported and pulls himself to stand holding onto furniture. He babbles and can say a few two-syllable words. He transfers toys and has a pincer grip. He was weighed in A&E and was 8.5 kg (charted as close to the 50th centile).

Drugs history: No known allergies. Sam has been given some paracetamol whilst unwell.

Social history: Sam is your first baby. You don't smoke but your husband, Sam's father, does. He smokes outside the house but does smoke in the car. You have a pet dog at home. No one else lives at home. Sam's father has a desk job with an insurance company and you have not yet returned to your job from maternity leave as a saleswoman in a department store.

Family history: You have asthma, which you have had since childhood. The baby's father is well and there is no other significant family history on either side. You have had a cold yourself in the past week, though no fevers.

If asked:

Ideas: You are very worried about Sam as his breathing scares you and it looks like he is unwell. He has been healthy up till now so this illness has worried you.

Concerns: You are worried Sam is developing asthma.

Expectations: You want to be reassured that Sam is not going to die and you want to know if this is a sign that he will develop asthma. You want to know if he needs antibiotics.

CLINICAL KNOWLEDGE AND EXPERTISE

The main differential diagnoses here are bronchiolitis, croup and pneumonia. The history is classical for bronchiolitis rather than croup as the cough is not barking and the baby is not having noisy breathing (or stridor) other than occasional wheeze, which can be present in bronchiolitis. More serious respiratory illness such as pneumonia is unlikely as the baby sounds as though he is relatively well (still feeding and active) and only had a low-grade fever. Pneumonia is also less likely in a previously healthy child who has had their vaccinations. There are no worrying features.

Bronchiolitis does not always require admission. If admitted, it is rare for children to require more intensive support than oxygen and hydration (by nasogastric feeds or intravenous fluids), but occasionally they can require non-invasive ventilation (CPAP—continuous positive airways pressure). Rarely, they can become seriously unwell and need invasive ventilation on a Paediatric Intensive Care Unit; this is more likely in children with other medical issues (for example, previous prematurity).

You may be asked to discuss whether Sam could be managed at home. It is important to describe how you would assess him (including respiratory rate, saturations, intercostal/sternal recession, tracheal tug, nasal flaring and head bobbing) as well as ensuring that he is feeding adequately and has good hydration (adequate capillary refill, absence of tachycardia, moist mucous membranes). In order to discharge safely, you should also 'safety-net', i.e., explain to the parents that they should always bring the child back if concerned. You should give them information about any specific signs and any other features that should prompt them to return. Giving parents an information leaflet about the condition is also useful.

2

⚠ WARNING

- Drowsiness, listlessness, floppiness
- Poor feeding, not producing wet nappies
- Presence of rash, high fevers or rapidly worsening features.

The presence of any of these features may point towards a more serious diagnosis, or a more severe case requiring hospital admission.

✓ How to excel in this station

Action	Reason	How
Listen and respond.	Parents are often distressed and emotional when their child has had to come to hospital, particularly for the first time.	Be empathetic, have open and kind body language and listen to, and address, their specific concerns.
Associated conditions.	Many parents worry about asthma when their child is admitted with wheeze.	Reassure parents that bronchiolitis is not associated with asthma. However, bronchiolitis can leave a child with a residual cough for weeks after the acute episode, so it is worth warning parents.
Ongoing management.	Demonstrate awareness of the risk assessment made on children with bronchiolitis that allows decisions to be made about their ongoing care.	By questioning Mum about feed and wet nappy frequency and volumes, make an assessment of the child's ability to feed. State that you would assess the child's hydration status, oxygen saturations and level of respiratory distress. Many children can be managed at home but some need admission for feeding support, oxygen or due to severe symptoms.
Offer more information.	Parents are often anxious.	Parents are often more reassured if they have more information (regardless of admission), so leaflets on the condition can be very helpful.

2

Common errors in this station

Common error	Remedy	Reason
Missing smoking cessation advice.	Briefly give smoking cessation advice to Mum (regarding Dad)	We should never miss an opportunity to give smoking cessation advice. It is important to mention briefly and politely that exposure to smoke (including on hands and clothes) can affect babies and that the health service can offer support if Dad would like to quit. Practice with a partner talking about this in a way that is not offensive or judgemental.
Suggesting antibiotics.	If Mum brings this up, politely explain they are not necessary.	Bronchiolitis is a viral infection and antibiotics will be ineffective, and used inappropriately could cause side effects such as allergy or diarrhoea.

STATION VARIATIONS

O Advanced

Wheeze in an older child

A case about an older child with wheeze could encompass many other aspects, such as explaining to parents the difference between viral-induced wheeze and early asthma in the pre-school age group, or the basic management priorities and escalation of treatment in early childhood asthma.

Further reading

Bronchiolitis: SIGN guideline 91. http://www.sign.ac.uk.

Douglas G., et al., Macleod's Clinical Examination, 13th edn (Churchill Livingstone, 2013), Ch. 15.

Many patient/parent information leaflets are available at http://www.patient.co.uk.

QS25 Asthma guidance covers diagnosis and management of asthma in children >12 months, young people and adults. http://guidance.nice.org.uk/QS25.

Persistent low mood

2.10

CANDIDATE INFORMATION

Background: You are a junior doctor in general practice seeing Bill Nightingale (52 years old), who has presented complaining of feeling very unhappy.

Task: Please take a history and in the final 2 minutes discuss the diagnosis and management with the examiner.

APPROACH TO THE STATION

The instructions give a strong indication that the focus is on a mood disorder. Before starting, consider what symptoms this might produce. Remember that mood is 'bipolar' or 'cyclothymic' and the different symptoms these might lead to. In either case, consider how you will determine the severity of the patient's condition.

Whilst good communication is always important, it is very important here due to the patient's vulnerability and state of feeling. How can you phrase some of the more difficult questions? What will your general approach be?

At the end you must discuss diagnosis and treatment. Look out for features that will help you be precise about the diagnosis. Bring to mind treatments that you know of before starting. That way you can be considering what seems appropriate as you proceed.

PATIENT INFORMATION

This script could be modified to suggest hypomania.

Name: Bill Nightingale   **Age:** 52 years   **Sex:** Male

Occupation: Unemployed

Opening statement: You often feel quite low — perhaps for the past 3 to 4 months This has got worse recently. Increasingly you're not able to focus on any work or jobs, and you think that is why you lost your most recent job.

If asked:

(Continued)

2

You often feel that things feel quite hopeless. Your sleep is poor — you often wake very early in the morning and you just turn over the thoughts that you have. These focus around ideas that your life has no purpose or direction. You used to be a passionate football fan — going to matches with a group of friends most weekends — but you feel like you've lost your enthusiasm now. You don't seem to enjoy the football much anymore, and being around the other guys makes you feel like 'a loser'. You find it fairly hard to enjoy anything, and you now spend most of your time around the house. You're not eating very well — you're less interested in food, and cooking is a huge effort.

Sometimes when you're lying awake, you wish you weren't alive. You've never made any plans to harm yourself; mostly the thought of your children makes you think that you could never do that. Thinking of them makes you feel a sense of guilt — you feel as though you've been a bad father. You don't experience any feelings of anxiety or panic. You have never had an episode of very elated or raised mood.

Previous medical history: Previous appendectomy, hypercholesterolaemia.

Meds: Simvastatin 40 mg at night.

Allergies: Nil.

Social history: You are unemployed. You lost your job as an aerospace engineer 2 years ago, and were previously married (separated 10 years ago).

You have two children in their late teens who live with their mother.

You are not currently in a relationship.

You have been actively looking for work ever since losing your job, but have only found temporary office work, which you don't enjoy — especially as most other people in this work are much younger than you.

You don't smoke. You drink a can or two of lager occasionally. You don't currently take any exercise, although you used to work out often in the gym. You live in a small flat which you've had for several years, but paying your bills has been gradually eating into your savings.

If asked:

Ideas: You are not sure what is wrong with you. You think that you might be depressed, but you feel that it is your fault.

Concerns: You are worried that you will always feel this way.

Expectations: You are hoping that the doctor will help you feel better, as you feel incapable of helping yourself.

CLINICAL KNOWLEDGE AND EXPERTISE

Depression is a condition characterised by low mood and loss of pleasure in most activities. It involves a combination of biological, social and psychological factors. A diagnosis of depression rests on the combination and severity of a range of psychological and biological symptoms, and the length of time they have persisted for. People whose symptoms do not meet this definition can still suffer from 'sub-threshold depressive symptoms'.

Diagnosing depression

Assessment should include the number and severity of symptoms, duration of the current episode and course of illness. Key symptoms include:
- Persistent sadness or low mood; and/or
- Marked loss of interests or pleasure;
- At least one of these, most days, most of the time for at least 2 weeks.

If any of the above present, ask about associated symptoms:
- Disturbed sleep (decreased or increased compared to usual);
- Decreased or increased appetite and/or weight;
- Fatigue or loss of energy;
- Agitation or slowing of movements;
- Poor concentration or indecisiveness;
- Feelings of worthlessness or excessive or inappropriate guilt;
- Suicidal thoughts or acts.

The combination of symptoms a person has can then be used to grade their depression:
- **Sub-threshold depressive symptoms:** Fewer than five symptoms of depression.
- **Mild depression:** Few, if any, symptoms in excess of the five required to make the diagnosis, and symptoms result in only minor functional impairment.
- **Moderate depression:** Symptoms or functional impairment are between 'mild' and 'severe'.
- **Severe depression:** Most symptoms are present, and the symptoms markedly interfere with functioning. Can occur with or without psychotic symptoms.

There are no specific investigations for depression; diagnosis is based on the history. Nonetheless, a validated depression scoring tool, such as the PHQ-9, should be used to document the severity of the condition, as this allows comparison to assess the effect of treatment. Management comprises a mixture of support, psychological interventions and medication, in a series of increasing 'steps', based on the degree of improvement which occurs (Fig. 2.10.1).

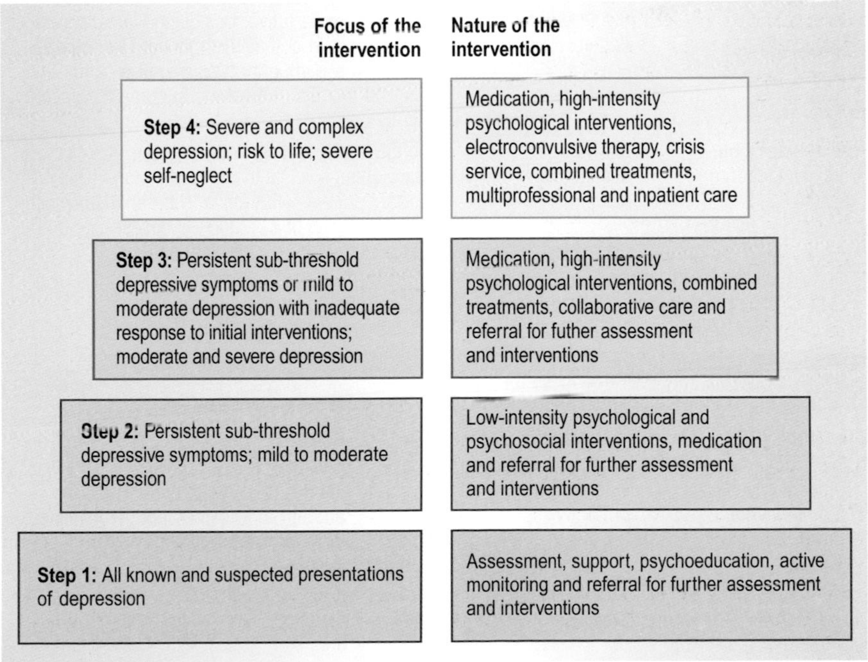

Focus of the intervention	Nature of the intervention
Step 4: Severe and complex depression; risk to life; severe self-neglect	Medication, high-intensity psychological interventions, electroconvulsive therapy, crisis service, combined treatments, multiprofessional and inpatient care
Step 3: Persistent sub-threshold depressive symptoms or mild to moderate depression with inadequate response to initial interventions; moderate and severe depression	Medication, high-intensity psychological interventions, combined treatments, collaborative care and referral for further assessment and interventions
Step 2: Persistent sub-threshold depressive symptoms; mild to moderate depression	Low-intensity psychological and psychosocial interventions, medication and referral for further assessment and interventions
Step 1: All known and suspected presentations of depression	Assessment, support, psychoeducation, active monitoring and referral for further assessment and interventions

Figure 2.10.1 Stepped care of depression (From NICE Guidance: *Depression in Adults*, with permission)

This patient has moderately severe depression with greater than five symptoms:
- Persistent low mood for 3–4 months;
- Hopelessness;
- Poor concentration;
- Reduced sleep;
- Anhedonia;
- Reduced appetite;
- Guilt;
- Suicidal ideation.

These have impacted on his function and it would be appropriate to start at step 2, progressing to step 3 if necessary. Importantly, his risk of suicide is low—he has not made any plans of self-harm, and has protective factors. Advice regarding sleep may help, and both his sleep and his mood may be aided by physical exercise.

 WARNING

- You must ask directly about suicide; including any plans about this (method, notes, previous attempts, etc.).

How to excel in this station

Action	Reason	How
Legitimise his feelings.	Builds relationship.	Actively listen, non-verbally encouraging him to continue. It has taken courage for him to come and he needs to feel safe and that his symptoms are valid and taken seriously.
Identify symptoms—severity and functioning.	Establishes diagnosis and degree.	Most of the symptoms required will come out if you encourage his narrative. Use closed questions to cover the rest in a sensitive manner. The duration and pattern are important for diagnosis, as is the impact on function. Use these to grade the severity of his illness.
Be certain about suicidal ideation.	Allows quantification of risk.	Although it may feel very intrusive, it is vital that you enquire about suicidal thoughts and plans. This is an important patient safety issue. This can then be used to judge his level of risk, and—if necessary—to put in place measures to keep him safe.

Common errors in this station

Common error	Remedy	Reason
Being judgemental in verbal or non-verbal communication.	Do not be judgemental or give any sense that he is to blame for his illness.	It will break down any trust or openness, and will undermine any attempt to empower him, which may form part of psychological interventions.
'Ticking off' a checklist of symptoms.	Listen to the patient's story and descriptive terms.	It will give you a clearer impression of symptom severity and impact on his life.

STATION VARIATIONS

⦿ Advanced

There is unlikely to be time in 10 min to perform a full mental state examination, but an advanced station could include all or part of it. A mental state exam involves describing the patient in terms of the following:

- **Appearance:** how they look or dress, their general body habitus and whether they're unkempt;
- **Behaviour:** the way they move or act; whether they're agitated, fidgeting or showing 'psychomotor retardation';
- **Speech:** whether speech is pressured, quick, slow, or very reluctant; the volume and clarity;
- **Mood:** whether their mood is low, neutral (euthymic) or elated;
- **Affect:** their ability to react to things that can change their mood – this may be blunted, normal or heightened;
- **Thought – form:** whether their thoughts seem to follow logical or linear patterns, whether the thoughts seem to get 'blocked' or whether there is erratic or 'knight's move' thinking;
- **Thought – content:** the ideas around which their thoughts revolve; these might be hopeless or persecutory ideas, grandiose or simply bizarre;
- **Perception:** whether they appear to be experiencing any unusual sensory experiences;
- **Cognition:** cognitive functioning – using mini-mental test or MMSE.

Further reading

PHQ-9 Questionnaire. http://www.patient.co.uk/doctor/patient-health-questionnaire-phq-9.

NICE guidance: Depression in Adults. http://guidance.nice.org.uk/CG90.

2

An injury whilst drunk

2.11

CANDIDATE INFORMATION

Background: You are a junior doctor in Accident and Emergency where Mr Arkwright has attended this evening with a sprained ankle managed by the nurse practitioner. She noted that Mr Arkwright smelt of alcohol, although he conversed sensibly. She remembered him presenting similarly with a laceration a few weeks ago so she has asked you to talk to him about his drinking.

Task: Please take a focused history of Mr Arkwright's alcohol use. Please include any health advice which you think may be relevant.

APPROACH TO THE STATION

Taking an alcohol history requires a different approach from more routine histories. Nonetheless, the 'history of presenting complaint' can still be applied by exploring:
- Quantity of alcohol the person drinks;
- Pattern of drinking throughout the day (or week);
- How it has changed over time;
- Associated important symptoms — the impact that alcohol is having on the person.

Consider the classification of the person's drinking once you have obtained this information.

You will need to provide health advice, which is likely to involve reducing consumption, so how can you approach this in a manner that will increase the chance of your advice being effective? Understanding the patient's perspective is likely to be important, so clarify this as you proceed.

PATIENT INFORMATION

The script could be modified to suggest alcohol dependence rather than harmful drinking.

Name: Fred Arkwright   **Age:** 33 years   **Sex:** Male

Occupation: Storeman

Instructions to patient (look annoyed): 'Hi Doctor, the nurse practitioner says I drink too much and I have to speak to you before I go home.'

Drinking history: Drink most days, usually 2–3 home-poured measures of whisky every evening (perhaps 1–2 inches in a glass) whilst relaxing watching TV. A bottle of whisky lasts about a week. If being honest, you remember that a year or two ago it would have lasted a fortnight or more, but you have drunk 'socially' for as long as you can remember.

As well as this, you like to go out for a drink with friends a few evenings a week — perhaps 3 or 4 pints. You usually still have a whisky when you get in. On Fridays, workmates head out for drinks with their pay as soon as the day is finished, and you often have 6 or 8 pints then — especially if the shop has been stressful, which it has been a lot recently. On Saturdays you usually lie in bed, feeling unwell, but you have never missed work due to drinking.

You enjoy drinking — part of having a good time — and you look forward to the evening drink. You feel in control of your drinking — you could stop if you wanted, but you have never wanted to. You never shake or tremble in the morning, and you have never had a fit or any hallucinations.

You are a sociable person, but over the past few months you have noticed that you feel a bit down at times, and sometimes you feel that the enjoyment has gone out of life. You have never seen your GP about this.

If asked: You will admit that you might get more done on Saturday if you didn't drink so much on Friday nights, but you don't mind this. Friday nights are the best part of the week. Your wife gets cross sometimes on Saturdays because of this, and you feel annoyed with her as a result but you never feel guilty or have thought that you need to cut down. You never drink in the morning.

Previous medical history: Hypertension; laceration to left arm due to falling against fence a month ago.

Drugs history: Bendroflumethiazide 2.5 mg od.

Allergies: Nil.

Social history: You are married, and have one son who is 14 years old. You work as above. You smoke 20/day. You do not exercise.

Ideas: You never really thought that drinking is problematic. You are unaware of a link between excess alcohol and hypertension, and equally do not know that alcohol can produce low mood or depression.

Concerns: You feel a bit embarrassed that people think you might be an 'alcoholic' and you are cross that it has been suggested. You accept that being drunk caused your ankle sprain, but this could happen to anyone. You have heard advice about 'not drinking too much', but you do not really know why not, although you know that 'alcoholics' can die from drinking. You do not think that anything bad will happen.

Expectations: Once you understand the impact and danger of alcohol on health, you are willing to accept the need to reduce alcohol intake. You do not want health to deteriorate. It might be hard to cut down though, especially as it is a main pleasure. You do not expect anything from the doctor in particular — a healthcare professional initiated the consultation — but it would be useful to know where you can get support.

2

CLINICAL KNOWLEDGE AND EXPERTISE

Alcohol misuse is very common and assessing a patient's use of alcohol and related symptoms is frequently encountered in OSCEs. Alcohol misuse can occur to differing degrees. Avoid using the term 'alcoholic'; it is technically meaningless as it has no precise definition and it is often felt to be pejorative by patients. Instead, classify the person's drinking and refer to it:

Hazardous drinking: *Regularly* drink more than the recommended daily amounts (5 units for men, 3 for women) or they drink more than the recommended weekly limit (21 units for men, 14 for women). Hazardous drinking places the individual at increased risk of liver disease, alcohol-related cognitive impairment, high blood pressure and some cancers, and can affect all body systems.

Harmful drinking: Drinking which causes actual physical or mental harm (e.g., liver disease or depression). It is not defined in terms of units, but occurs when hazardous drinking has produced harm. The definition of harm includes trauma sustained whilst under the influence of alcohol, or the presence of alcohol-related health conditions.

Alcohol dependence: This is a mix of physiological, psychological and behavioural features, which all relate to a very strong and persistent desire to drink. It can be diagnosed in people who have had three or more of the following in the past year:

1. Strong desire/compulsion to drink;
2. Difficulty controlling drinking — starting, stopping or amount;
3. Physiological withdrawal on stopping/reducing drinking (e.g., tremor, sweating, rapid heart rate, anxiety, insomnia, or less commonly seizures, disorientation or hallucinations) **or** drinking to stop or prevent withdrawal symptoms;
4. Being tolerant of alcohol — increasing amounts required for the same effect; doses that would harm or kill a non-tolerant user;
5. Neglect of other activities or alternative pleasures — due to time taken to obtain alcohol or recover from its effects;
6. Persistent drinking despite being aware of *overtly* harmful consequences — i.e., liver damage, depression or alcohol-related cognitive impairment.

One unit in the UK usually means a beverage containing 8 g of ethanol, e.g., a half pint of 3.5% beer or lager, or one 25 ml pub measure of spirits. A small (125 ml) glass of average strength (12%) wine contains 1.5 units. If the person has alcohol-related cognitive impairment, they may not be able to give a clear account and a history from a third party may be necessary. See Fig. 2.11.1.

Obtaining an alcohol history should involve establishing the amount and the pattern of drinking (moderate each day, or a lot on some days?). You should then carefully

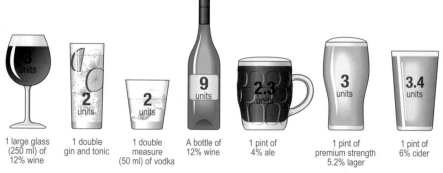

| 1 large glass (250 ml) of 12% wine | 1 double gin and tonic | 1 double measure (50 ml) of vodka | A bottle of 12% wine | 1 pint of 4% ale | 1 pint of premium strength 5.2% lager | 1 pint of 6% cider |

Figure 2.11.1 Units of alcohol in standard UK drinks

consider any evidence of harm—depressive symptoms, relevant medical conditions and any alcohol-related traumatic injuries. Next you should consider the impact on the individual's life and functioning, as well as specifically addressing the issues that would suggest alcohol dependence. An important part of the history is to explore why the person drinks, whether they perceive that it may be harmful, and if it is, to see whether they are willing to consider reducing it.

In this case, the patient has harmful drinking as he is drinking 50–60 units per week. Most probably either it is worsening his hypertension or it is the cause of it, as well as his low mood. Additionally, he has injured himself twice in the context of alcohol. Apart from feeling unwell on Saturdays, he shows no features of dependence.

 WARNING

2

- Harmful drinking may not be recognised until the patient presents with end-organ damage—it is important to utilise any opportunities to discuss excessive alcohol intake before alcohol-related health conditions develop.

✓ How to excel in this station

Action	Reason	How
Develop trust.	Developing a rapport with the patient is key to developing a management plan to reduce his drinking.	Make sure you do not seem to be 'having a go' at him. Show empathy towards his injury. Explain that he does not have to see you if he doesn't want to—it's just good practice when someone has injured themselves to discuss their alcohol use and promote healthy living. Gently explain that no one is trying to accuse him of anything, and that if he had gained that impression then you are sorry.
Promote health.	Opportunistic screening and intervention can have a beneficial impact for the patient.	Find out whether he knows that his drinking is harmful. Explain why this is, and discuss cutting down his consumption. Explain why this will make him feel better. Help him believe it is possible, and that support is available. Acknowledge his feelings (he might feel daunted or scared). Suggest he sees his GP for more support.

✗ Common errors in this station

Common error	Remedy	Reason
Failing to classify his drinking.	Find out how much he drinks (weekly), which will probably need some closed questions. Establish the impact on his function, and look for evidence of harm and dependence. Include the CAGE questions (see below), but try to make them conversational.	An accurate classification is the basis of an intervention and management plan.

2

STATION VARIATIONS

O Basic

The patient may not have any particular alcohol problems but has simply presented to A&E and you are asked to screen them. One approach is to use the **CAGE** questions:
1. Have you ever felt you should **C**ut down on your drinking?
2. Have people **A**nnoyed you by criticising your drinking?
3. Have you ever felt bad or **G**uilty about your drinking?
4. Have you ever had a drink first thing in the morning to steady your nerves or to get rid of a hangover (**E**ye opener)?

A total score of 2 or greater is considered clinically significant (sensitivity of 93% and a specificity of 76%).

Further reading

More detailed information on this subject is available from the NICE clinical guideline CG115: Alcohol dependence and harmful alcohol use. Available from http://www.nice.org.uk/CG115.

Physical examination

3

Introduction to examination skills

3.0

Clinical examination stations are certain to appear in an OSCE. These stations represent a good opportunity to get high marks, as they are easy to practise. We have covered many of the common examinations, but more detailed versions are covered in the *Macleod's Clinical Examination* text. We have adapted these examinations so that you should be able to complete them within the limited timescale of an OSCE.

The examinations will either be on normal individuals with no pathology or on patients with real disease. It is worth practising the systematic examinations on your colleagues so that these flow smoothly and expertly. The patients that are used in OSCEs tend to have a limited number of chronic and stable conditions. This is because the examiners will usually need a number of patients with similar signs who they can use for multiple examinations. It is also for this reason that acutely unwell patients are mostly not used. For example in a respiratory examination, if you hear crepitations they are much more likely to be due to someone having a chronic condition such as pulmonary fibrosis rather than pneumonia. This means that you should be sure to learn about diseases that commonly crop up in OSCEs – so that you can get top marks if these appear.

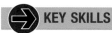 **KEY SKILLS**

There are several key skills for every clinical examination station:
1. Introduce yourself to the patient
2. Ensure good hand hygiene
3. Explain to the patient what you are going to do and ask their permission
4. Be systematic in your examination
5. Be wary of causing discomfort to the patient
6. Be systematic in your presentation, giving key clinical findings
7. Give a differential diagnosis and then the most likely diagnosis.

We have suggested a structure for clinical examinations that you should follow. Try to practise using this structure and using colleagues. Following this makes it less likely that you will miss things. As a general rule you should start a general examination at the hands, work up the arm to the neck, look at the face and then continue down the chest/abdomen and legs as appropriate.

Suggested structure for clinical examination (mnemonic PIPPAS):
* Present yourself to patient
* Inspection
* Palpation
* Percussion
* Auscultation
* Special tests.

Examining the patient with a murmur

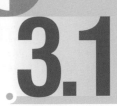

3.1

CANDIDATE INFORMATION

Background: Mrs Bendon is a 65-year-old woman who has been referred by her GP after a murmur was noticed during a routine check-up. Her only symptom is of occasional palpitations.

Task: Please examine the patient and present your findings, then discuss your differential diagnosis and the first-line tests that you would request.

APPROACH TO THE STATION

The station information is fairly vague and therefore could be used as the candidate information for any murmur. The history of intermittent palpitations may direct you to a valvular lesion that predisposes to atrial fibrillation—but bear in mind that palpitations are commonly reported even in people with structurally normal hearts. You will need to perform a full cardiovascular examination and report your findings. Valvular heart disease is commonly encountered in OSCEs as the patients tend to be clinically stable for long periods.

When examining the chest of female patients, you should keep their chest covered with a sheet for as long as possible. Alternatively, you could suggest that they keep their bra on but unfasten it so that you will be able to examine underneath it more easily. Ensure the patient is reclining at 45° (if comfortable) for the examination.

PATIENT INFORMATION

You should wear a top that is easy to remove and be prepared to strip to the waist (you may be able to keep your bra on but unfasten it, or be provided with a sheet to place over your chest). Then follow the instructions from the candidate during the examination.

CLINICAL KNOWLEDGE AND EXPERTISE

Cardiovascular examination
Introduction
- Introduce yourself, explain what you are about to do and obtain consent.
- Clean your hands prior to beginning.

Inspection

- Observe the patient from the end of the bed—do they look unwell or breathless?
- Start with the hands—look for clubbing and splinter haemorrhages.
- Face—look around the eyes for xanthalasma and a corneal arcus. Gently examine the conjunctivae for pallor or petechial haemorrhages. A malar flush is an uncommon finding suggestive of mitral stenosis. Look at the lips and tongue for central cyanosis.
- Neck—examine the JVP (see *Macleod's Clinical Examination*, Chap. 6 for a detailed explanation). Palpate the carotid pulse at this point.
- Chest—examine front and sides for scars (midline sternotomy scar or left thoracotomy scar for mitral valve repair).
- Inspect legs for peripheral oedema (this could be done at the end of the examination).

Palpation (Fig. 3.1.1)

3

- Palpate the pulses. Palpate both radial pulses simultaneously to check for radio-radial delay and to check the rate. Examine a central pulse for character.
- Palpate for a collapsing or water-hammer pulse by placing three fingers of your right hand loosely around the wrist, covering the radial area but not applying pressure. Support the elbow and check for any shoulder discomfort before lifting the patient's arm. If a collapsing pulse is present you will feel the sharp pulse in the radial area.
- Palpate the apex beat by placing your fingers flat on the chest parallel to the ribs in the 5th intercostal space mid-clavicular line.
- Examine for a heave by placing the heel of your hand firmly over the left parasternal position.
- Palpate for thrills by placing the flat of your fingers at the apex and then on both sides of the sternum.

Auscultation (Fig. 3.1.2)

- Listen at the apex, lower left sternal edge and upper right and left sternal edges first with the bell and then the diaphragm.
- Ask yourself whether the first or second heart sound is easily heard, loud or soft.
- Roll the patient onto their left side. Listen with the bell using light pressure at the apex, specifically the mid-diastolic low-pitch rumbling murmur of mitral stenosis.
- Sit the patient up and ask them to lean slightly forwards. Using the diaphragm, listen over the right and left upper sternal edges at end-expiration for the high pitched murmur of aortic regurgitation.
- Listen over the carotids on end-expiration and in the left axilla for radiation of any murmurs.
- If you hear a murmur, palpate the carotid pulse while you auscultate.

Special Tests

- Examine for pulmonary ocdema by auscultating the lung bases only (you could do this after examining for aortic regurgitation), and examine for dependent oedema in the lower legs and sacrum.
- Ask to check the blood pressure.

After finishing your examination, thank the patient and fit your findings together. This can be the hardest part of a cardiovascular examination, but be methodical— Table 3.1.1 may help. The asterisks show stable conditions that can easily be brought to OSCEs and those in bold are common.

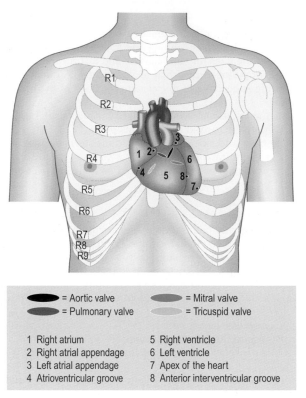

R1
R2
R3
R4
R5
R6
R7
R8
R9

3
1 2
4 5 8
6
7

= Aortic valve
= Pulmonary valve
= Mitral valve
= Tricuspid valve

1 Right atrium
2 Right atrial appendage
3 Left atrial appendage
4 Atrioventricular groove
5 Right ventricle
6 Left ventricle
7 Apex of the heart
8 Anterior interventricular groove

Figure 3.1.1 Surface anatomy of the chambers and valves of the heart (From Douglas G., et al., *Macleod's Clinical Examination*, 13/e (Churchill Livingstone, 2013) with permission.)

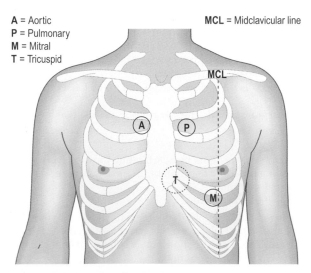

A = Aortic
P = Pulmonary
M = Mitral
T = Tricuspid

MCL = Midclavicular line

MCL

A P

T

M

Figure 3.1.2 Sites for auscultation (From Douglas G., et al., *Macleod's Clinical Examination*, 13/e (Churchill Livingstone, 2013) with permission.)

Present Your Findings

- Comment on any findings from your inspection.
- Comment on the heart sounds—S1 (closure of the mitral valve) and S2 (closure of the aortic valve).
- Describe any murmurs (systolic or diastolic, loud/harsh or soft, mid to late or pan), including where they were loudest and whether they radiate.
- Comment on any other tests and suggest a differential diagnosis.
- Suggest appropriate initial investigations—ECG and transthoracic echocardiography are reasonable initial investigations for possible valvular heart disease.

Table 3.1.1 Differential diagnosis of cardiac murmurs

Pathology	Murmur	Radiates to	Heart sounds	Other findings
Aortic stenosis*	Loud, ejection systolic murmur loudest over aortic area	Carotids	Soft or absent S2	Narrow pulse pressure, left ventricular hypertrophy
Aortic regurgitation	High-pitched, early diastolic murmur best heard at aortic area sitting forwards in end-expiration	—	—	Collapsing pulse and wide pulse pressure, displaced apex beat
Mitral stenosis*	Mid-diastolic rumbling, best heard at apex	—	Loud S1	Malar flush, atrial arrhythmias
Mitral regurgitation*	Pan-systolic, loudest at apex	Axilla	Runs up to S2	Possibly laterally displaced apex beat, atrial arrhythmias
Tricuspid regurgitation*	Pan-systolic, loudest lower left sternal edge	—	—	Giant V waves in JVP, pulsatile liver
Coarctation of the aorta*	Loud systolic murmur audible throughout praecordium	Throughout praecordium and heard over the back	—	Likely to have sternotomy scar. May have some residual radio-radial or radio-femoral delay.
Ventricular septal defect*	Pan-systolic (often loud), usually loudest lower left sternal edge	—	Usually normal	May have sternotomy scar if it has been surgically corrected.
Atrial septal defect*	—	—	Fixed splitting of S2	
Mechanical valves* **(either mitral or aortic)**	May or may not have flow murmur around relevant valve	—	Loud, mechanical valve click, often audible from end of bed	Usually midline sternotomy scar but possibly left thoracotomy. May have bruising from anticoagulation.

3

3

 WARNING

- Patients with valvular heart disease should be considered for surgery if they become symptomatic—i.e., if they complain of syncope, chest pain or increasing dyspnoea.

✓ How to excel in this station		
Action	**Reason**	**How**
Present your findings clearly.	Succinctly presenting your examination findings after completing the examination can turn a good performance into an excellent one.	When you practise examinations, also practise presenting your findings. Start with other tests that you would request and then present your findings methodically. It can be tricky to remember all the findings, but if you practise you will improve.
Good knowledge of the different patterns of valvular lesions.	It is difficult to approach an examination without an idea of what the different pathologies present with.	You will get good experience from a cardiology ward or clinic. You can also listen to recordings of heart sounds and murmurs online. If you have not had much exposure to clinical signs, then at least ensure the basic examination is polished.

✗ Common errors in this station		
Common error	**Remedy**	**Reason**
Not treating the patient with dignity and respect, nor giving clear instructions or being polite.	Introduce yourself and explain the examination. Ensure the patient is comfortable and if female, cover their chest or suggest they leave their bra on but unfastened.	Remember the essential aspects of good communication skills—make good eye contact, have a reassuring manner and explain what you are going to do clearly. It is better to run short of time and ensure the patient is comfortable and not distressed than to finish and have upset the patient.
Poor technique or disordered examination.	Practise the examination and be methodical. Gain experience from clinical practice and from observing others where appropriate.	This is a frequently encountered examination so the examiner will be expecting it to be slick.

STATION EXTENSIONS

⦿ Advanced

You may be asked to perform a cardiovascular examination combined with data interpretation of an ECG and possibly an echocardiograph report.

Further reading

Douglas G., et al., Macleod's Clinical Examination, 13th edn (Churchill Livingstone, 2013), Ch. 6.

Peripheral arterial examination

3.2

CANDIDATE INFORMATION

Background: You are a doctor in the general surgical clinic. Mr Bidwai (70 years old) has pain in his legs whilst walking and more recently in bed at night. He has a past history of type 2 diabetes, hypertension and ischaemic heart disease. He smokes 20 cigarettes/day.

Task: Please examine him to establish a diagnosis and discuss the immediate tests you would request with the examiner.

APPROACH TO THE STATION

The history is suggestive of peripheral arterial disease (see Table 3.2.1), especially with the multiple risk factors. After your focused examination, remember to leave enough time (2 min) to discuss investigations (see Table 3.2.2). If a real patient is used, then comment on findings as you proceed.

Table 3.2.1 Symptoms of peripheral arterial disease	
Intermittent claudication	Pain in calf, thigh or buttocks when walking; typically relieved with rest.
Nocturnal pain	Wakes patient and relieved by hanging legs out of bed or walking; suggestive of severe disease.
Erectile dysfunction	Often an early sign of peripheral arterial disease (ask in history).
Ulceration	Signs of severely ischaemic limbs and poor wound healing is also common.

Table 3.2.2 Immediate tests to be requested	
Blood tests	FBC, U + E, lipids. LFT if considering statin therapy.
ABPI	Ankle-brachial pressure index—an ABPI of <0.9 is predictive of atherosclerosis.
Duplex ultrasound	Allows evaluation of all the vascular beds.
ECG	Screen for cardiovascular disease—looking for LVH, LBBB and other markers.
Angiography	Not usually first-line investigation. Can be digital subtraction angiogram, CT angiogram or MR angiogram.

3

PATIENT INFORMATION

Name: Mr Bidwai   **Age:** 70 years   **Sex:** Male

Occupation: Retired

For a simulated patient (usually a male) you should remove your trousers and be covered on an examination couch.

CLINICAL KNOWLEDGE AND EXPERTISE

Examination of the peripheral arterial system

Introduction
- Gain permission to examine patient and explain what you are about to do.
- Clean your hands prior to beginning.

Inspection
- Start with hands—look for tobacco staining.
- Face—look for xanthelasma.
- Scars—look for scars on the abdomen (aortic aneurysm repair), groin (angiography) or medial aspect of thighs (bypass grafting).
- Ulcers—comment on arterial ulcers (punched out, usually over medial malleoli) or venous (anterior aspect of shin, associated with venous eczema and skin changes).
- Skin changes—loss of hair and skin thinning.
- Feet—examine dorsum and plantar aspects and between toes for ulcers.
- Feel for the skin temperature in the feet.

Palpation (Fig. 3.2.1)
- Measure (or say you would) the blood pressure in both arms.
- Palpate the major pulses—radial, carotid, aortic, femoral, popliteal and dorsalis pedis.
- Check for radio-femoral delay after palpating radial pulse—explain this to the patient.
- Check for capillary refill time over big toe.

Auscultation
- Listen over the aorta, carotid and femoral arteries for bruits.

Special tests
Buerger's test—With patient lying on their back, raise their feet to 45° for 2 minutes. Then sit the patient on the edge of the bed with legs down. A positive test (peripheral arterial disease) occurs when legs initially go pale when raised then hyperaemic (red) when down.

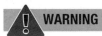 **WARNING**

Acute limb ischaemia—
The following suggest the requirement for urgent assessment (the 6 P's): pallor, perishing cold, pulseless, paresthesia, paralysis, pain on squeezing muscle.

Figure 3.2.1 Position of major arteries for palpation (From Douglas G., et al., *Macleod's Clinical Examination*, 13/e (Churchill Livingstone, 2013) with permission.)

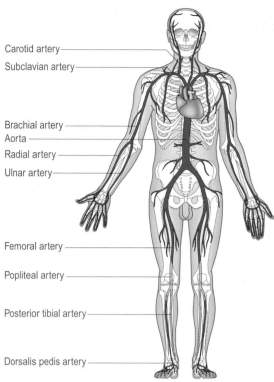

Carotid artery

Subclavian artery

Brachial artery

Aorta

Radial artery

Ulnar artery

Femoral artery

Popliteal artery

Posterior tibial artery

Dorsalis pedis artery

3

Critical limb ischaemia—

Pain at rest, non-healing ulcers and gangrene require urgent vascular assessment.

✓ How to excel in this station

Action	Reason	How
Look confident and follow a system for the examination.	This means you are less likely to miss something important and helps the examiner to see you know what you are doing.	Follow the systematic approach to examination as discussed above.
Explain to patient what you are doing.	In this examination you will be examining sensitive areas such as the patient's groin.	Explain to the patient what you are doing especially when examining sensitive areas such as the groin.
Discuss why you are requesting tests.	This shows the examiner you understand why tests are appropriate.	For example, 'I would like to check the U + E to look for any possible signs of renovascular disease.'

✗ Common errors in this station

Common error	Remedy	Reason
Forgetting to present all findings.	Present your findings in the order that you examined them.	This gives you a good structure and means you are less likely to miss important findings.

3

STATION EXTENSIONS

⭕ Advanced

You may be asked to use a Doppler machine to detect the pulses or to complete the ABPI, so familiarise yourself with these investigations. You may also be asked to look at an angiogram and comment on lesions.

⭕ Basic

You may be asked about the treatment of peripheral arterial disease including prevention.

Further reading

Douglas G., et al., Macleod's Clinical Examination, 13th edn (Churchill Livingstone, 2013), Ch. 6.

European Society of Cardiology, Peripheral Artery Diseases Guidelines. Available at http://www.escardio.org.

Examining the breathless patient

3.3

CANDIDATE INFORMATION

Background: Mr Rodgers is 76 years old and has been referred to the clinic due to increasing breathlessness. He stopped smoking 6 years ago (50 pack-years). He used to work as a builder and retired 15 years ago.

Task: Please examine him and discuss with the examiner your differential diagnosis and first-line tests.

APPROACH TO THE STATION

You should think of the most common differential diagnoses and look specifically for these. Most candidates can do the basic respiratory exam but the best will tailor this to the history. In an OSCE it is most likely that a real patient will have chronic disease with stable signs. In this case the likely differential would be between chronic obstructive pulmonary disease, lung fibrosis and cardiac failure, so show the examiner that you are looking for features of these.

PATIENT INFORMATION

You should wear a T-shirt and be prepared to strip to the waist. Then follow the instructions from the candidate during the examination.

CLINICAL KNOWLEDGE AND EXPERTISE

Respiratory examination
Introduction
- Gain permission to examine patient and explain what you are about to do.
- Clean your hands prior to beginning.

Inspection

3

- Start with hands—look for tobacco staining, finger clubbing and a flap (indicates CO_2 retention).
- Look for central cyanosis in the tongue and lips.
- Neck—examine the JVP, which may be raised in cor pulmonale or fixed in superior vena cava obstruction. Examine the patient for lymphadenopathy.
- Chest—examine front, back and sides for scars (lobectomy/pleural drain scars).
- Look for hyper-expansion and poor or unequal chest wall movement.
- Count the respiratory rate and look for accessory muscle use.
- Inspect for peripheral oedema (end of the examination).

Figure 3.3.1 illustrates the signs you will find in the common respiratory diseases.

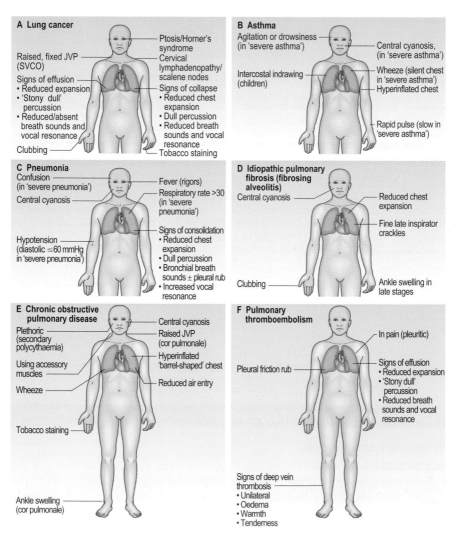

Figure 3.3.1 Signs of common respiratory diseases (From Douglas G., et al., *Macleod's Clinical Examination*, 13/e (Churchill Livingstone, 2013) with permission.)

Figure 3.3.2 Surface anatomy of the posterior chest wall for examination

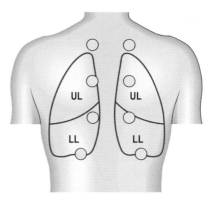

3

Palpation

- Palpate trachea for deviation.
- Chest expansion—usually best seen on the posterior chest wall.
  Divide the chest into three zones—upper, middle and lower (see Fig. 3.3.2).
- Tactile vocal fremitus—place hands on both sides of the chest and ask patient to say 99—repeat three times down the posterior chest wall.

Percussion

- Percussion—percuss four areas down the back and front of the chest. Pay special attention to lung bases—is there unilateral dullness suggesting an effusion or collapse?

Auscultation

- Listen with either bell or diaphragm in the zones as above. Are there any added sounds (crepitations or wheezes)? Pay special attention to the lung bases—are there crepitations? Are they unilateral/bilateral, coarse or fine?

Special tests

- State you would check oxygen saturations using a pulse oximeter.
- You may be asked to check peak flow so be prepared to do so.

Common tests that you would request (and justify your suggestions) would include: pulse oximetry, chest X-ray, full blood count (erythrocytosis), spirometry (see Fig. 3.3.3; obstructive, restrictive patterns), peak flow variability (asthma), full pulmonary function testing (including flow volume loops—see Fig. 3.3.4) with reversibility and transfer factor.

 WARNING

- Lymphadenopathy on examination may suggest lung cancer and you should ask the patient about haemoptysis and weight loss.
- If a patient is breathless or centrally cyanosed at rest, this would indicate severe respiratory disease.

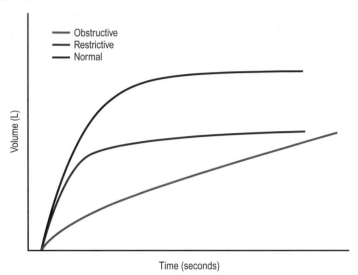

Figure 3.3.3 Spirometry patterns

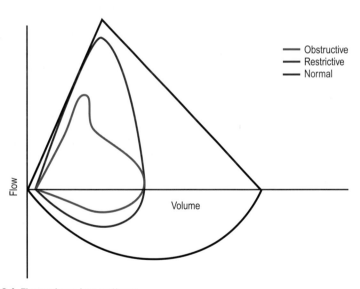

Figure 3.3.4 Flow volume loop patterns

✔	How to excel in this station		
Action	**Reason**		**How**
Give a differential diagnosis.	This shows examiner you have breadth of knowledge and have considered alternative diagnoses.		Give a differential diagnosis and then state which you feel is most likely and why (based on the clinical signs that you can find).

How to excel in this station—cont'd

Action	Reason	How
Tailor further investigations to most likely diagnosis.	This shows examiner you are not just requesting a set list of 'routine' investigations.	For example, if clinically the patient has pulmonary fibrosis then state that you would like to perform lung function tests to look for a restrictive pattern of lung disease and a high resolution CT scan to look for honeycombing and the pattern of fibrosis.

✗ Common errors in this station

Common error	Remedy	Reason
Running out of time.	Practise the examination. Focus on examining the patient's chest from the back.	You are more likely to pick up clinical signs on the patient's back, so if you are pressed for time, focus your examination here.
Percussing poorly.	Practise on yourself.	Percussion is a learned skill and examiners will be able to tell if you are not experienced in performing it.

3

STATION EXTENSIONS

○ Advanced

You may be presented with a chest radiograph or some pulmonary function tests (including a flow volume loop) to interpret after examining the patient. As with your physical examination, you should comment in a structured manner. Radiograph interpretation is discussed in further detail in station 7.2.

○ Basic Pulmonary Function Testing

Calculate the FEV1/FVC—this is called the FEV1%.
FEV1% >70 suggests restrictive lung disease (such as fibrosis).
FEV1% <70 suggests obstructive lung disease (the lower the figure the more severe the obstructive disease).

Further reading

American Thoracic Society guidelines. Available at http://www.thoracic.org/ statements.
Douglas G., et al., Macleod's Clinical Examination, 13th edn (Churchill Livingstone, 2013), Ch. 7.
Japp, A., Robertson, C., Macleod's Clinical Diagnosis (Churchill Livingstone, 2013), Chapter 12, 'Dyspnoea'.

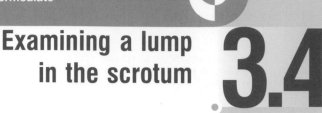

Examining a lump in the scrotum

3.4

CANDIDATE INFORMATION

Background: You are a junior doctor in a general practice and are seeing Mr Mark Davison (25 years) who is complaining of a scrotal lump.

Task: Please examine Mr. Davison's groin and scrotum. You are not required to take a history.

APPROACH TO THE STATION

This station requires examination of the groin and external genitalia, as well as some clinical knowledge regarding scrotal and testicular lumps. Furthermore, as this is an intimate examination, good communication, gaining appropriate consent and establishing a rapport are essential to perform well.

This station may involve a simulated patient for you to explain briefly the examination and gain consent. Occasionally the examiner may take on this role. You will then perform the examination on a specialised model, but will be instructed to continue to explain what you are doing as if it were a real patient. These models can usually be set up to have any scrotal or testicular pathology, or can be set up as a normal examination.

The examiner will ask you to present your findings and may ask some brief questions on causes of scrotal swellings or an appropriate initial management plan.

PATIENT INFORMATION

Name: Mr Mark Davison   **Age:** 25 years   **Sex:** Male

Communication: You consent to the examination and are cooperative with it. You agree to a chaperone. You have noticed a painless lump in your scrotum which has been there for a week.

If you are asked: You cannot 'move' or 'reduce' the swelling.

CLINICAL KNOWLEDGE AND EXPERTISE

Examination of the scrotum and groin (Fig. 3.4.1)
Introduction
- Introduce yourself, and explain briefly what you plan to do.
- Ask for consent and offer a chaperone.

Figure 3.4.1 Scrotum and contents (From Douglas G., et al., *Macleod's Clinical Examination*, 13/e (Churchill Livingstone, 2013) with permission.)

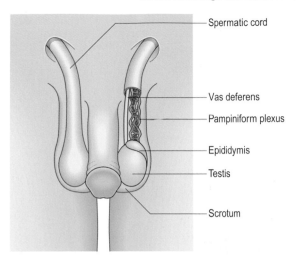

Spermatic cord

Vas deferens

Pampiniform plexus

Epididymis

Testis

Scrotum

3

- Clean your hands and put on a pair of gloves.
- Examination of the scrotum is best performed with the patient standing. You will also need to examine the groin so this must be visible—explain that you will need to examine the lower abdomen to the upper thigh. Allow the patient privacy to undress.
- Check with the patient whether there is any pain or tenderness before you start.

Inspection

- Look at the scrotum and groin. Are there any obvious areas of swelling? Are there any previous surgical scars? Is there any redness?

Palpation

- Palpate the scrotum gently, using both hands (thumb and forefingers). Check that both testes are present in the scrotum; if not, examine the inguinal canals.
- With each testis in turn, immobilise one side by placing one hand behind it, and use the index finger and thumb to palpate the entire body of the testis, and then the cord structures and epididymis at the top of each testis.
- If you palpate a swelling, try to ascertain whether it is separate to the testis or part of it, or part of the epididymis. If you cannot get 'above' the swelling, it may be an inguinal hernia.
- Finally, palpate both groins for any swelling and for inguinal lymph nodes which may be present in epididymitis (but remember that testicular tumours spread to the para-aortic nodes).

Auscultation

- You should auscultate any scrotal swelling for bowel sounds as it may be an inguinal hernia.

Special tests

- Using a torch, shine the light through any scrotal swellings. Hydrocoeles and larger epididymal cysts will transmit the light and transilluminate, whereas other swellings will not (Fig. 3.4.2).

3

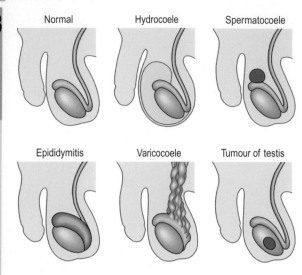

Normal | Hydrocoele | Spermatocoele

Figure 3.4.2 Swellings of the scrotum (From Douglas G., et al., *Macleod's Clinical Examination*, 13/e (Churchill Livingstone, 2013) with permission.)

Epididymitis | Varicocoele | Tumour of testis

- If you suspect an inguinal hernia, ask the patient if they can reduce (push back or move) the swelling, and if not, try and reduce it yourself. If it is reducible, then once reduced place your fingers over the deep inguinal ring and ask the patient to cough to see if it is contained.

Comparison of examination findings for different scrotal pathologies

Table 3.4.1 Comparison of examination findings for different scrotal pathologies			
Type of scrotal swelling	**Types/Causes**	**Features**	**Special tests**
Hydrocoele	Idiopathic or secondary to other pathology.	Separate to testis but may overlie it and prevent examination of it—can be very large.	Transilluminates
Varicocoele	Most usually idiopathic but note can be a rare presentation of a renal cell carcinoma due to obstruction of the testicular vein.	Separate to testis and may feel like part of cord structure (but caused by varicosities in the spermatic vein).	—
Epididymitis	Commonly due to STI (sexually transmitted infections) but can be secondary to urinary tract infections.	Usually tender uniform swelling of epididymis.	Examine inguinal nodes
Epididymal cyst	—	Separate to testis, benign.	Transilluminates
Inguinal hernia	Indirect or direct—but only indirect is likely to extend into the scrotum.	May be reducible. Unable to 'get above' the swelling.	Auscultation Try to reduce Cough test
Testicular tumour	Teratoma Seminoma Remember that an undescended testis increases the risk of testicular cancer.	Part of the testis, may feel firm and irregular. Cannot tell the difference between them clinically but teratomas tend to affect a younger age group.	-

WARNING

- Testicular torsion is an emergency. Any male presenting with acute scrotal or lower abdominal pain and scrotal swelling should be referred to the urology department immediately.
- Remember that testicular cancer affects males of all ages. Scrotal swellings should be further investigated by ultrasound in the majority of cases.
- A hydrocoele may be idiopathic, but can be secondary to a testicular tumour, and its presence will usually impair clinical examination of the testis. Ultrasound is mandatory.

✔ **How to excel in this station**

Action	Reason	How
Professional and respectful approach.	The patient may be nervous about an intimate examination; you must behave professionally and put the patient at ease.	Remember the essentials of good communication—make good eye contact, have a reassuring manner and explain clearly what you are going to do. Offer the patient privacy to undress and always offer a chaperone for intimate examinations.
Good knowledge of the different scrotal pathologies.	It is difficult to approach an examination without an idea of what the different pathologies feel like.	Read about the different pathologies. Practise the examination in a skills lab where you can examine models with a range of different pathologies. You can also get relevant experience in a urology or sexual health clinic.

✖ **Common errors in this station**

Common error	Remedy	Reason
Poor communication/consent, unable to establish rapport.	Understand that good communication is a central element.	Intimate examinations when performed inappropriately or without a chaperone can be a cause of complaints and even litigation.
Poor technique or disordered examination.	Practise the examination and be methodical. Gain experience from clinical practice and from observing others where appropriate.	This is an important examination but not encountered as frequently as others. It will be obvious if you have little clinical knowledge of the anatomy and relevant pathologies.

STATION VARIATIONS

◐ ◑ Basic–Intermediate

A digital rectal examination or breast examination is frequently encountered, both of which require a similar approach, with similar considerations of communication and consent. Refer to *Macleod's Clinical Examination* (rectal examination, pp. 207–8; breast examination, pp. 239–42) for the clinical knowledge, and you can use this station (and adapt the mark-sheet) to practise your general approach to intimate examinations.

Further Reading

Douglas G., et al., Macleod's Clinical Examination, 13th edn (Churchill Livingstone, 2013), Ch. 10. The male genital examination provides further detail about male genital examination and the various pathologies.

Examining the patient with liver disease

3.5

CANDIDATE INFORMATION

Background: David Hall is a 46-year-old man who has been referred to the outpatient clinic with abnormal liver function tests. He drinks 30–40 units of alcohol a week. He has also noticed some recent weight loss.

Task: Please examine him and then discuss with the examiner your differential diagnosis and your first-line tests.

APPROACH TO THE STATION

After reading the above you should think of the most common differential diagnoses and look out specifically for these. A standard abdominal examination is straightforward; however, the candidate information suggests that you should tailor this towards liver disease. In an OSCE it is most likely that a real patient would have chronic disease with stable signs. In this case, there is a heavy alcohol history, but also weight loss. As well as alcoholic liver disease, a gastrointestinal malignancy with liver metastasis should be high on the list of differentials. You should consider all causes of chronic liver dysfunction including fatty liver disease (alcoholic or non-alcoholic), viral hepatitis and potentially congestive cardiac failure, so look for their features and demonstrate this to the examiner.

PATIENT INFORMATION

You should wear a T-shirt and be prepared to strip to the waist. Then follow the instructions from the candidate during the examination.

CLINICAL KNOWLEDGE AND EXPERTISE

Examining a patient with liver disease
Introduction
• Gain permission to examine patient and explain what you are about to do.
• Clean your hands prior to beginning.

Inspection

- Look at the patient from the end of the bed—are they noticeably jaundiced or cachectic, or is there obvious abdominal distension? Are there any visible tattoos (risk factor for viral hepatitis)?
- Move to the hands—look for finger clubbing, leukonychia, palmar erythema and a liver flap (asterixis).
- Face—look at the sclerae for signs of jaundice and the conjunctiva for pallor (possible GI malignancy).
- Neck—examine the JVP, which may be raised in congestive cardiac failure. Examine the patient for lymphadenopathy in the left supra-clavicular fossa only (see diagram).
- Chest—have a brief look for spider naevi and gynaecomastia.
- Abdomen—look for spider naevi, caput medusa (enlarged veins around the umbilicus indicative of portal hypertension) and distension. It is helpful to crouch at the bedside and look across the abdomen, which can help to identify organomegaly or masses even before palpating the abdomen. Comment on any scars, herniae or stomas.
- Inspect legs for peripheral oedema (this can be done at the end).

Figure 3.5.1 shows signs of chronic liver disease.

3

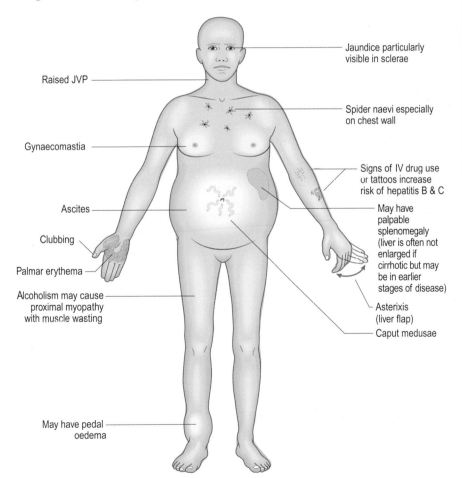

Figure 3.5.1 Signs of chronic liver disease (From Douglas G., et al., *Macleod's Clinical Examination*, 13/e (Churchill Livingstone, 2013) with permission.)

3

Palpation

- Ask the patient whether they have any tenderness. If they do, palpate this area last and check with the patient if they are in discomfort; stop if they are.
- Palpate the nine areas of the abdomen first superficially, then more deeply, whilst looking at the patient's face. Try to keep your hand flat on the abdomen and bend your hand rather than poking your finger tips in.
- Palpate for organomegaly, this time with your hand tilted so that you are palpating mainly along the index finger. For the liver, start in the right iliac fossa gently palpating upwards on inspiration and moving sequentially upwards. For the spleen, use the same technique starting in the right iliac fossa and moving diagonally towards the left hypochondrium.
- In a standard examination you would also ballot the kidneys.
- Palpation may be difficult if the abdomen is very distended or in the presence of ascites.

Percussion

- Percuss the liver from the lower ribs to below the level that you felt a liver edge on palpation. If you could not feel a liver edge then percuss downwards until the note changes (becomes tympanic).
- If the abdomen is distended, percuss horizontally across the abdomen at the level of the umbilicus to assess for dullness in the flanks. If there is dullness, proceed to test for shifting dullness.

Auscultation

- In a standard abdominal examination you would listen for renal bruits, but this is not as relevant here. In this case, you may want to perform a liver scratch test (see further reading).

Special Tests

- A standard abdominal examination would finish with a request to perform examination of the groin and external genitalia for hernias, and a PR examination.

 WARNING

- Any history of weight loss should prompt you to consider malignancy as a differential diagnosis. Some GI malignancies (such as pancreatic cancer) present late, often with metastatic disease.
- If a patient has signs of liver cirrhosis and portal hypertension they need to undergo screening for oesophageal varices as these can cause life-threatening upper GI bleeding.

How to excel in this station		
Action	**Reason**	**How**
Focus your examination.	This shows the examiner you are adapting your examination based on your clinical knowledge.	Look specifically for signs of liver disease and concentrate on these.
Establish a rapport with patient.	This demonstrates you have good communication skills and respect for the patient.	Tell the patient what you are going to do during the examination and check with them that it is alright to proceed.

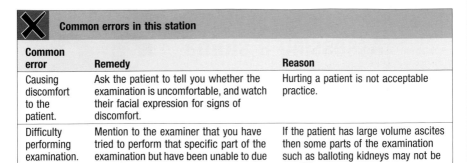

Common error	Remedy	Reason
Causing discomfort to the patient.	Ask the patient to tell you whether the examination is uncomfortable, and watch their facial expression for signs of discomfort.	Hurting a patient is not acceptable practice.
Difficulty performing examination.	Mention to the examiner that you have tried to perform that specific part of the examination but have been unable to due to ascites.	If the patient has large volume ascites then some parts of the examination such as balloting kidneys may not be possible.

STATION VARIATIONS

3

⬤ Basic

A standard abdominal examination, usually on a healthy volunteer.

⬤ Intermediate

Other focused abdominal stations could include renal disease or haematological disease. Think about the ways in which you would adjust your clinical examination to make it particularly relevant to these systems.

⬤ Advanced

As well as the examination above, you may be asked questions at the end about investigation and management of the patient. Basic investigation of patient presenting with liver disease would include:

- Imaging—such as an ultrasound
- Bloods—bilirubin, liver enzymes (ALT, AST, Alk phos, GGT), INR and prothrombin time, albumin, full blood count, U+E
- Autoantibodies—antimitochondrial antibody, anti-smooth muscle antibody, anti-nuclear antibody
- Screening for other diseases—immmunoglobulins, ferritin and transferrin, α_1-antitrypsin, ceruloplasmin, α-fetoprotein
- Screening for infection—hepatitis B and C, cytomegalovirus, Epstein–Barr virus, HIV.

Further Reading

Douglas G., et al., Macleod's Clinical Examination, 13th edn (Churchill Livingstone, 2013), Ch. 8.
Macleod's Clinical Diagnosis, Chapter 19, 'Jaundice'.

Assessing a stoma

3.6

CANDIDATE INFORMATION

Background: You are attached to the colorectal surgical team. Mr. Geoffrey Ford (59 years old) is currently an inpatient following recent abdominal surgery. The staff nurse has asked you to review him as he is complaining of a reduction in output from his new stoma.

Task: Assess Mr Ford's stoma and present your findings.

APPROACH TO THE STATION

This station is asking you to assess the patient's stoma with no information as to the operation. This indicates that not only should you comment on the appearance and health of the stoma, you should also establish the stoma type; look at the appearance of the stoma and where it has been positioned on the abdomen. Having a stoma fitted can have a huge psychological impact in terms of body image and requires a significant adjustment, especially in the first few weeks, so any examination should be undertaken with care and sensitivity.

PATIENT INFORMATION

Be prepared to lie on a couch with your stoma (with bag fitted) exposed. You will have a sheet to cover your abdomen. Listen to the candidate and then give consent. The candidate is not expected to take a history from you.

CLINICAL KNOWLEDGE AND EXPERTISE

A stoma is an opening in the skin, allowing the connection of a hollow organ to the outside; with a bag attached for the organ contents to drain. Most commonly this is gastrointestinal (colon, ileum), although urostomies are required in some cases of invasive bladder or prostate cancer. Stomas may be permanent or temporary, with the intention of closing the latter at a later date.

Assessment of a stoma

Introduction

- Introduce yourself and gain consent.
- Wash hands and apply gloves.
- Ensure that the patient is appropriately exposed (ideally this would be nipples to knees—but to preserve dignity would normally just expose abdomen).

Inspection (Table 3.6.1)

- *From the end of the bed:* Look for abdominal scars, stoma position and whether the patient appears unwell (unlikely in OSCE) and any other indicators of systemic disease.
- *Looking at the stoma:* Note appearance (flush with skin or has a spout?), health (colour should be pink/red and appear moist and glistening), stoma contents (comment if absent) and colour, consistency and volume.

Palpation

- Check whether the patient is in any pain—both asking and reviewing patient's face for discomfort.
- Palpate abdomen for any surrounding tenderness, masses or the presence of parastomal hernias.
- In addition you should percuss the abdomen and auscultate for bowel sounds (indicating a functioning bowel).

Special tests

For completion you should offer to perform a digital stomal examination using the index finger with gloves and lubricant (not expected in the OSCE).

Problems with stomas

Although these are unlikely to feature within the OSCE, it is important to comment on their presence or absence to demonstrate that you are aware of possible complications including:

- Erythema, rash or ulceration;
- Bleeding or fissuring;
- Parastomal hernias;
- Stomal prolapse, retraction or necrosis;
- Separation of the mucocutaneous edge;
- Narrowing or obstruction of the stoma lumen;
- Diarrhoea or constipation; and
- Iatrogenic injury, e.g., resulting from rubbing of clothing.

Table 3.6.1 Differences between a colostomy and an ileostomy		
Stoma	Colostomy	Ileostomy
Surface	Mucosa sutured to and flush with skin	Spout appearance, proud from skin
Location	Usually in the left iliac fossa	Usually in the right iliac fossa
Contents	Brown solid formed stool, intermittently present	Green liquid stool, continuously present
Indications	Colorectal carcinoma, diverticular disease	Inflammatory bowel disease, familial adenomatous polyposis coli

3

✓ How to excel in this station

Action	Reason	How
Demonstrate knowledge.	Show an awareness of stoma types and how to differentiate between these and demonstrate knowledge of possible complications.	An excellent candidate will comment on findings systematically throughout their examination before summarising, including what type of stoma the patient has and why.
Treat patient with dignity and respect.	Acknowledge that this can be an intimate and sensitive examination with stomas having a profound effect on confidence and body image.	Ensure the patient's comfort throughout and explain each stage of the examination to ensure continuing consent. Remember to cover the patient at the end.

✗ Common errors in this station

Common error	Remedy	Reason
Accidentally cause pain to the patient.	Check with the patient prior to starting whether they have any pain and recheck throughout verbally and through checking the patient's expressions.	The skin surrounding any stoma can be sensitive, especially early postoperatively although the stoma mucosa itself doesn't have any nerve endings—which can make it prone to injury.
Inadequate exposure of the stoma itself.	Ask the patient if they would be able to remove their stoma bag after inspection of the patient at the end of the bed.	Fear and embarrassment about asking the patient to remove their stoma bag, but without doing so, it is not possible to assess stoma health and check for any complications.

Further Reading

http://www.fastbleep.com/medical-notes/surgery/8/56/284.

For further information on stomas; http://www.patient.co.uk/doctor/Stoma-Care. htm (not expected in the OSCE).

Examining vision

3.7

CANDIDATE INFORMATION

Background: You are a doctor in a general practice. Mr Martin Peters is 45 years old and has come in for a routine examination as part of his heavy goods vehicle licence renewal, which includes having to test his vision.

Task: Please examine Mr. Peters' vision using the equipment provided (see Patient Information).

APPROACH TO THE STATION

This station requires you to examine vision thoroughly, not just testing the patient's visual acuity. Clues to the examiner's expectations can be the equipment provided and that no past medical history is given indicates that the examiner may wish to focus on a complete examination rather than identification of specific signs.

Fundoscopy can be uncomfortable for a patient, especially if performed repeatedly, and adequate explanation and consent should be obtained. You should assess vision with and without any visual aids required and, if their glasses are not available, a pinhole in a piece of card can be used to correct refractive errors.

Pitfalls in examining vision can occur if there is a lack of comprehension or understanding and it can be difficult to perform such tests on a confused patient or a child with limited attention. The examination relies upon the candidate having a good level of vision and deficiencies within the candidate's own visual fields could affect the accuracy of the test. Ideally candidates should remove their own glasses (if worn) when using the ophthalmoscope and use the dial provided to correct for their visual impairment prior to performing fundoscopy.

PATIENT INFORMATION

It is not necessary to have any abnormalities for this examination; however, should glasses normally be worn, they should be available for use.

Equipment:
- Snellen chart
- Pen torch
- Ophthalmoscope
- Large headed pin (if available)

3

CLINICAL KNOWLEDGE AND EXPERTISE

Examination of vision

Introduction

- Introduce yourself and confirm the patient's identity.
- Gain consent and explain the need for a darkened room with the use of a bright light that may be 'dazzling but not damaging'.
- Check whether the patient requires glasses and that they are available.

Inspection

- Examine the eyes externally to look for any indicators of pathology, e.g., proptosis, lid retraction, ptosis, asymmetrical pupils at rest.

Visual acuity

- Examination should be performed with the patient's glasses both on and off.
- The Snellen (or LogMar) chart should be used 6 m away from the patient.
- Ask the patient to cover one eye with their hand and read the lowest line possible on the chart before switching eyes.
- If the patient is not able to make out any of the letters on the chart, then assess their ability to count fingers, see hand movement or distinguish between light and dark.

Visual fields

- Sit directly across from the patient, about a metre away, so that your eyes are level with theirs.
- Ask the patient to cover one eye with a hand and cover your eye directly opposite their covered one, i.e., the contralateral eye to theirs.
- Ask the patient to stare directly ahead into your eye at all times—to detect any unwanted eye movement.
- Extending your arm outwards, wiggle your index finger in each of the four outer quadrants of their visual field; ask the patient to say 'yes' when they see your finger move and bring it in from the periphery inwards until it is seen.
- If sensory inattention is suspected, ask the patient to stare forwards at you with their eyes open whilst testing both visual fields at the same time.
- Use the hat pin to detect the patient's blind spot (and your own) by asking the patient to cover an eye as before (and you do the same) and focus on your eye then, holding the pin laterally, move it horizontally and inwards until it disappears and reappears in your vision.

Pupillary reaction (to light and accommodation)

- Using a pen torch, compare the size and shape of each pupil.
- Asking the patient to stare straight ahead, shine the light from the side directly at each pupil and look for constriction of both pupils (direct and indirect reflexes).
- Test accommodation by asking the patient to fix on a point in the distance, then quickly focus on your finger close to their nose—look for constriction of both pupils.

Eye movements (Fig. 3.7.1)

- Note any convergent or divergent squint.
- Hold your index finger vertically and, whilst asking the patient to keep their head still, slowly move your finger in the shape of an H to assess each ocular muscle.
- Look for nystagmus and ask the patient about any diplopia.
- Remember that nystagmus can be normal on extreme gaze.
- If diplopia is detected, establish the direction and ask the patient to close one eye to confirm whether it is binocular.
- The direction that the diplopia is worse in corresponds with the direction of action of the affected muscle.

Figure 3.7.1 Examining eye movement

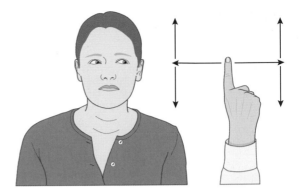

Fundoscopy

- Ensure a darkened room.
- State that you would want to dilate the pupils for best visualisation of the fundus – unlikely in an OSCE (unless already done).
- Remember to adjust the dial to correct for your own refractive error before starting if removing your glasses.
- Test for the red reflex by standing back from the patient and shining the ophthalmoscope at each eye whilst looking through it; any abnormalities would appear opaque.
- Examine the patient's left eye using your left eye, holding the ophthalmoscope in your left hand, and vice versa, whilst asking the patient to stare at a point in the distance.
- Get as close as you can to the patient without knocking heads and do not forget to breathe!
- Adjust the dial until the fundus comes into focus then follow the path of a blood vessel to the optic disc and assess the disc and surrounding retina and arteries for any abnormalities such as haemorrhages or scarring.

Colour vision (if required)

- This can be assessed using Ischihara plates if provided. If not provided, still state that you would test it for completeness.

 WARNING

- Sudden visual loss, or sudden onset of a visual field defect, should be regarded as a medical emergency and prompt immediate referral.
- New onset impairment of red-green colour vision can be an early sign of optic nerve damage before visual acuity is lost and should warrant urgent ophthalmology assessment.

✔	**How to excel in this station**		
Action	**Reason**		**How**
Know how to use the equipment.	Fumbling around with an ophthalmoscope is a waste of valuable time and also looks unprofessional and unprepared.		Fundoscopy is a difficult skill to master (including for qualified doctors). The key is to practise repeatedly on colleagues or patients.

(Continued)

3

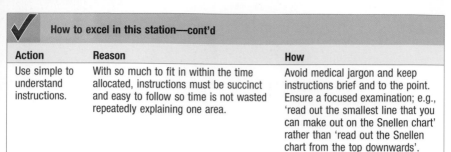

Action	Reason	How
Use simple to understand instructions.	With so much to fit in within the time allocated, instructions must be succinct and easy to follow so time is not wasted repeatedly explaining one area.	Avoid medical jargon and keep instructions brief and to the point. Ensure a focused examination; e.g., 'read out the smallest line that you can make out on the Snellen chart' rather than 'read out the Snellen chart from the top downwards'.

Common errors in this station

Common error	Remedy	Reason
Running out of time.	Practise breaking down the visual examination into sections and work out how long to allow for each to ensure all are completed within the time.	The tendency can be to focus too much on one aspect of the examination and not allow enough time to complete a full assessment.
Forgetting one section entirely.	Work systematically through the sections remembering that each is testing a different cranial nerve (II, III, IV and VI) and check that each has been assessed before finishing—talk through them aloud if needed.	In the rushed panic of the exam situation it can be possible to forget sections of such a complex assessment entirely, thus leaving the exam incomplete.

STATION EXTENSIONS

⭘ Advanced

To add clinical signs to a simulated patient, abnormal fundoscopy photographs could be provided with the candidate being asked to describe the findings (or use a patient with diabetic eye disease). Alternatively, the examiner may provide a normal fundoscopy photograph, so do not try to identify abnormalities that are not actually there in an attempt to impress!

Further Reading

Macleod's Clinical Examination, Chapter 12: 'The Visual System; Examination of Vision'.

Lower limb sensory examination

3.8

CANDIDATE INFORMATION

Background: You are a junior doctor in Accident and Emergency. Mrs Elsie Jacobs (84 years old) has a history of ischaemic heart disease and type 2 diabetes. Her carer has brought her in with a puncture wound in the sole of her right foot. Mrs Jacobs is not aware of injury and admits that she has not had a lot of feeling in the soles of her feet for a couple of years.

Task: Please perform a sensory examination on Mrs. Jacobs' lower limbs, focusing on the history of diabetes and present your findings.

APPROACH TO THE STATION

You are told about the background diabetes, making it likely that sensory examination will reveal a peripheral neuropathy in a 'stocking' distribution (Fig. 3.8.1). The examination should focus on eliciting the relevant signs and assessing the severity and extent of the neuropathy. Vibration sense is often the first to be affected in diabetes and this must not be missed through time pressures. You must use a systematic process: working up the lower limbs comparing one side with the other whilst testing the different sensory modalities.

PATIENT INFORMATION

The key assessment is the methodical approach, thus making simulated patients useful even without clinical signs to elicit. A simulated patient may be briefed to assume a pattern of sensory loss typical of a peripheral diabetic neuropathy.

Suggested briefing for sensory loss
- Absent vibration sense over the great toe and ankle (preserved over tibial tuberosity and anterior iliac spine if tested — simulated patient will be instructed where these are).
- Reduced sensation of light touch extending from the feet up to the mid-calf bilaterally.
- Reduced sensation of pinprick touch extending from the feet up to the mid-calf bilaterally.
- Normal joint position sense in the great toes.
- Reduced temperature sensation over feet bilaterally.

3

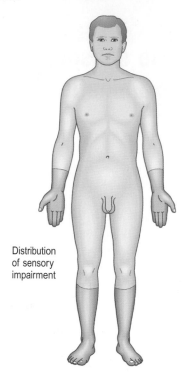

Distribution
of sensory
impairment

Figure 3.8.1 Illustration of glove and stocking distribution of neuropathy (From Douglas G., et al., *Macleod's Clinical Examination*, 13/e (Churchill Livingstone, 2013) with permission.)

CLINICAL KNOWLEDGE AND EXPERTISE

Peripheral neuropathy can be divided into acute and chronic presentations that can be symmetrical or affect several nerves (mononeuritis multiplex). Most peripheral neuropathies are chronic and develop slowly over several months, with sensory neuropathies starting distally. Diabetes is the commonest cause of chronic peripheral neuropathy in the western world but, in the absence of diabetes, other differentials should be considered, especially alcohol — through direct nerve damage or through an associated nutritional deficiency (see Box 3.8.1).

Diabetic peripheral neuropathy is common (20–40% of diabetic patients). It often coexists with peripheral arterial disease with high risk of complications such as ulceration, deformity or amputation. Those particularly at risk include older people, patients with poor vision, smokers, patients with a long history of diabetes and those with poor self-care or footwear.

Box 3.8.1 Predominant causes of sensory neuropathy
• Diabetic neuropathy • Thiamine deficiency (alcohol) • Malignancy (paraneoplastic syndrome), e.g., breast or lung carcinoma • Leprosy (very rare in the developed world) • Sarcoidosis (rare) • Amyloidosis (rare) • Uraemia • Hereditary sensory neuropathies

Examination of the sensory system

Introduction
- Introduce yourself and gain informed consent.
- Explain that you may be discussing your findings with the examiner during the examination.
- Wash your hands.
- Ensure that the patient is adequately exposed — with the lower limbs fully visible and any clothing removed.

Inspection
- Inspect the lower limbs, commenting on signs of muscle wasting, peripheral vascular disease (hair loss and dusky skin colour), ulceration or joint deformity, e.g., Charcot's joint.
- Comment on additional findings present such as insulin injection sites in the tops of the thighs or any walking aids visible next to the bed.

Light touch
- Use a small piece of clean cotton wool provided.
- Ask the patient to look away or close their eyes.
- Working your way up the lower limbs, comparing one leg with the other, touch each leg sequentially and ask the patient to comment each time they feel the touch.
- Use a dabbing rather than stroking motion and time each touch irregularly to avoid anticipation by the patient.
- Confirm any areas of reduced or absent sensation.

Superficial pain (pinprick)
- Use a fresh neurological pin and dispose of it in the sharps bin provided.
- Explain to the patient the need to assess pinprick and demonstrate normal sensation over the sternal edge.
- Ask the patient to report whether the sensation is sharper or blunter than normal whilst moving systematically up the limbs, comparing limb with limb.

Vibration sense (see Fig. 3.8.2)
- Use the 128-Hz tuning fork provided and hit it against your hand or the examination couch.
- Demonstrate normal vibration sense by placing the tuning fork on the sternum and checking that the patient feels a buzzing sensation (Fig. 3.8.2).
- Place the tuning fork on the tip of each great toe and ask the patient to confirm whether they can feel the vibration.
- If impairment is evident, move up to the medial malleolus, then the tibial tuberosity before the anterior iliac spine, stopping when normal sensation is felt.
- If answers are equivocal, ask the patient to tell you when the vibration stops and then you hold the tuning fork prongs.

Joint position sense (proprioception)
- Demonstrate what this involves to the patient with their eyes open initially.
- Hold the distal phalanx of the great toe at the sides and move it up and down, confirming this with the patient.
- With the patient's eyes closed ask them to confirm whether subsequent small movements in a random order are 'up' or 'down'.
- Do not press on the top or bottom of the toe when performing this to avoid giving any pressure clues.
- Compare each side with the other.

3

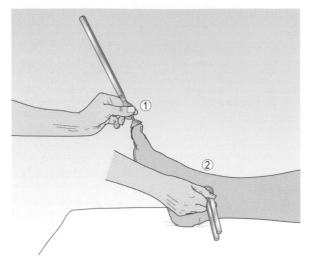

Figure 3.8.2 Picture of doctor applying tuning fork to medial malleolus (From Douglas G., et al., *Macleod's Clinical Examination*, 13/e (Churchill Livingstone, 2013) with permission.)

Temperature

- Often missed due to time but is worth mentioning or attempting to perform a basic assessment.
- Touch the patient with a cold object, e.g.,+ a tuning fork, and ask if it feels cold over sequential parts of the lower limbs, moving upwards.

Special tests

- Offer to assess gait and Romberg's test when standing (patient sways when standing with eyes closed, suggesting posterior column disease).
- Thank the patient and ensure that they are adequately covered up.
- Wash hands or apply alcohol hand gel.
- Present findings concisely to the examiner, focusing on important positive findings rather than a long list of negatives.

 WARNING

- Assessing pinprick sensation can be uncomfortable. Ensure that the patient has consented and understands what will happen so as to avoid any distress or embarrassment.
- Diabetic peripheral neuropathy can often coexist with peripheral arterial disease and you must offer to check the pedal pulses and assess the peripheral vascular system to complete the lower limb examination.
- Injury to a high risk diabetic foot leads to increased ulceration risk, which if infected can lead to amputation. All diabetic feet should be closely examined for any new injury, ulceration, swelling or dusky discolouration, which must prompt urgent referral.

✓ **How to excel in this station**

Action	Reason	How
A systematic approach to the examination.	A fluid, well-rehearsed and organised approach demonstrates competence to the examiner and also ensures that you are less likely to miss out important components.	Work methodically through the different sensory modalities, comparing one limb with the other before moving on to the next stage.
Explanation to the patient of the examination process.	The sensory examination can be confusing and good explanation throughout can mean that it progresses more smoothly.	Ensure that normal sensation is demonstrated for each modality at the beginning of each component, e.g., by touching the sternum.

✗ **Common errors in this station**

Common error	Remedy	Reason
Influencing the patient's answers through suggestion.	Give the patient their response instructions at the start of each component and ask them to respond without prompting, with their eyes closed. Time your touch irregularly, thereby minimising anticipation.	The patient may be eager to please, or worried about not getting the answer correct and just answer 'yes' if asked the question 'Can you feel this?'
Running out of time during the examination.	Do not take a history, as this is not necessary. Keep the examination succinct and present your findings during the examination if needed.	A laborious sensory examination can be tedious for both the examiner and the patient, and patient fatigue can result in inconsistent results from having to concentrate hard. A focused concise examination is preferable.

Further Reading

Hughes, R., 2002. Peripheral neuropathy. BMJ 324, 466–469.

Macleod's Clinical Examination, Section 11, 'The Nervous System: The Sensory System'.

Neurological Examination of the Lower Limbs. http://www.patient.co.uk/doctor/Neurological-Examination-of-the-Lower-Limbs.htm.

Willison, H.J., Winer, J., 2003. Clinical evaluation and investigation of neuropathy. J. Neurol. Neurosurg. Psychiatr. 74, ii3–ii8.

3

Limb weakness

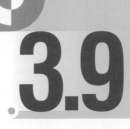

3.9

CANDIDATE INFORMATION

Background: Mr Smith has left arm weakness.

Task: Please examine him and discuss with the examiner your differential diagnosis and initial investigations.

Approach to the station

The main distinction is between weakness secondary to an upper motor neurone (UMN) and that to a lower motor neurone (LMN) lesion. This will provide a differential diagnosis and guide your investigations. The initial inspection is key as it can provide important clues as to which lesion is present — you can then examine for features that confirm this. For example, if the arm is held in flexion and there is obvious leg weakness (with extension), it is likely to be upper motor neurone (most likely a stroke).

PATIENT INFORMATION

This case will utilise a real patient with physical signs rather than a simulated patient.

CLINICAL KNOWLEDGE AND EXPERTISE

This station requires a full neurological examination of the upper limbs and, if time allows, some focused quick examination of other aspects of neurological examination. It is important to do your examination systematically and compare both sides as you go along — for example, examine tone on the left and then the right before moving on to examining power. When examining, you should decide whether the weakness is unilateral or bilateral and if it is an UMN or a LMN lesion (Table 3.9.1).

Table 3.9.1 Differentiating between upper motor neurone (UMN) and lower motor neurone (LMN) lesions

Domain	UMN lesion	LMN lesion
Inspection	Pyramidal pattern weakness	Flaccid weakness, prominent wasting
Tone	Increased—clasp knife spasticity	Decreased
Power	Reduced	Reduced—usually focally (depending on site of lesion)
Reflexes	Increased	Reduced/absent
Sensation	If sensory disturbance is present, usually entire limb is affected	Either a peripheral sensory loss or a dermatomal sensory reduction may be present

Introduction

- Gain permission to examine patient and explain what you are about to do.
- Clean your hands prior to beginning.

Inspection

- General inspection—look for other pathological signs such as facial droop or ipsilateral leg weakness. Listen to the patient's voice when you introduce yourself—is there any dysarthria or dysphasia? Do they have any walking aids near them, which would suggest lower limb weakness as well?
- Look for posture—is the arm held in flexion at elbow and wrist (pyramidal pattern suggesting UMN lesion)?
- Compare both sides—is there any muscle wasting or are any fasciculations present?

Tone

- Hold arm at the wrist and assess tone in the wrist and then the elbow. Compare the sides.
- Clasp knife increase in tone suggests an upper motor neurone lesion.
- Cog wheel (or 'lead pipe') increases are seen in extrapyramidal lesions (e.g., Parkinson's disease).

Power

- Again compare left to right. Grade using the MRC power rating (see Table 3.9.2). Myotomes tested are in brackets.
- Test shoulder abduction (C4), then adduction (C5).
- Elbow flexion (C6), then extension (C7).
- Wrist flexion (C7), then extension (C6).
- Finger abduction (T1).

Reflexes

- Biceps (C5)—put thumb in biceps tendon and observe for elbow flexion.
- Supinator (C6)—strike supinator tendon on lateral side forearm and observe for elbow extension.
- Triceps (C7)—strike triceps tendon just above elbow on posterior surface and observe for elbow extension.

Coordination

- Examine finger to nose coordination at the extremes of reach, looking for pass pointing.
- Pyramidal drift—ask patient to hold both arms out in front of them, palms up and then close their eyes—if the arm pronates, the test is positive, suggesting an upper motor neurone lesion.

Table 3.9.2 MRC power table	
Grade	Power
1	No movement
2	Flicker of movement
3	Movement with gravity eliminated
4	Movement against gravity, not resistance
5	Normal power

3

Special tests

- You may wish to examine the median, radial and ulnar nerves—this is detailed in station 3.12.
- You should say you would like to examine the rest of the neurological system including cranial nerves and lower limbs. In this station you could quickly look for signs of upper motor neurone weakness of the face (facial drooping on right) and the leg.

Stroke is a very common disease with a consistent persistent pattern of weakness and therefore the most common form of unilateral weakness that will appear in OSCEs. You should therefore know about common patterns of stroke so you can gain extra marks (Fig. 3.9.1). The Bamford classification subdivides stroke into the following clinical presentations:

1. *Total anterior circulation stroke* (TACS)—all three of (1) arm weakness, (2) homonymous hemianopia and (3) cortical dysfunction (dysphasia/ apraxia).
2. *Partial anterior circulation stroke* (PACS)—2/3 of the above or cortical dysfunction by itself.
3. *Lacunar stroke* (LACS)—limited motor/sensory deficits without cortical dysfunction.
4. *Posterior circulation stroke* (POCS)—cerebellar dysfunction/visual defects/brainstem events.

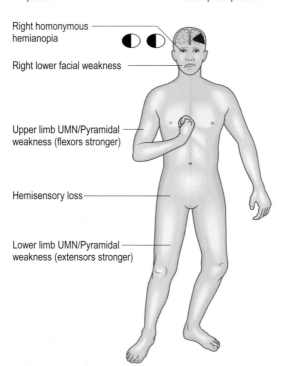

Left sided cerebral infarct

Dominant hemisphere
(right handed)
- Dysphasia
  (expressive/receptive)
- Aphasia

Non-dominant hemisphere
(left handed)
- Neglect
- Apraxia
- Visuospatial problems

Right homonymous hemianopia

Right lower facial weakness

Upper limb UMN/Pyramidal weakness (flexors stronger)

Hemisensory loss

Lower limb UMN/Pyramidal weakness (extensors stronger)

Figure 3.9.1 Clinical features of total anterior circulation stroke

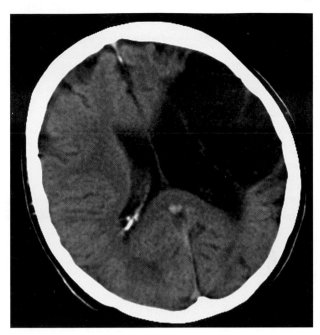

Figure 3.9.2 CT scan showing old right middle cerebral artery (MCA) infarct (From Perkin GD, *Atlas of Clinical Neurology*, 3/e (Saunders, 2011) with permission.)

3

⚠ WARNING

- A sudden onset of weakness may mean a stroke or TIA and requires urgent assessment.
- In a younger person, sudden onset of stroke following trauma caused by neck rotation or extension may mean a carotid artery dissection.
- A mixture of upper and lower motor neurone signs (usually bilaterally) could mean motor neurone disease — fasciculation is a prominent feature. Examine for speech and swallowing difficulties.

✓ How to excel in this station

Action	Reason	How
Be confident testing reflexes.	It is easy for examiners to tell whether you have practised your skills on real patients.	Practise testing left- and right-sided reflexes standing on one side of the bed. Practise with a real tendon hammer and remember the key is to let the hammer fall onto the tendon under gravity rather than hitting it forcefully.
Look for risk factors for stroke.	This demonstrates that you are aware of the risk factors for stroke and you know how to examine for them.	Feel pulse for atrial fibrillation, check blood pressure and listen to carotid arteries for a bruit.

3

Common errors in this station		
Common error	**Remedy**	**Reason**
Examining only one side.	Examine both sides, comparing one side to the other.	You would not want to miss bilateral weakness.
Being unsystematic.	Follow the structure suggested above and stick to it.	Neurological examination can be complex so following the structure means you are unlikely to miss something important.

STATION VARIATIONS

● Intermediate

You may be asked to assess lower limb weakness instead—do this following the same pattern and decide: is it unilateral or bilateral and is it a UMN or LMN lesion?

● Advanced

You may be asked to comment on a CT or MR scan—this is similar to commenting on an X-ray (see station 7.2). Compare the sides and look for the obvious abnormality. Remember in stroke the infarct will be on the contralateral side to the clinical signs.

Further Reading

Macleod's Clinical Examination, Chapter 11, 'The Nervous System'.
Macleod's Clinical Diagnosis, Chapter 22, 'Limb weakness'.
NICE stroke guidelines. http://www.nice.org.uk/cg68.

The patient with a tremor 3.10

CANDIDATE INFORMATION

Background: You are a junior doctor in the neurology clinic. The referral for this patient is as follows:

'Mr Herron presents with a 6-month history of a tremor in his right hand and some difficulty walking. He is not taking any medication currently. He wonders if he may have Parkinson's disease?'

Task: Examine the patient and discuss your diagnosis with him.

APPROACH TO THE STATION

There are two parts to this station—a focused neurological examination and then a discussion that may involve breaking bad news—leave adequate time for both. You should have a clear idea of the differential diagnosis so that you focus on positive features. The main differential is between Parkinsonism, essential tremor and other less likely causes (see Table 3.10.1). You must consider which cause of Parkinsonism is most likely based on your examination (see Table 3.10.2). A diagnosis of idiopathic Parkinson's disease (IPD) is based on the triad of bradykinesia, rigidity and tremor.

Table 3.10.1 Differential diagnosis of tremor					
	Location	**Timing**	**Frequency**	**Symmetry**	**Other signs**
Parkinson's disease	Hands or legs	Worse at rest	Coarse	Presents asymmetrically	See Table 3.10.2
Essential tremor	Hands	Worse on action	Coarse	Usually bilateral	Head titubation (nodding)
Hyperthyroidism	Hands	Ever present	Fine	Bilateral	Goitre, tachycardia; see station 3.11
Cerebellar	Arms	Worse on action/ intention (end of movement)	Usually fine	Depends on site of lesion— can be either	Ataxia, dysdiadochokinesia, nystagmus

Table 3.10.2 Parkinsonian syndromes (* = Parkinson's plus syndromes)

Parkinsonism syndrome	Pattern	Specific history	Specific signs
Idiopathic Parkinson's disease (IPD)	Asymmetrical tremor and signs	Asymmetry. Initial leg tremor suggests IPD.	Bradykinesia, rigidity and tremor
Vascular Parkinsonism (VaP)	Lower body Parkinson's, gait dyspraxia	History of vascular disease	Lack of tremor
Multiple systems atrophy (MSA)*		Autonomic neuropathy, urinary symptoms, lack of response to levodopa	Postural hypotension
Progressive supranuclear palsy (PSP)*	Truncal rigidity and increased tone	Early falls, lack of response to levodopa	Gaze palsy
Dementia with Lewy bodies (DLB)*		Early cognitive impairment, more severe psychiatric side effects with levodopa	Cognitive impairment
Drug-induced Parkinsonism	Total body rigidity	Antipsychotic drugs, metoclopramide	Lack of tremor

PATIENT INFORMATION

This station will normally use a real patient with a tremor disorder. The candidate will examine you and should ask you to walk as part of this.

CLINICAL KNOWLEDGE AND EXPERTISE

This is a focused version of a neurological examination (see station 3.9). Examining sensation is not required, but assessing function including gait is key.

Introduction
- Gain permission and explain what you are about to do.
- Clean your hands prior to beginning.

Inspection (Fig. 3.10.1)
- General inspection — look for hypomimia (lack of facial expression), use of walking aids. Look for any dyskinesia (may be a side effect of levodopa).
- Look for tremor (see Table 3.10.1).
- Check eye movements (PSP) and for nystagmus (cerebellum).
- Listen for low volume monotonous speech.

Tone
- Check tone for cogwheel rigidity in Parkinson's disease. Bring this out by asking the patient to tap their other hand on their knee.
- Check for tone in lower limbs.

Power
- Briefly examine power — should be normal.

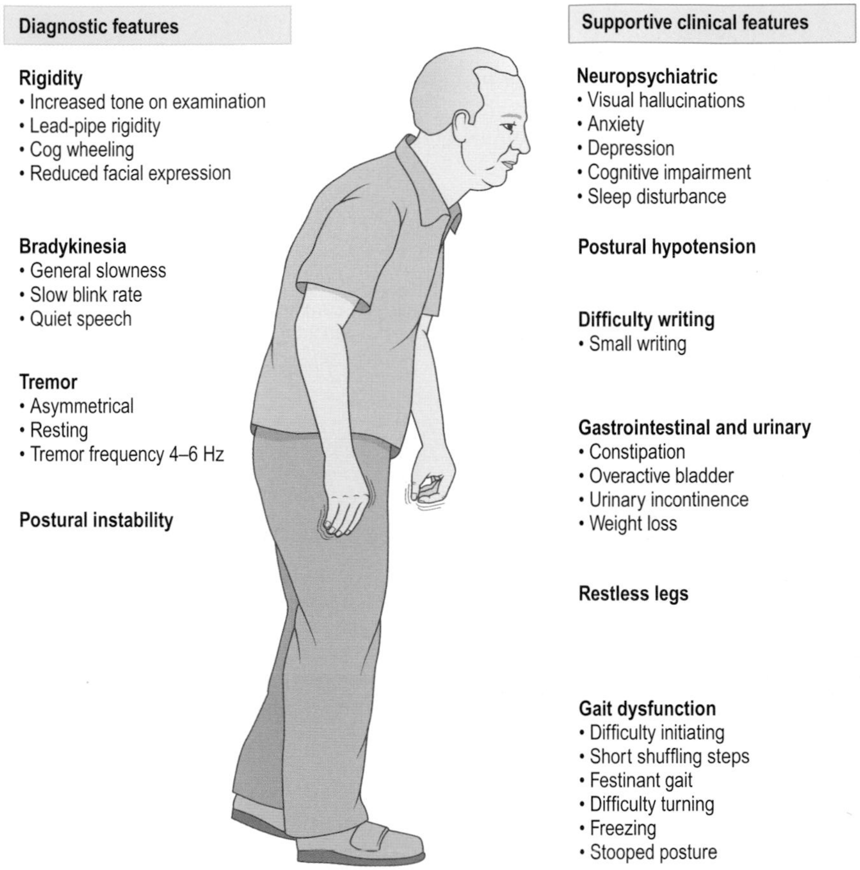

Diagnostic features

Rigidity
• Increased tone on examination
• Lead-pipe rigidity
• Cog wheeling
• Reduced facial expression

Bradykinesia
• General slowness
• Slow blink rate
• Quiet speech

Tremor
• Asymmetrical
• Resting
• Tremor frequency 4–6 Hz

Postural instability

Supportive clinical features

Neuropsychiatric
• Visual hallucinations
• Anxiety
• Depression
• Cognitive impairment
• Sleep disturbance

Postural hypotension

Difficulty writing
• Small writing

Gastrointestinal and urinary
• Constipation
• Overactive bladder
• Urinary incontinence
• Weight loss

Restless legs

Gait dysfunction
• Difficulty initiating
• Short shuffling steps
• Festinant gait
• Difficulty turning
• Freezing
• Stooped posture

3

Figure 3.10.1 Clinical features of idiopathic Parkinson's disease

Reflexes
• Check upper limb reflexes—should be normal.

Coordination
• Examine the tremor—ask patient to do finger/nose coordination. Is tremor worse at rest or on action?
• Look for bradykinesia—ask patient to rapidly tap index finger and thumb together. Also look for a progressive reduction in amplitude—both suggest idiopathic PD.
• Ask patient to write a sentence—look at grip (can they pick up the pen?) and at writing (typically smaller than normal in idiopathic PD).
• Examine gait—ask patient to walk a short distance, turn around and walk back. Look for arm swing, difficulty turning, bradykinesia, shuffling gait, freezing, festinant gait (Parkinsonism).

Special Tests
Say you would screen for non-motor features of Parkinson's disease by enquiring about falls, mood and sleep disorders, testing cognition (see station 3.18) and checking postural BP.

3

 WARNING

- Look for signs and symptoms of Parkinson's plus syndromes (see Table 3.10.2 — these patients deteriorate more rapidly) — where patients have signs of Parkinson's but also evidence of other system involvement.

✓	How to excel in this station	
Action	**Reason**	**How**
Ask about non-motor signs.	Demonstrates breadth of knowledge as these can often have a significant impact on quality of life.	Comment that you would like to ask about mood, sleep disturbance and test cognitive function.

✗	Common errors in this station	
Common error	**Remedy**	**Reason**
Not examining gait.	Examine gait—ask the patient to walk a short distance and then turn around.	Gait abnormalities are a key feature of Parkinsonism.
Not focusing the examination.	Follow the focused neurological examination described above.	Shows that you can apply your knowledge practically.

STATION VARIATIONS

◐ Advanced

You may be asked to comment on the treatment options for Parkinson's disease (Table 3.10.3).

Table 3.10.3 Treatment options for Parkinson's disease	
Patient and carer support	Specialist nurses, charities (e.g., Parkinson's UK) and sources of information about disease and prognosis
Multidisciplinary management	Physiotherapy, occupational therapy, social work, speech and language therapy, Parkinson's disease specialist nurses
Levodopa	Usually combined with a peripheral dopa-decarboxylase inhibitor to reduce systemic side effects
Dopamine agonists	Usually used in younger patients. Include pramipexole, ropinirole, rotigotine
COMT inhibitors	Entacapone: Used for reduction in 'off time' (dopamine effects wearing off before next dose due)
Apomorphine	Subcutaneous infusion used in severe disease
Anti-cholinesterase inhibitors	Rivastigamine—used if cognitive impairment ± hallucinations
Surgery	Deep brain stimulation in severe treatment resistant cases

Further Reading

Macleod's Clinical Examination, Chapter 11, 'The Nervous System'.
Parkinson's UK, website: http://www.parkinsons.org.uk/for-professionals.aspx.
Movement Disorders Society, website: http://www.movementdisorders.org.

Thyroid status and neck examination

3.11

Background: You are a junior doctor in a general practice. Ms Megan Cross (27 years old) is attending because of weight loss and heat intolerance.

Task: Please examine Ms Cross' thyroid status, including examination of her neck. You are not required to take a history.

APPROACH TO THE STATION

This station requires examination of the neck, but also specifies assessment of the thyroid status. The examination should therefore commence at the hands and progress as per the recommended outline. Before you reach the neck, you should have already elicited the patient's thyroid status.

In this station the patient is a young woman and the background information given highlights weight loss and heat intolerance. These are frequent features of hyperthyroidism (see Table 3.11.1) and Graves' disease is common in this age group. However,

Table 3.11.1 Clinical findings in hypo- and hyperthyroidism	
Hypothyroidism	**Hyperthyroidism**
Lethargic	Agitated and restless
Dressed warmly, cool to touch	Dressed coolly, warm and sweaty to touch
Dry, coarse skin	Hand signs Thyroid acropachy (looks like clubbing) Onchyolysis Palmar erythema (common) Fine tremor (common)
Bradycardia	Tachycardia, possible atrial fibrillation
Recent weight gain	Recent weight loss
Hair dry and coarse, may be alopecia and loss of the outer third of the eyebrow	Hair loss
Slow relaxing reflexes	Proximal myopathy (mostly subclinical)
Croaking speech (voice change common)	Eye signs Lid lag (common) Lid retraction Exophthalmos (Graves) Ophthalmoplegia (rare—severe)
± Goitre	± Goitre

3

Table 3.11.2 Types of thyroid enlargement	
Type of thyroid lesion	**Causes**
Diffuse enlargement	Graves' disease (common) Hashimoto's thyroiditis De Quervain's thyroiditis Anaplastic carcinoma
Single nodule	Simple cyst Benign adenoma Follicular or papillary carcinoma
Multinodular	Toxic multinodular goitre (hormone excreting) Non-toxic multinodular goitre (non-hormone excreting)
Tender goitre	Thyroiditis Anaplastic carcinoma

it is important to evaluate the patient carefully and link her thyroid status with the thyroid gland examination, as she could have a toxic multinodular goitre (see Table 3.11.2 for differential diagnosis of a goitre).

PATIENT INFORMATION

Name: Megan Cross   **Age:** Approximately 20–30 years   **Sex:** Female

Findings: Patient with goitre

CLINICAL KNOWLEDGE AND EXPERTISE

Clinical findings in hypo- and hyperthyroidism are summarised in Table 3.11.1 and the causes of the main thyroid enlargements are in Table 3.11.2.

Figure 3.11.1 shows the appearance of a goitre.

Examination of thyroid status and the neck
Introduction
- Introduce yourself, explain briefly and gain consent.
- Clean your hands prior to beginning.
- Ensure the patient is seated comfortably with space for you to stand behind.
- Uncover the patient so the neck is exposed to the clavicles.

Inspection
- Inspect and comment on agitation, flushing, hair loss, dress, body habitus, lesions or scars in the neck and exophthalmos.
- Inspect the shins for pretibial myxoedema.
- Inspect the neck, looking for masses or lumps, enlargement of the thyroid gland or scars from surgery (classic 'necklace' scar — thyroidectomy).
- Give a glass of water and ask the patient to take a small amount and swallow when directed. Stand in front and observe the neck while they swallow. A goitre should ascend on swallowing.
- Ask the patient to protrude their tongue. A thyroglossal cyst is a midline lesion that ascends on protrusion of the tongue.
- Inspect the eyes for lid retraction and exophthalmos (look down on the patient from behind their head, the eyes should not be visible beyond the supra-orbital ridge).

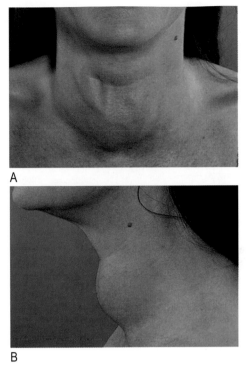

Figure 3.11.1 Goitre (From Douglas G., et al., *Macleod's Clinical Examination*, 13/e (Churchill Livingstone, 2013) with permission.)

Palpation

- Examine the hands, commenting on skin temperature and presence or absence of palmar erythema, onycholysis or thyroid acropachy.
- Ask the patient to hold their hands out flat—lay a piece of paper over them to demonstrate a fine tremor.
- Take the pulse, noting the rate and rhythm.
- Check the power of shoulder abduction as a simple marker of proximal myopathy. Ask the patient to cross their arms and stand from the chair.
- Elicit the ankle reflexes and comment if they appear slow-relaxing.
- Test eye movements for ophthalmoplegia and test for lid lag—follow your finger vertically up and then down.
- Examine the neck from behind—feel gently with the fingertips.
- Feel for lymph nodes (see Fig. 3.11.2), examine in the following order and comment on size, consistency and mobility:
  - Begin with your fingers touching under the chin and move simultaneously on each side (submental nodes).
  - Continue to under the angle of the jaw (submandibular nodes).
  - Feel anterior to the tragus (parotid nodes), just above this (pre-auricular nodes) and posterior to the pinnae (posterior auricular nodes).
  - Palpate at the base of the skull (occipital nodes).
  - Palpate down each side of the neck using the sternocleidomastoid muscle as a guide (anterior cervical chain in front of the muscle and posterior cervical chain behind).
  - Finally, feel in the supraclavicular notch (supraclavicular nodes).

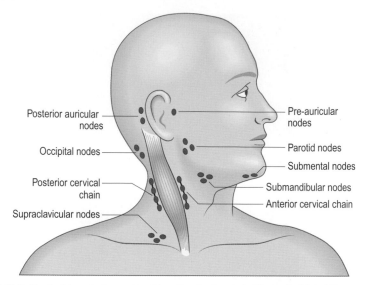

Figure 3.11.2 Cervical lymphadenopathy (From Douglas G., et al., *Macleod's Clinical Examination*, 13/e (Churchill Livingstone, 2013) with permission.)

- Palpate the thyroid gland, feeling both lobes (the central isthmus is rarely palpable). Comment on shape, consistency, nodularity and tenderness.
- Again ask the patient to swallow some water, while palpating if the gland is fixed — suggestive of invasive carcinoma.

Auscultation
- Standing in front, listen for a bruit over each side of the thyroid gland, which can occasionally occur with increased blood flow (Graves' disease).

Percussion
- Percuss down from the sternal notch; a dull note may indicate a retrosternal goitre but this is a poor physical sign.

⚠ WARNING

- A patient in (new) atrial fibrillation is at risk of embolus and needs immediate consideration of anticoagulation.
- Carcinoma of the thyroid gland must be considered if a nodule is stony hard or the thyroid gland is fixed — urgent referral is required.
- A hoarse voice and bovine cough may indicate recurrent laryngeal nerve palsy — complication of thyroid surgery or carcinoma of the thyroid.

 How to excel in this station

Action	Reason	How
Recognise Graves' disease.	An advanced candidate can distinguish the signs of Graves' disease from those of hyperthyroidism.	Clinical signs specific to Graves' disease Exophthalmos and eye disease Pretibial myxoedema (rare infiltrative dermopathy) Thyroid acropathy.

How to excel in this station—cont'd

Action	Reason	How
Identify complications.	Demonstrates multi-level knowledge of the features of Graves' disease, and the complications if untreated.	Exophthalmos can lead to chemosis, conjunctivitis, corneal ulceration and ophthalmoplegia. Graves' eye disease may require cosmetic surgery. Atrial fibrillation can lead to emboli and stroke. Osteoporosis Complications in pregnancy Thyrotoxic crisis.

3

Common errors in this station

Common error	Remedy	Reason
Misdiagnosis of the thyroid status.	Consider clinical features together; remember the patient (OSCE) may be euthyroid.	A patient on treatment for Graves' disease who is euthyroid may still have a goitre and eye signs. Similarly, a patient with Graves' disease may be hypothyroid (treatment complication).
Causing pain to the patient.	Explain what you are doing and palpate gently at all times.	Examination of the thyroid and the neck can be uncomfortable.

STATION VARIATIONS

○ Basic

'Please examine the neck'

If the information specifically requests examination of the neck only, introduce yourself, check the patient is comfortable and consents and then begin inspection of the neck.

There are a number of common neck lumps (see Table 3.11.3) and you should be able to give a differential diagnosis. The site of the lump in the neck is often an important clue to the aetiology.

Remember that the patient may have a goitre even if you are not asked to examine the thyroid status, as many patients with a goitre become euthyroid while on treatment.

Table 3.11.3 Causes of neck swellings	
Midline	Goitre (ascends on swallowing) Thyroglossal cyst (ascends on protrusion of tongue) Submental lymphadenopathy Enlarged parathyroid gland (extremely rare)
Lateral	Lymphadenopathy—consider malignancy, especially in adults Salivary gland enlargement, secondary to an impacted stone or tumour Parotid gland enlargement Other benign lesions—lipoma, sebaceous cyst In children—cystic hygroma, branchial cyst

3

Table 3.11.4 Interpreting thyroid function tests			
	Low free T4	**Normal free T4**	**High free T4**
Low TSH	Secondary hypothyroidism (very rare)	Subclinical hyperthyroidism	Hyperthyroid
Normal TSH		Euthyroid	
High TSH	Hypothyroid	Subclinical hypothyroidism	Secondary hyperthyroidism (very rare)

TSH, thyroid stimulating hormone.

⦿ Advanced

Examination station combined with interpretation of thyroid function tests

You may be asked to interpret thyroid function tests. The normal ranges vary between laboratories and will be provided with the question.

At undergraduate level, you are likely only to be asked to identify the biochemical patterns highlighted in bold (see Table 3.11.4).

Further Reading

MacLeod's Clinical Examination, Chapter 5, 'The Endocrine System'.

Examination of the hands

3.12

CANDIDATE INFORMATION

Background: Mrs O'Hanlon is a 65-year-old woman who presents to her GP with painful and swollen hands.

Task: Please examine her hands and then speak to the examiner about the most likely diagnosis and investigations you would perform to confirm this.

APPROACH TO THE STATION

This is a common station as there are many patients with chronic stable hand signs. Look for the following:
- *Number of joints involved*: One joint involved is a mono-arthritis, 2–4 joints suggest an oligoarthritis and 5+ suggest a polyarthritis.
- *Pattern of arthritis*: Is it symmetrical or bilateral, and which joints are affected?
- *Extra-articular features*: Eye, skin and nail, genital changes.

In an OSCE the most common conditions would be osteoarthritis, rheumatoid arthritis or a seronegative (such as psoriatic) arthritis. As well as looking for signs that point to the diagnosis, you should examine the function of the hands, as this is what causes disability.

PATIENT INFORMATION

You should wear a T-shirt or shirt and be prepared to bare your elbows.

CLINICAL KNOWLEDGE AND EXPERTISE

Introduction
- Gain permission to examine patient and explain what you are about to do.
- Clean your hands prior to beginning.
- Get patient to place their hands in a comfortable position — on a pillow if available.

Inspection
- General inspection — look for alopecia (may suggest seronegative arthritis), check ears for gouty tophi and check skin for psoriasis or vasculitis.
- Inspect the hands — look for swelling and comment on symmetry and position (see Fig. 3.12.1).

Rheumatoid arthritis

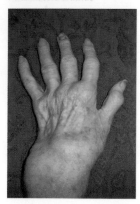

Osteoarthritis

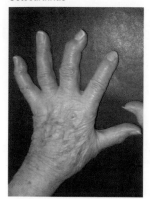

A

Polyarthritis

Bilateral symmetrical MCP/ PIP swelling

Rheumatoid nodules

Swan neck deformity

Soft tissue swelling

Radiological changes

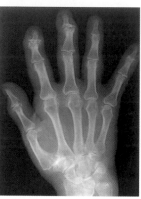

B

Oligo/ polyarthritis

Bilateral, asymmetrical DIP swelling

Hebedens and Bouchards nodes

Bony swelling

Radiological changes

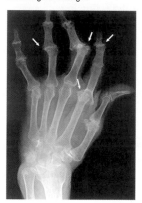

C

Juxta-articular osteopaenia

Bony erosions

Joint space narrowing

Subluxation

D

Subchondral sclerosis

Joint space narrowing

Osteophyte formation

Figure 3.12.1 Comparison of rheumatoid arthritis and osteoarthritis in hands (Part D from Weiss S, *Hand Rehabilitation*, 2/e (Mosby, 2005) with permission.)

- Look for typical deformities—swan neck or boutonniere.
- Examine nails for vasculitic lesions and psoriatic changes (pitting/ridging/ onycholysis).
- Look at elbows for rheumatoid nodules (indicate seropositive rheumatoid arthritis).

Palpation
- Palpate each joint gently, feeling for swelling or bony deformity—do this systematically—MCP, PIP, DIP.

Special Tests

Functional Tests
- Test grip strength ('grip my finger').
- Test function—writing ability.
- Test function—ask to do up buttons on shirt.
- Ask to pick something up off table (pen, for example).

Motor Function of Nerves
- Radial—test wrist extension against resistance.
- Median—test thumb abduction.
- Ulnar—abduct extended fingers against resistance.

3

Sensory function of nerves
- Radial—dorsal aspect of hand between 1st and second metacarpals.
- Median—palmar aspect of hand, thumb, index, middle and half of ring finger.
- Ulnar—palmar aspect of hand, little and half of ring fingers.

The basic investigations for this lady should include the following in this setting. Further investigations would be done in specialist clinics following referral, and may include aspiration of synovial fluid ± MRI scanning of joints.
- FBC, U + E, bone profile (to check for associated conditions or extra-articular manifestations of rheumatological disease)
- ESR/CRP (to screen for inflammation)
- Rheumatoid factor or CCP antibodies (to screen for rheumatoid arthritis)
- X-ray of hands/feet (to look for radiological evidence of joint disease (see Fig. 3.12.1).

WARNING

- A single hot swollen joint with systemic signs of infection needs urgent investigation to exclude septic arthritis (usually including joint aspiration and gram staining).
- NSAIDs have many side effects including cardiovascular events, gastric irritation/ulceration and renal failure.

✓	How to excel in this station	
Action	**Reason**	**How**
Comment on classification criteria for inflammatory arthritis.	This shows that you have wider knowledge of the subject and that you have read guidelines.	See American College of Rheumatology classification in Further Reading section.
Ask about difficulty in function.	This shows you are assessing function and understanding how the person's arthritis affects their day-to-day life.	Ask if there any specific tasks that the person finds difficult. Show understanding that this may have an effect on their quality of life.
Comment on the X-ray systematically.	Doing so means you do not miss anything and shows you are being thorough.	Use a systematic approach to commenting on X-rays, similar to that detailed in station 7.2; e.g., 'This is an AP X-ray of the left hand. Penetration is adequate. The main features are... this suggests....'.

3

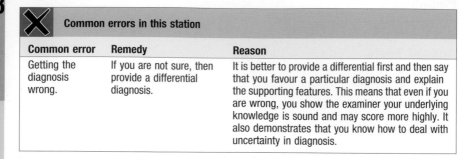

Common errors in this station

Common error	Remedy	Reason
Getting the diagnosis wrong.	If you are not sure, then provide a differential diagnosis.	It is better to provide a differential first and then say that you favour a particular diagnosis and explain the supporting features. This means that even if you are wrong, you show the examiner your underlying knowledge is sound and may score more highly. It also demonstrates that you know how to deal with uncertainty in diagnosis.

Table 3.12.1 Treatment options for rheumatoid arthritis

Multidisciplinary management	Occupational and physiotherapy
Analgesics	Paracetamol, NSAIDs or COX-2 inhibitors if required
Steroids	Oral or intramuscular—for rapid control of disease flares
Disease-modifying anti-rheumatic drugs (DMARDs)	E.g., methotrexate, azathioprine, leflunomide, gold—require drug monitoring
Biological agents	TNF-α inhibitors, e.g., infliximab, etanercept, adluminab
Surgery	Joint replacements and fusion surgery

STATION VARIATIONS

● Advanced

You may be asked to comment on treatment options for rheumatoid arthritis; list these in order (Table 3.12.1).

Further Reading

American College of Rheumatology classification criteria for rheumatic diseases. http://www.rheumatology.org.

Macleod's Clinical Examination, Chapter 14, 'The Musculoskeletal Examination'.

NICE guidance on Rheumatoid arthritis. http://www.nice.org.uk.

Knee examination

3.13

CANDIDATE INFORMATION

Background: You are a junior doctor working in Accident and Emergency. Mr. Keith Bryce is a 59-year-old builder and has a painful left knee in the absence of any recent trauma or injury. He thinks it might be swollen. Normally, he is well with no past medical history and takes no regular medications.

Task: Examine Mr. Bryce's knee and present your finding to the examiner.

APPROACH TO THE STATION

Examination of a knee joint is a popular OSCE station, and although it is probable that candidates will be asked to examine a normal joint, it is important to have a systematic and methodical approach that demonstrates good anatomical and pathophysiological knowledge. You must ensure that examination covers not only the tibiofemoral and patellofemoral components, but also the muscular and ligamentous structures.

If there is an abnormal knee joint within the OSCE, osteoarthritis is likely to be the cause and there may be clues at other joints, e.g., the hands, although remember that osteoarthritis can coexist with an inflammatory arthropathy. Other causes of knee pain and swelling are listed in Table 3.13.1. You should not take a history, as this is not required and would only waste time. With any joint examination you should offer to examine the joints above and below to exclude referred pain as the possible cause. It is also important to compare with the corresponding opposite joint (although in osteoarthritis, both may be abnormal).

Table 3.13.1 Causes of knee pain and swelling	
Trauma	Fracture, ligament or meniscal injury
Arthritis	Reactive inflammatory arthropathy, osteoarthritis, gout, pseudo-gout
Infection	Septic arthritis, osteomyelitis, gonorrhoea
Tumour	Malignant, e.g., osteosarcoma, or benign, e.g., osteochondroma (unlikely in OSCE)

3

PATIENT INFORMATION

Name: Mr Keith Bryce   **Age:** 59 years   **Sex:** Male

Communication: You are happy for the examination, but should not discuss any background history with the candidate even if asked.

Examination findings: The information for the candidate indicates that your left knee might be mildly swollen. You are mainly tender around the inside of the knee along the joint line (you should express discomfort). You can move the knee fully.

CLINICAL KNOWLEDGE AND EXPERTISE

Examination of the knee
Introduction
- Introduce yourself, confirm the patient's identity and obtain consent.
- Expose the knee fully. Use a blanket or towel to maintain the patient's dignity.
- Wash hands or apply alcohol hand-gel.
- Check whether he/she has any pain currently and get him/her to point to the most painful area so that you can proceed with most caution around this area.

Inspection
- Ensure adequate exposure of both knees extending up to quadriceps muscles and down to calves.
- Comment on any muscle wasting evident—in particular, around the quadriceps—and compare sides.
- Comment on the joint position at rest (legs should be relaxed and fully extended with knees resting on the couch) and any deformity visible; e.g., fixed flexion deformity or genu varus/valgus.
- Comment on any swelling and its position relative to the knee joint—is it generalised or localised?
- Comment on erythema or skin changes (e.g., psoriasis) or scars/signs of previous surgery.

Palpation
- Check for pain again and start the examination away from any painful area.
- Comment on any temperature difference between the two knees.
- Describe any swelling—soft or hard, localised or generalised?
- Palpate for an effusion using the patellar tap or ripple test (Fig. 3.13.1). First empty the suprapatellar pouch by sliding your left hand down the thigh to the patella. Fix in that position and tap on the patella to feel it 'floating' on top of the effusion (patellar tap), or massage the fluid out of the medial joint then watch it re-accumulate when stroking the lateral joint (ripple test).

Movement
- Get the patient to flex and extend the knee as far as possible and establish if it is painful and estimate the maximal range.
- Move joint passively through its range whilst feeling for crepitus over the joint (may be audible) and taking care that the patient is not in pain.

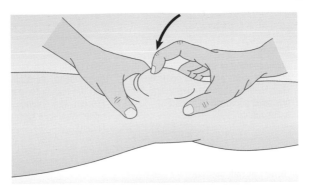

Figure 3.13.1 Testing for effusion using the patellar tap (From Douglas G., et al., *Macleod's Clinical Examination*, 13/e (Churchill Livingstone, 2013) with permission.)

3

Stability
- Assess the cruciate ligaments with the knee flexed at 90° and the sole of the corresponding foot planted flat on the bed with the quadriceps relaxed. Hold the knee with both hands (thumbs facing towards you) and try to pull the lower leg towards you then push it backwards — excess movement would indicate laxity.
- Assess the lateral ligaments by holding the patient's lower leg into your side to stabilise, then use both hands to apply valgus then varus force and look for opening up of the joint or discomfort.

Special tests
You may wish to discuss these tests although they would not be appropriate for this case and may cause discomfort.
- *Patellar apprehension test*: Push the patella laterally whilst the knee is fully extended, then attempt to flex the knee slowly — resistance by the patient suggests instability or previous dislocation (Fig. 3.13.1).
- *Meniscal provocation test*: Flex the knee fully and externally rotate the foot; then extend the knee and listen/feel for a clunk and discomfort before repeating with the foot held in internal rotation when the knee is flexed and extended (Fig. 3.13.2).

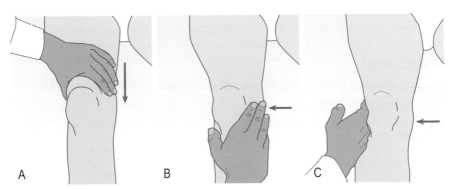

A   B   C

Figure 3.13.2 The ripple test (From Douglas G., et al., *Macleod's Clinical Examination*, 13/e (Churchill Livingstone, 2013) with permission.)

3

 How to excel in this station

Action	Reason	How
Demonstrate knowledge.	Understanding of the underlying anatomy of the knee and common abnormalities shows a methodical, well-practised approach to a joint examination.	Talk to the examiner throughout the examination, describing each aspect and the reason for performing it. Present your findings systematically rather than as a long list of negative findings.

Common errors in this station

Common error	Remedy	Reason
Causing pain to the patient during the examination.	Ensure that you have discussed with the patient prior to starting where the pain is located and palpate very gently around this area initially, constantly checking the patient's face for discomfort.	The examiner will watch closely for you considering the patient's comfort at all times, especially during an examination of an abnormal joint that can be extremely tender. It is important to adapt any examination around the patient if painful.

Box 3.13.1 Treatment options for osteoarthritis (in order)

- Activity and exercise
- Weight loss where appropriate
- Analgesia—paracetamol and topical NSAID
- Consider NSAID and COX-2 inhibitors (but risk of cardiovascular disease needs careful consideration)
- Intra-articular joint injections
- Consider referral for joint replacement

STATION VARIATIONS

Intermediate

Examiners will often ask candidates in OSCEs to discuss common X-ray findings in osteoarthritis of the knee. These are listed for the hands in Fig. 3.12.1 in station 3.12.

Advanced

You may be asked to discuss treatment options for osteoarthritis (see Box 3.13.1).

Further Reading

Macleod's Clinical Examination, Chapter 14, 'The Musculoskeletal System', pp. 388–392.

http://www.arthritisresearchuk.org/health-professionals-and-students/student-handbook/the-msk-examination-rems/examination-of-the-knee.aspx.

Shoulder examination

3.14

CANDIDATE INFORMATION

Background: You are a junior doctor working in general practice. Mrs Annabelle Hayes (48 years old) is a hairdresser who is complaining of a painful and stiff right shoulder for the past fortnight, which is affecting her ability to work. She denies any trauma to the arm and is right-handed. She is on hormone replacement therapy, but is otherwise fit and well and takes no other medications.

Task: Examine Mrs Hayes' shoulder and present your findings.

APPROACH TO THE STATION

Painful shoulders are very common and can be debilitating, especially in this case where her occupation relies on raising her arms and the pain is affecting her dominant arm. Shoulder pain can be referred, most commonly from the cervical spine, so it is important to exclude this and you should offer to examine the neck. As with other examination stations, it is not necessary to take a history and, although you may be presented with a normal shoulder to examine, you should take into account the patient's background when examining. Also be mindful that any joint examination may cause pain and you should check for this throughout.

Should an abnormal shoulder be used during the OSCE, the most likely diagnosis would either be degenerative disease or adhesive capsulitis (frozen shoulder), but you should still utilise the examination to exclude other possible pathologies, such as impingement syndrome, tendonitis and polyarthropathies. If the last is suspected, you should offer to examine other joints or look for clues in the hands and other exposed joints.

When differentiating between intra-articular disease and a focal tendonitis it is important to assess whether pain is reproduced throughout all movements (as with generalised degeneration) or just one plane. As this patient has a job that involves repetitive movement, one may anticipate the diagnosis of tendonitis, but it is important to remember that pathologies can coexist and there may also be a degree of osteoarthritis or impingement.

PATIENT INFORMATION

Name: Mrs Annabelle Hayes **Age:** 48 years **Sex:** Female

Communication: You are happy for the examination. You should not discuss any background history with the candidate even if asked. You do not require a chaperone.

3

> **Examination findings:** You do not have any pain when the shoulder is being examined. If the candidate examines your neck movement, then this causes the pain (not bad) and also you have some tingling over the shoulder.

CLINICAL KNOWLEDGE AND EXPERTISE

Examination of the shoulder
Introduction
- Introduce yourself and confirm the patient's identity.
- Obtain consent for the examination.
- Wash hands or apply alcohol hand-gel.
- Ensure that the patient is exposed from the waist (with bra on) and offer a chaperone.

Inspection
- You should examine the patient from the front, side and back and with the patient leaning up against a wall (position and symmetry of the scapulae).
- Inspect for any asymmetry between the sides, scars, swelling, deformity or muscle wasting.

Palpation
- Feel over the joint for any warmth suggesting inflammation.
- Palpate pain, swelling and crepitus around these joints: shoulder girdle starting medially at the sternoclavicular joint, along the clavicle to the acromioclavicular joint, around the spine of the scapula, then the anterior and posterior glenohumeral joint.

Movement
- Movements should be active before passive and you should estimate degrees of movements of both. All planes should be covered including:
- Flexion (arm comes forward);
- Extension (arm goes backwards with elbow bent to 90°);
- Abduction (arm goes out to side and above head); note the amount that the corresponding scapula has to move on the chest wall to facilitate abduction;
- Adduction (arm goes across front of chest);
- Internal rotation (arm rotates inwards and goes up back);
- External rotation (arm tucks into side with elbow flexed and hand moves outwards).
- Ask the patient to abduct the arm from the side of the body against resistance, whilst comparing one side with the other. An inability or pain can indicate a rotator cuff problem.

Function
- Ask the patient to put their arms behind their head then switch to put arms behind back to touch the lower shoulder blades.

Special tests (see Fig. 3.14.1)
There are multiple special tests for assessing the different functions of the shoulder, with a variety of names. Learn a few well and understand what they are testing rather than get overwhelmed by trying to master too many.
- *Impingement test* — First check for any 'painful arc' between 60 and 120° of abduction of the shoulder. Next, with the patient's arm flexed at 90°, and elbow also flexed at 90°, push down on the patient's wrist, thus internally rotating the shoulder and look for pain.
- *Apprehension test* — Glenohumeral instability: lie the patient on their back with the arm hanging over the edge of the bed with the elbow flexed at 90°. After abducting

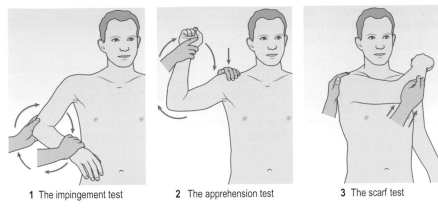

1 The impingement test   2 The apprehension test   3 The scarf test

Figure 3.14.1 Special tests for the shoulder

3

the arm to 90°, attempt to externally rotate the arm whilst pushing with the other hand anteriorly on the glenohumeral joint. If there is instability the patient will actively resist this.

- *Scarf test* – Flex the elbow to 90°, then push the arm towards the opposite shoulder so it appears to wrap like a scarf around the neck. Ask about pain around the stretched acromioclavicular joint.

Completion of the examination
- Offer to examine the cervical spine and any other appropriate joints.
- Thank the patient and ensure that they are appropriately covered.
- Present your findings in a concise summary. Do not just reel off a long list of negative findings.

✓	How to excel in this station	
Action	**Reason**	**How**
Demonstrate knowledge.	Articulate what is being tested for at each stage of the examination rather than just working through with no demonstrable understanding of the anatomy or underlying pathology.	Explain to the examiner what is being examined and why. This demonstrates that you have understanding of the reasons for each element. Review the different individual tests for the muscles of the rotator cuff to gain extra marks in a more advanced station (see Station Variations).

✗	Common errors in this station	
Common error	**Remedy**	**Reason**
Trying to examine through clothing.	Offer the patient a chaperone and explain to them the necessity to remove upper clothing prior to examining the shoulder.	It is easy to feel embarrassment when asking a patient to remove their upper clothing, but you must visualise the area fully to detect deformity and abnormality of the joint.

3

STATION VARIATIONS

○ Advanced

Demonstrate or discuss how a candidate would assess the individual muscles within the rotator cuff to look for suspected pathology. Examples of how to do this include:

- *Supraspinatus* — Flex arms at 30° with thumbs pointing downwards. Ask the patient to flex further against resistance and look for pain or reduced power.
- *Infraspinatus/Teres minor* — Hold elbows into chest wall whilst flexed at 90°. Ask the patient to externally rotate the arms against resistance and look for pain or reduced power.
- *Subscapularis* — With the elbows in the same position as previously, ask the patient to internally rotate the arms against resistance and look for pain or reduced power.

Further Reading

Macleod's Clinical Examination, Chapter 14, 'The Musculoskeletal System: The Shoulder'.

Obstetric examination

3.15

CANDIDATE INFORMATION

Background: You are a junior doctor in a general practice. Miss Lewis was seen routinely by the midwife last week and noted to have a slightly high blood pressure. The midwife has asked Miss Lewis to return to clinic for a further check-up.

Task: Please perform a complete obstetric examination on Miss Lewis.

APPROACH TO THE STATION

Obstetric examination is a useful skill for anyone who will work in primary or emergency care. However, being familiar with palpating a women's abdomen and finding the foetal heart takes practice. Take every opportunity to examine pregnant women when on your obstetric rotation and in primary care. It may be possible to spend a day with the community midwives, and this can be invaluable. In this station you need to demonstrate a confident and systematic examination of a pregnant woman, have a good bedside manner and demonstrate an awareness of important obstetric conditions not to be missed. Make sure you leave a couple of minutes after your examination to present your findings to the examiner. The case information should suggest the possibility of pre-eclampsia, and it is important to demonstrate to the examiner that you have considered this and are examining for the various features.

PATIENT INFORMATION

Name: Miss Jane Lewis **Age:** 31 years **Sex:** Female

Communication: You consent to the examination and are cooperative with it. You are currently 34 weeks pregnant in your first pregnancy. You have no headache or swelling. Foetal movements are normal.

Examination Findings: BMI is calculated at 23. There are no visible marks on the abdomen. Fundal height measures at 35 cm. Amniotic fluid volume appears normal. The foetus is in a longitudinal lie with the head as the presenting part. The head is not engaged (5/5ths palpable). The foetal heart is easily auscultated at 140 and regular. Blood pressure is 115/72 (booking blood pressure was 110/68). There is no peripheral oedema. Urinalysis demonstrates no protein, blood, leucocytes, nitrites or ketones.

3

CLINICAL KNOWLEDGE AND EXPERTISE

Obstetric examination

Equipment
- Tape measure
- Pinard's stethoscope or Doppler foetal heart monitor.

Examination

Introduction
- Introduce yourself, explain briefly what you plan to do and gain consent for the examination.
- Clean your hands prior to beginning.
- Measure the patient's height and weight and then calculate her BMI (kg/height in m^2).
- Ensure the patient is comfortably on a bed or examination couch in a semi-recumbent position and exposed from the rib case to the pubic bone. Ensure you maintain the patient's privacy and dignity.

Inspection
- Inspect the abdomen for distension compatible with pregnancy, striae, linea nigra, scars and visible foetal movements.
- Inspect for oedema; in pre-eclampsia this is often generalised but particularly affects the hands and face.

Palpation
- Measure the symphysis-fundal height over 24 weeks by palpating the fundus of the uterus and then measuring from the symphysis pubis to the fundus (with the blank side of the tape measure facing up). Compare the measurement to gestation (see Table 3.15.1).
- Palpate the abdomen noting the position of the foetal parts. Palpate either side of the uterus to get an impression for which foetal parts are lying on each side (a fullness on one side is often the back). Then palpate the lower uterus and feel for the foetal head—ballot gently between your hands. Be aware of the possibility of a multiple pregnancy.
- While palpating the abdomen, try to assess the amniotic fluid volume. Excessive fluid (polyhydramnios) may lead to large measurements for dates and difficulty in palpating parts, while too little fluid (oligohydramnios) is associated with small measurements and more obvious foetal parts on palpation.
- Distinguish the lie (the relationship between the foetus and the long axis of the uterus; see Fig. 3.15.1):
  - *Longitudinal*—the buttocks and head are palpable at each end of the uterus (either cephalic, if the head is in the pelvis, or breech, if the buttocks are in the pelvis).
  - *Transverse*—the foetus lies across the uterus and the pelvis is empty.
  - *Oblique*—the head or buttocks will be palpable in one of the iliac fossae.

Table 3.15.1 Interpretation of symphysis-fundal height	
Gestation	**Symphysis-fundal height**
12–14 weeks	Uterus becomes palpable
20–24 weeks	Fundus should be palpable at the level of the umbilicus
24+ weeks	Symphysis-fundal height in centimetres should match gestational age ± 3 cm Causes of large for dates—multiple pregnancy, polyhydramnios, obesity Causes of small for dates—oligohydramnios, intrauterine growth restriction

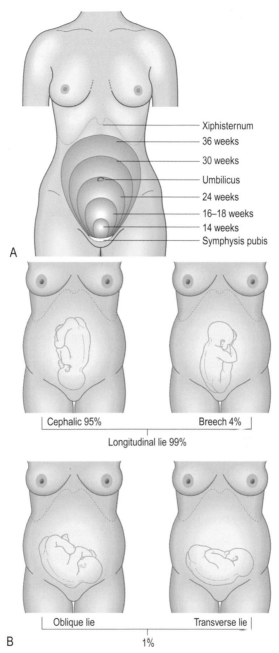

3

Figure 3.15.1 Symphysis-fundal height and foetal lie (From Douglas G., et al., *Macleod's Clinical Examination*, 13/e (Churchill Livingstone, 2013) with permission.)

3

- Distinguish the presentation, warning the patient that this part of the examination can be a little uncomfortable. Palpate just above the symphysis pubis to find which foetal part is occupying the lower segment of the pelvis.
- Estimate engagement of the head, described as 5ths palpable above the pelvic brim.

Auscultation
- Auscultate with a Pinard's stethoscope (over 28 weeks) or Doppler foetal heart rate monitor (over 14 weeks) over the anterior shoulder of the foetus. This is usually palpable between the foetal head and the umbilicus. The foetal heart rate should be between 110 and 160/min and regular.

Special tests
- Record a blood pressure.
- Review the patient's urine dipstick result if available. Offer an opportunity to give a urine sample prior to commencing the examination, as it can be uncomfortable with a full bladder.

 WARNING

- It is mandatory for all health professionals to be aware of the warning signs of pre-eclampsia and to refer urgently for further obstetric assessment if suspected. Features of pre-eclampsia include *hypertension* (compared to booking BP), *headache, oedema* and *proteinuria*.
- Decreased foetal movements or an abnormal (or absent) foetal heart rate should be taken very seriously and the patient should be urgently referred for further obstetric assessment.

✓ How to excel in this station		
Action	**Reason**	**How**
Be reassuring.	Particularly first-time mothers can find obstetric examinations stressful and uncomfortable, especially if it is hard to locate the foetal heartbeat.	Have a polite and calm bedside manner. Talk to the patient throughout the examination and explain what you are doing. Warn that parts of the examination may be uncomfortable (this is particularly true when you are feeling for the presenting part and engagement).
Demonstrate obstetric knowledge.	An excellent student will not only be technically able to perform the examination but also have an awareness of the relevance of the examination findings.	Learn the importance of a high or low BMI in pregnancy, a small or large symphysis-fundal measurement and the suggestion of oligo- or polyhydramnios. Be aware of important conditions such as gestational diabetes, pre-eclampsia and the risks of multiple pregnancies.

Common errors in this station		
Common error	**Remedy**	**Reason**
Failure to maintain dignity.	Draw the curtain around the bed and avoid interruptions. Offer privacy to undress. Place a sheet over any visible underwear. Ask patient permission for any extra observers.	It is important to demonstrate that your patient's privacy and comfort are paramount to you.

STATION VARIATIONS
3

O Advanced

Features of pre-eclampsia

Following your examination, an examiner may ask you what you would think if you found the following features:

- Proteinuria 2+ on urine dipstick
- Blood pressure 145/90 (booking blood pressure 110/70).

State that you are concerned about pre-eclampsia (BP over 140/90 or rise of 30 mmHg systolic and 15 mmHg diastolic from booking BP). Pre-eclampsia can progress to HELLP syndrome (**h**aemolysis, **e**levated **l**iver function tests and **l**ow **p**latelets) or eclampsia, which are both potentially life-threatening, and therefore this patient would need urgent transfer to a hospital obstetric team for further assessment and investigation.

Further Reading

Macleod's Clinical Examination, Chapter 10, 'Reproductive Medicine', especially the section regarding 'Obstetric Examination'.

Newborn examination

3.16

CANDIDATE INFORMATION

Background: You are a junior doctor completing a Paediatrics rotation and have been asked to complete a discharge newborn examination on Grace.

Task: Complete a newborn examination of the baby or on the manikin. Communicate with the accompanying parent or carer and the baby/manikin.

APPROACH TO THE STATION

Identifying and being confident of what is 'normal' in a newborn is an important skill in primary care or Paediatrics. All babies have a check at around 8 weeks of life, normally by their GP, and most of this is very similar to the newborn examination (though it does include a few extra elements).

Many medical schools include the newborn examination as a key OSCE skill and assessment may be on a baby or a manikin. When examining a baby, it is important to handle him/her appropriately, and you may be asked not to examine the hips or to examine a model of the hips, as this can be uncomfortable. It is important to have a systematic approach so you do not omit anything important and to have good communication with the parent, and handle the baby competently and confidently. It is obvious when you have never picked a baby up before! The focus for medical students is recognising 'normal findings'. Further information has been provided about primitive reflexes (see Table 3.16.1), and although it is not necessary to demonstrate all of these in a routine newborn examination, it is important to be familiar with them. More detailed information on examination of the hips has also been included (see Table 3.16.2 and Fig. 3.16.1).

Table 3.16.1 Primitive reflexes	
Rooting reflex	Elicit by lightly stroking the cheek; the infant will turn their head to that side.
Sucking reflex	Elicit by placing gentle pressure on the hard palate with a finger while examining the mouth.
Grasp reflex	Hands and feet will grasp in response to gentle pressure—lost by 2–4 months.
Stepping reflex	A baby will step if lowered onto a hard surface—lost by 2 months.
Aysmmetrical tonic neck reflex (ATNR)	In response to head rotation, the baby will extend their arm on that side and the other will flex—lost by 6 months.

Table 3.16.1 Primitive reflexes—cont'd	
Moro reflex	Head is gently released from grasp and allowed to drop 2–3 cm—upper limbs abduct and extend symmetrically. An aysmmetric response may suggest hemiparesis (central, e.g., CP, or peripheral, e.g., brachial plexus injury)—lost by 6 months.
Plantar reflex	Bilaterally upgoing until approximately 12 months.
Galant reflex	When newborn is in ventral suspension, stroking one side of the spine causes spinal flexion on that side—may not be lost until 5 years old, but it is hard to elicit in a larger child.

3

Table 3.16.2 Examination of the hips	
Barlow manoeuvre	• This examines for a dislocatable hip—examine the hips separately. • Stabilise the pelvis with one hand by placing your thumb on the pubis symphysis and your fingertips on the sacrum. • With your other hand, hold one hip and knee flexed at 90° with thumb on the medial femoral condyle and middle finger tip on the greater trochanter, and try to push the hip posteriorly. • If there is a click, you have dislocated the hip. • Repeat on the other side.
Ortolani manoeuvre	• This aims to reduce a dislocated hip. • Again, examine the hips separately and stabilise the pelvis with one hand. • With the other hand, use the same grip as above, then lift the femoral head forward with the middle finger while abducting the thigh with your thumb. • If there is a clunk, you have reduced a dislocation. • Repeat on the other side.

Barlow manoeuvre

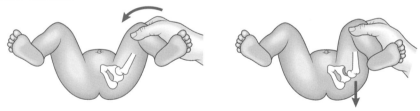

Adduct the hip while directing light pressure posteriorly, to try to dislocate a dislocatable hip

Ortolani manoeuvre

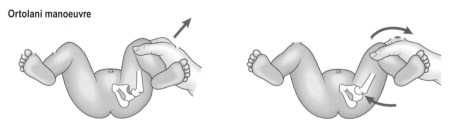

Perform immediately after Barlow manoeuvre. Flex the hips while abducting the leg, to try to relocate a dislocated hip

Figure 3.16.1 Examination of the hips

3

Name: Grace Hill   **Age:** 36 hours   **Sex**: Female

Background: Born by a normal vaginal delivery and normal pregnancy, Grace is feeding well and has passed meconium and urine. There are no particular concerns from the midwives or from Mum, who is with Grace and is happy to consent to the examination. As this is her first baby, please explain what you are doing throughout.

CLINICAL KNOWLEDGE AND EXPERTISE

Equipment required
- Tape measure
- Ophthalmoscope
- Tongue depressor
- Pulse oximetry machine.

Examination
The newborn examination is unlike most other examinations as rather than following the normal approach of inspection, palpation, percussion, auscultation (IPPA), it is performed in a top-to-toe manner.

Introduction
- Introduce yourself to the parents, briefly explain what you are going to do and gain consent. Explain your actions as you progress through the examination.
- Wash your hands.
- Ask parents to strip baby down to the nappy, if not already done so.

Inspection
- General inspection of the baby.
- Note any dysmorphic features.
- Note the colour of the baby (jaundice, plethora, pallor or cyanosis).
- Note the posture and activity.

Top-to-toe Examination (Fig. 3.16.2)
- If the baby is quiet initially, listen to the heart sounds and feel for the femoral pulses—difficult if the baby is crying.
- *Head*—measure the head circumference; note the shape, the size of the fontanelles and the sutures.
- *Face*—look for dysmorphic features or facial asymmetry and check the ears for abnormalities and pre-auricular pits or tags.
- *Eyes*—note any obvious abnormalities (e.g., coloboma, ptosis) and check for a red reflex in both eyes (retinoblastoma and congenital cataract).
- *Mouth*—examine within the mouth; particularly check the palate is intact. Use a torch and tongue depressor to visualise the palate and uvula. Check the rooting and sucking reflexes.
- *Neck*—examine for any swellings or lesions.
- *Chest*—listen for heart sounds (if not already performed) and breath sounds. Note any respiratory distress (tachypnoea, recession, nasal flaring or grunting) and murmurs. Perform pulse oximetry if a machine is provided (easiest to measure at the wrist or foot in a newborn).

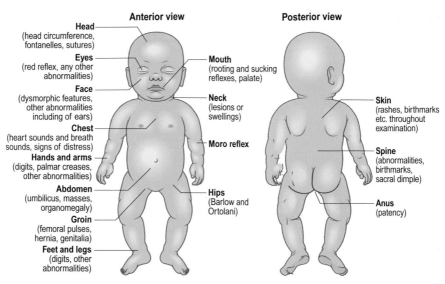

Anterior view

Head
(head circumference,
fontanelles, sutures)

Eyes
(red reflex, any other
abnormalities)

Face
(dysmorphic features,
other abnormalities
including of ears)

Chest
(heart sounds and breath
sounds, signs of distress)

Hands and arms
(digits, palmar creases,
other abnormalities)

Abdomen
(umbilicus, masses,
organomegaly)

Groin
(femoral pulses,
hernia, genitalia)

Feet and legs
(digits, other
abnormalities)

Mouth
(rooting and sucking
reflexes, palate)

Neck
(lesions or
swellings)

Moro reflex

Hips
(Barlow and
Ortolani)

Posterior view

Skin
(rashes, birthmarks
etc. throughout
examination)

Spine
(abnormalities,
birthmarks,
sacral dimple)

Anus
(patency)

Figure 3.16.2 Summary of examination of the newborn

- *Skin* — throughout the examination note any rashes, birthmarks or naevi.
- *Abdomen* — inspect the umbilical stump for redness or discharge. Palpate the abdomen for organomegaly or masses; it is normal to be able to palpate a spleen tip and 1-cm liver edge.
- *Hands and arms* — examine the hands and arms, including the axillae, particularly noting the skin condition, number of digits and the palmar creases.
- *Groin* — palpate the femoral pulses (if not done), which is difficult to do if the baby is crying, so you may have to ask parents to help settle the baby. Note any hernias. Check for normal genitalia. In boys, palpate the testicles bilaterally. Check for a patent anus.
- *Feet and legs* — examine the feet and legs, particularly the skin condition and number of digits.
- *Spine* — turn the baby over and examine the spine and back, particularly for any abnormalities, birthmarks or hair patches in the lumbar region, which suggests spina bifida occulta. Also examine for any sacral dimple.
- *Moro reflex* — return the baby onto their back and perform a Moro reflex: hold baby in a semi-seated position with their bottom on the cot and one hand on their back and one behind their head. Gently drop the head support about 2–3 cm, which should elicit the Moro reflex. Never hold the baby in the air or out of the cot to perform a Moro reflex.
- *Hips* — Warn parents that the baby may cry as it can be slightly uncomfortable. First, inspect for asymmetrical skin folds or limited abduction, then perform the Barlow and Ortolani manoeuvres (see Table 3.16.2).

Completion

- Explain to the examiner that you would like to document your examination, and plot the baby's weight and head circumference on an appropriate growth chart.

3

 ⚠ WARNING

Hip examination is used to diagnose developmental dysplasia of the hips (DDH). However, even a technically perfect examination can miss some babies affected; therefore, any baby with risk factors should also be offered a routine hip ultrasound scan within 6 weeks of birth. Risk factors include breech presentation, first degree relative with DDH or fixed talipes. A missed diagnosis of DDH can lead to delayed walking, limp and arthritis.

✓ How to excel in this station		
Action	**Reason**	**How**
Good communication.	Demonstrates respect for patient and parents. Puts the parents at ease and empowers them to ask questions.	Gain verbal consent and explain actions throughout. Warn of discomfort/distress when checking the Moro reflex and examining the hips. Ask the parents if they have any questions.

✗ Common errors in this station		
Common error	**Remedy**	**Reason**
Unsystematic approach.	Examine from head-to-toe.	Systematic and structured approach gives parents confidence and prevents missing things out.
Baby anxiety	Practise handling babies.	It is always obvious when someone is notably anxious and handles babies awkwardly. This does not instil any confidence with the parents and demonstrates that you have not engaged fully with your Paediatric placement.

STATION VARIATIONS

○ Advanced
- Combination of examination station with communication station.
- Combined with a communication station such as 'breaking bad news'; for example, if you were told that the examination demonstrated multiple features of trisomy 21 (Down syndrome).
- Combined with a communication skill station to discuss investigation and management; for example, if the baby was noted to be obviously jaundiced.

Further Reading
Macleod's Clinical Examination, Chapter 15, 'Babies and Children'.

Examination of a child with lymphadenopathy

3.17

CANDIDATE INFORMATION

Background: You are a doctor in training on a Paediatric placement and have been asked to examine a boy (10 years old) who has been sent to clinic with possible cervical lymphadenopathy.

Task: Please examine Harry's reticulo-endothelial system and present your findings to the examiner.

APPROACH TO THE STATION

This station requires a thorough examination, involving the neck and cervical lymph nodes, but also looking for lymphadenopathy at other sites (axilla and groin) and examination of the liver and spleen.

Cervical lymphadenopathy in children is very common and most are due to a benign cause (see Table 3.17.1), requiring no further investigation or treatment. However, a thorough examination is essential to look for evidence of a haematological malignancy, a systemic condition or any red flag features (see below). If any of these are present, or the lymphadenopathy is generalised (enlargement in more than two non-contiguous groups), the patient needs urgent referral to a specialist team, and further investigation (see Fig. 3.17.1 for examination summary).

Table 3.17.1 Lymphadenopathy causes and investigation	
Causes of localised lymphadenopathy (enlargement of nodes in one group or contiguous groups)	• Localised infection, e.g., abscesses, cellulitis, URTI, ear infection, oral and dental infections. • Kawasaki disease. • Lymphadenitis (infection and inflammation of the lymph nodes themselves). • Axillary lymphadenopathy may occur secondary to vaccinations. • Inguinal lymphadenopathy may occur secondary to nappy rash.
Causes of generalised lymphadenopathy	• *Viral*—URTI, measles, varicella, rubella, hepatitis, HIV, EBV (Epstein–Barr virus) and CMV (cytomegalovirus). • *Bacterial*—TB, brucellosis, septicaemia. • *Protozoal*—toxoplasmosis. • *Rheumatological conditions*—sarcoidosis, JIA (juvenile idiopathic arthritis), SLE (systemic lupus erythematosus).

(*Continued*)

Table 3.17.1 Lymphadenopathy causes and investigation—cont'd	
	• *Storage diseases*—Gaucher's, Niemann-Pick. • *Malignancy*—leukaemia, lymphoma, neuroblastoma. • *Drugs*—phenytoin, carbamazepine, allopurinol. • *Hyperthyroidism.* **NB:** Any of these conditions can also cause localised lymphadenopathy.
Investigations	• No investigations are required for localised lymphadenopathy if there are no red flags and the cause is apparent. • *First-line investigations*—Full blood count, blood film, C-reactive protein (CRP), erythrocyte sedimentation rate (ESR), monospot (EBV screening ± send EBV serology) and liver and renal function. • *Second-line investigations*—Chest X-ray, further serology (for example, for EBV, CMV and toxoplasmosis), lactate dehydrogenase (LDH) if malignancy is suspected, and ultrasound of the node(s). • *Third-line investigations*—US-guided lymph node biopsy (normally performed by the ENT surgeons), full rheumatology blood screen and CT scan as appropriate.

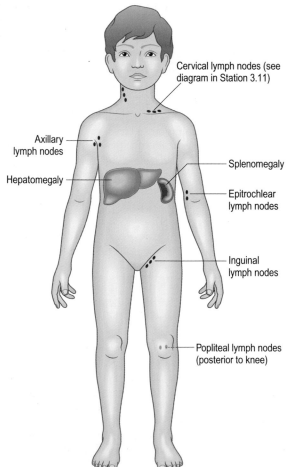

Figure 3.17.1 Summary of the lymphoreticular examination

Cervical lymph nodes (see diagram in Station 3.11)

Axillary lymph nodes

Hepatomegaly

Splenomegaly

Epitrochlear lymph nodes

Inguinal lymph nodes

Popliteal lymph nodes (posterior to knee)

PATIENT INFORMATION

Name: Harry Morris   **Age:** Approximately 10 years   **Sex:** Male

Findings: Bilateral scattered, less than 1-cm cervical lymph nodes (or non-detectable). No other positive findings.

CLINICAL KNOWLEDGE AND EXPERTISE

Introduction
- Introduce yourself, explain briefly and gain consent.
- Clean your hands.
- Ensure the patient is lying comfortably on a couch at 45°, and that there is space to stand behind patient to examine their neck.
- Uncover the patient so the neck, chest and abdomen are exposed.

3

Inspection
- Generally inspect, noting whether the child looks well grown or cachectic, and any pallor or jaundice.
- Inspect the neck for any visible masses or nodes.
- Note any rashes that may be related to an infectious cause, and any petechiae or purpura that may indicate a haematological cause.

Palpation
- Examine the hands, particularly noting pallor.
- Stand behind to palpate for cervical lymphadenopathy (for a full description see neck and thyroid examination, station 3.11).
- Examine for lymphadenopathy at–
  - Axillary (armpits)
  - Epitrochlear (ante-cubital fossae)
  - Inguinal (groin creases)
  - Popliteal (behind the knee).
- If you palpate any lymph nodes, comment on site, size (in cm), consistency (hard or fluctuant), fixation to underlying tissues and tenderness.
- Lie the patient flat and palpate the abdomen for hepatosplenomegaly or other abdominal masses (e.g., neuroblastoma) (see station 3.4 for more detail on abdominal examination).

Special tests
- Examine the ears, nose, throat and inside the mouth with an otoscope and tongue depressor as the most common cause of lymphadenopathy is due to mild infection.

 WARNING

- Generalised lymphadenopathy may still be due to a benign condition such as EBV; however, it is more worrying, often has a systemic cause and should be investigated.
- Lymph nodes over 2 cm, or that are firm or fixed are all red flag features and should be investigated, as are non-tender lymph nodes.
- Lymph nodes at some sites, particularly supraclavicular, epitrochlear and the posterior cervical chain, may be due to more serious causes and should be investigated further.

3

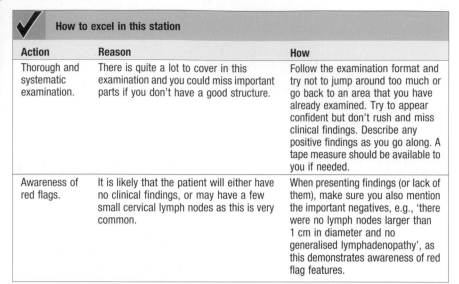

✓ **How to excel in this station**

Action	Reason	How
Thorough and systematic examination.	There is quite a lot to cover in this examination and you could miss important parts if you don't have a good structure.	Follow the examination format and try not to jump around too much or go back to an area that you have already examined. Try to appear confident but don't rush and miss clinical findings. Describe any positive findings as you go along. A tape measure should be available to you if needed.
Awareness of red flags.	It is likely that the patient will either have no clinical findings, or may have a few small cervical lymph nodes as this is very common.	When presenting findings (or lack of them), make sure you also mention the important negatives, e.g., 'there were no lymph nodes larger than 1 cm in diameter and no generalised lymphadenopathy', as this demonstrates awareness of red flag features.

✗ **Common errors in this station**

Common error	Remedy	Reason
Missing the cause.	Examine for potential causes as well as signs of lymphoreticular inflammation, particularly if you find a localised lymphadenopathy.	You could lose marks despite a good examination of the lymphoreticular system and a perfect description of lymphadenopathy, for example in the right inguinal region, if you had failed to note cellulitis on the leg.

STATION EXTENSIONS

⭘ Basic

Examine the head and neck

You may just be asked to examine the cervical lymph nodes and the head and neck for causes of lymph node enlargement. Follow the examination laid out in station 3.11 and then examine carefully for causes of lymph node enlargement. Remember to examine the eyes (conjunctivitis), the nose (coryzal symptoms), the throat (tonsillitis), the mouth (dental abscess, oral ulcers, lesions or thrush) and ears (otitis media); also make a note of any skin rashes, cellulitis or head lice infestations.

Further Reading

Macleod's Clinical Examination, Chapter 3, 'The General Examination', section 'The Lymph Nodes'.

Macleod's Clinical Examination, Chapter 15, 'Babies and Children', section 'The Physical Examination', specifically 'Examination of the Lymph Nodes'.

Testing cognitive function

3.18

CANDIDATE INFORMATION

Background: You are the junior doctor on an acute medical ward and have been asked by the nurse to assess 85-year-old Mrs Smith, admitted 2 days ago with a chest infection. The nurse is concerned that Mrs Smith is confused. Mrs Smith's son/daughter is also present and you can get further information from them.

Task: Please assess Mrs Smith for confusion. You may also speak to their relative. You should then explain to the examiner what the diagnosis is and give supporting information.

APPROACH TO THE STATION

The best way to assess cognitive function or level of confusion is to use standardised tests, e.g., abbreviated mental test score (AMTS), the 6CIT, Mini-Cog and the Mini mental state examination. Due to OSCE time constraints it would usually be worth using one of the shorter tests such as the AMTS or 6CIT. You would then need to consider whether the confusion is new or worse than normal (i.e., does the patient have a delirium?) or is this chronic cognitive impairment, so take a short focused history from a family member or carer.

PATIENT INFORMATION

Name: Mrs Smith **Age:** 85 years **Sex:** Female

Presenting symptom: Confusion

Opening statement: I don't feel very well, where am I?

Other symptoms (if asked): You were admitted 2 days ago because of a chest infection. You have been disorientated and confused. If the candidate asks, you have not had any memory problems. You should appear drowsy and easily distractible during the test.

The candidate should ask you some questions — these will depend on which test they apply. You should answer questions about time and place incorrectly. You should also display distractibility; for example, if asked to count from 20 to 1 you should stop at 13 and start counting upwards again. You should aim to answer approximately half of questions incorrectly.

3

For patient's relative: Your parent is not usually confused. They became unwell with a cough and green sputum 5 days ago. The general practitioner visited, diagnosed a chest infection and prescribed antibiotics but your parent got worse — very drowsy and wouldn't eat or drink much. They also became confused and started talking about their partner who had died 20 years ago. Sometimes they are less confused but this comes and goes. You are worried, as they don't know where they are.

CLINICAL KNOWLEDGE AND EXPERTISE

You should use a standardised test such as the AMTS or mini COG to assess for confusion (Box 3.18.1).

If you diagnose confusion, you need to determine whether this is new or worse than normal — if so, the person may have a delirium. Delirium is important as it is linked to excess morbidity and mortality, longer length of stay and increased chances of institutionalisation. It can also be a very distressing experience for patients and their relatives. Steps should be taken to re-orientate the person, treat underlying disease, optimise the environment, encourage nutrition and hydration, bladder and bowel function.

Delirium should be diagnosed using the *confusion assessment method* (Box 3.18.2).

More detailed tests of cognitive function can be used, especially if you want to diagnose dementia. These usually cover several different areas such as executive function, visuo-spatial function, memory and more. Examples of these are the Montreal Cognitive assessment (MoCA), the mini mental state examination (MMSE) and the Addenbrookes cognitive examination III (ACE III). Clock drawing tests are often used in these more detailed tests.

Box 3.18.1 Abbreviated mental test score—score 1 point for correct answer. A score of 8+ is normal

Age
Time (to nearest hour)
Give address to test recall at end (ask patient to repeat)
Year
Place (name)
Identification of two people
Date of birth
When was the 1st/ 2nd World War?
What is the name of the current monarch?
Count backwards from 20 to 1 (all the way)
Ask address for recall

Box 3.18.2 The confusion assessment method

For delirium to be diagnosed, features 1 *AND* 2 must be present plus *either* 3 or 4 (all are present in this case).
1. Acute onset and fluctuating course—did the confusion come on or worsen acutely? Does it fluctuate throughout the day?
2. Inattention—is the person easily distractible or having difficulty following conversations/ instructions (e.g., on the 20–1)?
3. Disorganised thinking—is their conversation rambling or not making sense? Do they switch subjects quickly?
4. Altered conscious level—drowsy (most commonly) or agitated (or fluctuating between these two states).

WARNING

- Do not assume confusion is chronic — a witness history is absolutely key.
- Delirium is more common in people who have dementia so do not miss it as it is a sign of underlying illness.

	How to excel in this station	
Action	**Reason**	**How**
Be sensitive and tactful.	Delirium is a very distressing condition for patients and their relatives.	Acknowledge that the person may be feeling confused and that this may be upsetting for them and for their relative, but that it should hopefully improve.

	Common errors in this station	
Common error	**Remedy**	**Reason**
Not using a standardised test.	Use one of the tests described above,	Standardised tests have been validated for use in these circumstances.
Diagnosing dementia.	Use the confusion assessment method.	An acute deterioration in the context of infection with an altered level of consciousness is delirium rather than dementia.
Running out of time.	Use a shorter test such as AMTS.	MMSE is a more sensitive and specific test for diagnosing cognitive impairment but it takes longer to administer than you will probably have in an OSCE setting.

3

STATION VARIATIONS

○ Intermediate

An alternative station — longer history of confusion and you are asked to assess a patient. In this instance you may need to know how to perform a clock drawing test or use a longer test such as the MMSE or a Montreal Cognitive assessment (MoCA).

○ Advanced

Consider the risk factors for delirium or discuss with the examiner about steps taken to prevent delirium — these are discussed in more detail in *Macleod's Clinical Diagnosis* (see Further Reading).

You could also be asked to explain to the patient's relative why their parent is confused and discuss prognosis (that most people will recover but some may be left with a cognitive deficit).

Further Reading

Macleod's Clinical Diagnosis, Chapter 8, 'Confusion: Delirium and Dementia'.
Helping you to assess cognition: a practical toolkit for clinicians — Alzheimer's Society (UK) available from http://www.alzheimers.org.uk.
NICE guideline CG 103 Delirium. Available from http://www.nice.org.uk.

Breast lump examination

.3.19

Background: You are a junior doctor in a general practice. Mrs Janice Clarke (42 years old) discovered a lump in her right breast last week. She has not noticed any discharge from the nipple or lumps elsewhere. She has no family history of breast cancer and is normally well with no history of breast lumps. She has a copper IUD and is around day 21 in her menstrual cycle. She took the combined oral contraceptive pill for 10 years prior to having children and breast-fed her two children (now 10 and 12). She doesn't take any regular medications.

Task: Examine Mrs Clarke's breasts and present your findings.

Approach to the Station

A patient with a breast lump is common and you must be able to differentiate between those that are more likely benign and those that warrant urgent investigation. Although it is highly improbable that there would be a woman with a breast lump in the OSCE, you must discuss features more indicative of malignancy and exclude these during examination. Any breast examination must examine both the affected breast and the contralateral breast together with the surrounding axillary and supra-clavicular lymph nodes. You must preserve the patient's privacy and dignity and ensure consent. You should know the common causes of breast lumps (see Table 3.19.1) and how to differentiate between these on examination, commenting that triple assessment with ultrasound, mammography and fine needle aspiration may be necessary to confirm the diagnosis. Certain 'red flag' signs are vital not to miss (see Warning section below).

Table 3.19.1 Common benign causes of breast lumps	
Benign causes of breast lumps	**Clinical features on examination**
Fibroadenoma	Non-tender mobile lump with rubbery consistency
Fat necrosis	Firm irregular fixed mass tethered to overlying skin in area of previous trauma or surgery
Fibrocystic change	Firm smooth, well defined lump—may be uncomfortable on palpation or irregular nodularity of the breast without a defined lump
Breast abscess (very unlikely in OSCE)	Tender erythematous lump with associated fever and systemic features of infection. Often in lactating women

PATIENT INFORMATION

Name: Mrs Janice Clarke   **Age:** 42 years   **Sex:** Female

Communication: You are happy for the examination and (*if asked*) you do not have any pain in the breasts or around the lump. You do not require a chaperone.

Examination findings (manikin): A 2-cm smooth mobile lump in the upper outer quadrant of the right breast that is fluctuant and non-tender on palpation. There are no overlying skin or nipple changes and no expressible nipple discharge. There are no palpable lumps in the left breast and no axillary or supraclavicular lymphadenopathy.

CLINICAL KNOWLEDGE AND EXPERTISE

Examination of patient with a breast lump (may be volunteer and a manikin)

Introduction

- Introduce yourself and confirm the patient's identity.
- Obtain consent and offer a chaperone.
- Ensure that the patient is undressed to the waist.
- Ask the patient to point where they have noticed any lumps prior to inspection.
- Wash hands or apply alcohol hand-gel.
- Ensure privacy and dignity throughout.

Inspection

- Get patient sitting upright on a chair or the side of a bed, initially resting hands on thighs to relax the pectoral muscles.
- Inspect each breast, comparing for asymmetry or tethering of the skin, localised swelling, skin changes and nipple changes.
- Repeat inspection with hands on hips (tensing pectorals), above head (stretching pectorals) and sitting allowing the breasts to hang forwards.

Palpation

- Ask the patient to lie supine with head on a pillow and arm under her head on the side to be examined.
- Ensure patient is comfortable prior to and during examination.
- Palpate the breast using the flat palmar surface of your fingers, pressing against the chest wall.
- Palpate around the whole of the breast clockwise, taking care to palpate underneath the nipple and up to the Tail of Spence.
- For any lump describe size, shape, consistency, mobility, location and skin changes.
- Palpate the nipple between thumb and index finger and gently massage the breast towards the nipple to express any discharge.
- Examine the other breast (may not be allowed in OSCE).

Lymph node palpation

- Warn about possible discomfort prior to palpating the axillae.
- Patient sitting facing you and support her arm at the wrist with your opposite hand whilst using your other hand to palpate around the axilla, pressing into the chest wall.

3

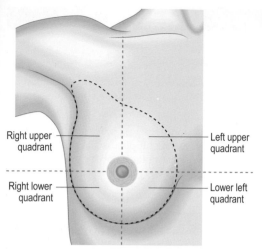

Figure 3.19.1 The four quadrants of the breast

Right upper quadrant

Left upper quadrant

Right lower quadrant

Lower left quadrant

- Palpate both the supraclavicular fossae and the cervical chain.

A complete description of any palpable breast lump is essential in an OSCE and to guide referral in clinical practice with an indication of the degree of urgency. When describing any lump it is important to record:

- *Size* — estimate diameter of lump in cm
- *Site* — in relation to four quadrants of the breast, e.g., right upper outer quadrant (Fig. 3.19.1)
- *Shape* — smooth and well-demarcated or irregular
- *Consistency* — e.g., hard, rubbery, fluctuant
- *Position* — superficial or deep within breast tissue
- *Degree of attachment* — e.g., mobile, tethered, fixed to skin or chest wall.

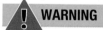 **WARNING**

Red flag features of a breast lump which may indicate cancer include:
- A hard, fixed, immobile lump
- Puckering, dimpling or tethering of the overlying skin
- Changes to the overlying skin, e.g., peau d'orange (lymphoedema of the breast) or eczema of the nipple (Paget's disease)
- Retraction or new inversion of the nipple
- Lymphadenopathy (usually hard and fixed)
- Blood-stained nipple discharge (can be tested for using dipstick if not clinically obvious).

✓	How to excel in this station	
Action	**Reason**	**How**
Demonstrate knowledge.	Awareness of important features indicative of malignancy and able to differentiate between possible causes of breast lumps.	An excellent candidate will work through the examination systematically, commenting on positive and negative findings before presenting a succinct summary.

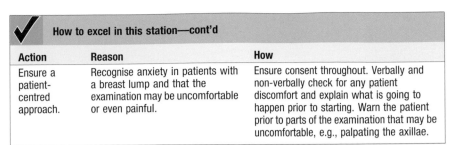

✔ How to excel in this station—cont'd		
Action	**Reason**	**How**
Ensure a patient-centred approach.	Recognise anxiety in patients with a breast lump and that the examination may be uncomfortable or even painful.	Ensure consent throughout. Verbally and non-verbally check for any patient discomfort and explain what is going to happen prior to starting. Warn the patient prior to parts of the examination that may be uncomfortable, e.g., palpating the axillae.

✘ Common errors in this station		
Common error	**Remedy**	**Reason**
Trying to take a history from the patient.	Limit any verbal communication to confirming identity, obtaining consent and checking throughout the examination that they are comfortable.	This is an examination station with the salient history already provided. Although it can feel unnatural to examine without taking a history first, this is not the expectation here—so time will be lost without gaining additional marks.
Not ensuring privacy and dignity.	Ensure consent prior to examination and that curtains are properly drawn. Cover the patient as soon as finished and prior to presenting findings.	It can be easy to forget the patient within the stress of the exam situation but remember that this is an intimate examination—treat the patient with dignity and respect.

STATION VARIATIONS

● Intermediate

Other intimate examinations that you can be asked to perform in an OSCE include rectal examination and speculum examination. These will likely be on manikins in the OSCE Follow the same principles of consent and preserving patients dignity.

(See also station 3.18, testing cognitive function)

Further Reading

Macleod's Clinical Diagnosis, Part 2: Assessment of Common Presenting Problems; 5: Breast Lump.

Macleod's Clinical Examination, Section 10 'The Reproductive System: The Physical Examination of the Breast'.

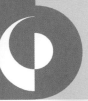

Practical skills

Introduction to practical skills

This chapter gives you an overview of the stations that have a practical skill element. There are obviously many other practical skills that you could be asked to perform, but our aim is to provide the basic principles of how to approach this style of OSCE station, rather than provide an exhaustive list.

In these stations you will be asked, for a non-painful procedure, to perform the skill on an actual or simulated patient (such as in the ECG station). Alternatively, there may be a simulated patient with a manikin nearby (for a potentially painful procedure). In these situations the manikin may be draped and in an appropriate position, so as to simulate 'real life'– for example, a venepuncture manikin arm draped next to the patient with their arm hidden, or a piece of fake skin draped over a patient's leg for the suturing station. If you are performing the procedure on a manikin, you must still talk to the simulated patient as though you are performing it on them. Good communication skills are mandatory.

➡ KEY SKILLS

There is a practical skill at the heart of each station and it is imperative you spend enough time in the clinical skills lab or on the wards, practising these skills on manikins, on other students or on real patients (once you are competent), until you feel comfortable. Certain practical elements are applicable to almost all of the stations:
- Good hand-washing technique;
- Appropriate personal protective equipment use (for example, gloves ± aprons or gowns);
- Aseptic non-touch technique (see station 4.2 for further information); and
- Safe disposal of sharps and appropriate disposal of clinical waste.

In addition, there are other recurrent themes applicable to all stations that are closely linked to competence in a practical skill. A flawless practical procedure alone is not enough to pass these stations. So remember to always pay attention to the following:
- Introduce yourself appropriately and check that the patient is happy for you to perform the procedure.
- Always ensure the patient's privacy and dignity are maintained.
- Demonstrate good communication skills — explain the procedure as you perform it, be empathetic and kind, answer patient's questions, etc.

Finally, remember to practise in groups of at least two people (preferably three), so you can all take turns as the simulated patient, the student and the examiner (using the marksheets provided with the eBook). It is difficult to remember to communicate normally with the simulated patient on exam day if you have never practised it!

Recording an ECG

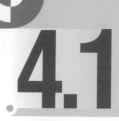

4.1

CANDIDATE INFORMATION

Background: You are a junior doctor in general medicine and have been asked to record an ECG on Mr Albert Brown, who has complained of chest pain to the nursing staff.

Task: Record an ECG and then discuss the interpretation of an ECG with the examiner. You are not expected to take a history from the patient.

APPROACH TO THE STATION

This is an important procedure as although technicians often complete ECG recordings during the day, it is still a common task for doctors to perform out-of-hours. You need to be comfortable recording and interpreting ECGs (see Fig. 4.1.1 and Table 4.1.1 for advice regarding ECG interpretation). This station requires practical knowledge, communication with the simulated patient and a systematic approach to the interpretation of an ECG. There are multiple books available on ECG interpretation but practice using ECGs of real patients is potentially more useful.

Depending on your level, an ECG given to you in an OSCE may be completely normal. However, as you progress you are more likely to be asked to interpret an abnormal ECG and comment on what management you might initiate. Clinically, remember it is always better to ask for a second opinion on an ECG that you are not sure about than to 'hope for the best' and ignore something that is potentially serious.

PATIENT INFORMATION

Name: Mr Albert Brown **Age:** 74 years **Sex:** Male

You have had some pain in your chest over the past few hours. A nurse has informed you that a doctor will come and perform an ECG. You have had one of these in the past and are familiar with the procedure. You are happy to consent and cooperate with the procedure today.

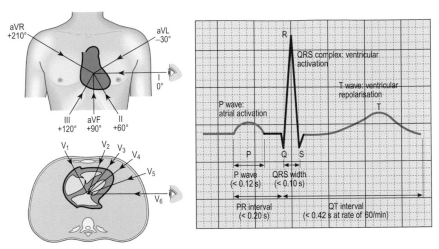

Figure 4.1.1 Normal ECG complex and surface anatomy (From Douglas G., et al., *Macleod's Clinical Examination*, 13/e (Churchill Livingstone, 2013) with permission.)

4

Table 4.1.1 ECG interpretation	
Elements of the ECG	**Interpretation**
Rate	If the rhythm looks regular, divide 300 by the number of large squares between two successive QRS complexes. If irregular, divide 900 by the number of large squares between four successive QRS complexes. A normal adult heart rate is 60–100/min, or 3–5 large squares between successive complexes. A heart rate <60 and >100 is described as bradycardic and tachycardic, respectively.
Rhythm	Mark out the regularity of a few complexes on a separate piece of paper by marking the edge at every R wave. If you then move this along the strip it is possible to see whether the rhythm is regular (e.g., do your marks still correspond to the R waves?). If the rhythm is irregular, look at the strip as a whole to look for a regularly irregular pattern or whether it is irregularly irregular.
Axis	To determine the axis, it is best to plot the relative depolarisation of leads I and aVf. If the S wave is greater than the R wave in lead I, there is right axis deviation. If the S wave is greater than the R wave in lead II—left axis deviation.
Detecting abnormalities	*P wave*—should be present before each QRS complex in sinus rhythm. *PR interval*— <5 small squares (0.2 s); if higher, it suggests a heart block. *QRS complex*—QRS complex width <3 small squares (0.12 s) is normal ('narrow complex'). Width >0.12 s is abnormal ('broad complex'). *QT interval*—normal is 0.38–0.42 s and must be corrected for the rate (corrected QT = $QT/\sqrt{RR}$). Abnormalities may be congenital or due to electrolyte disturbance or toxins. *ST segment*—elevation or depression above or below the baseline suggests ischaemia. *T wave*—may be inverted (suggestive of previous ischaemia, but is a normal variant in leads V1 and aVr, and sometimes in leads V2 and V3), small (hypokalaemia) or peaked (hyperkalaemia).

4

CLINICAL KNOWLEDGE AND EXPERTISE

Equipment

- ECG machine
- Electrode stickers
- Razor to remove excessive hair (if required)
- Alcohol wipes to remove visible dirt/grease (if required).

Procedure

1. Introduce yourself, briefly explain the procedure and gain verbal consent.
2. Wash your hands (or use hand sanitiser) prior to starting the procedure.
3. Patient should be lying comfortably with their chest, wrists and ankles exposed.
4. Enter the relevant patient information into the ECG machine prior to commencing the procedure.
5. Inform the patient of what you are doing as you go along and warn that the electrode stickers may be cold. Place the electrode stickers (see Fig. 4.1.2 and Table 4.1.2 for further information) and ensure good contact between the skin (must be clean and dry) and the sticker. If the skin is dirty, clean with an alcohol wipe prior to placing the sticker. Excessive hair may need to be shaved off (confirm consent prior to doing this).
6. Attach the leads to the electrode stickers.
7. Check good contact of the stickers and lead attachment and ask the patient to remain still while recording the ECG.
8. If the reading is unsatisfactory, check all leads and electrode stickers and ask the patient to lie still again prior to a further recording.
9. If the recording is satisfactory, remove the leads from the stickers and neatly store away on the ECG machine. Ask the patient if they would like you to remove the stickers, or if they would like to do it themselves. Warn that it can be slightly uncomfortable to remove the stickers, especially if they are on a hairy area.
10. Discuss the interpretation of the ECG with the examiner.

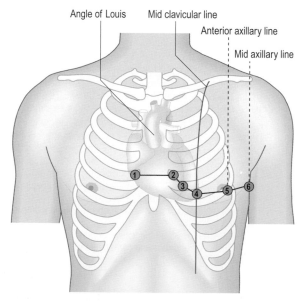

Figure 4.1.2 Placement of chest electrodes

Table 4.1.2 Placement of ECG electrodes

- Attach the limb leads to the four limbs, preferably placing on the bony prominences of the wrist and ankle. However, if not possible (e.g., amputation, dressings, etc.) place at the next most distal bony prominence. Limb leads are normally coloured and placed as follows. A useful pneumonic for remembering is 'Ride Your Green Bike'.
  - Red—right upper limb
  - Yellow—left upper limb
  - Green—left lower limb
  - Black—right lower limb
- Position the chest leads as follows:
  - V1 Fourth intercostal space at right sternal border
  - V2 Fourth intercostal space at left sternal border
  - V3 Midway between V2 and V4
  - V4 Fifth intercostal space in the mid-clavicular line
  - V5 Anterior axillary line at same horizontal level as V4
  - V6 Mid-axillary line at same horizontal level as V4 and V5

4

⚠ WARNING

- If a patient is extremely unwell or collapsed, you can check a basic recording via a defibrillator and defibrillator pads (available on a resuscitation trolley).
- It is essential that you can identify arrest rhythms (asystole, ventricular tachycardia, ventricular fibrillation and pulseless electrical activity). Further information on the identification and the management of these can be found in the *Advanced Life Support* handbook.
- ECGs that have been recorded must always be checked and signed prior to being filed in the notes, in order to avoid missing potentially life-threatening conditions, such as arrhythmias and myocardial infarctions.

✓ How to excel in this station

Action	Reason	How
Practical skill.	Demonstrate familiarity and confidence with the procedure.	Be able to place the electrodes quickly and accurately and be familiar with the calibration and normal layout of an ECG.
Systematic approach to ECG interpretation.	Avoids missing any of the fundamentals, even if there is an obvious abnormality.	Have a systematic approach to reporting an ECG (a system is given above but you can establish your own routine, as long as it covers all the basics and you appear competent).

✗ Common errors in this station

Common error	Remedy	Reason
Poor communication.	Confirm consent prior to commencing and maintain communication with the patient throughout.	Good communication demonstrates your respect for the patient and their comfort. It can put the patient at ease in a situation that may be alien or awkward.

(Continued)

4

Common error	Remedy	Reason
Missing obvious ECG abnormalities.	Learn the most common and potentially serious abnormalities (see below). Practise interpretation of ECGs regularly.	As you progress, and certainly once qualified, it will not be sufficient to discuss only the basics of an ECG (e.g., rate and rhythm). It is important to recognise common abnormalities, particularly those with potentially serious or life-threatening consequences.

Common errors in this station—cont'd

STATION VARIATIONS

O Basic

Record an ECG without data interpretation; follow instructions for the procedure as above.

O Advanced

The station may be made suitable for more advanced students by requiring them to demonstrate a systematic approach to ECG interpretation and recognise potential abnormalities. Appearing confident and recognising more complex abnormalities requires practice and skill. An advanced station could include ECGs of the following:

- Sinus tachycardia
- Sinus arrhythmia
- ST elevation myocardial infarction
- Non-ST elevation myocardial infarction, including posterior myocardial infarction
- Right and left bundle branch block
- Atrial fibrillation and atrial flutter
- Supraventricular tachycardia
- Ventricular tachycardia
- Arrest rhythms—asystole, ventricular tachycardia, ventricular fibrillation
- 1st, 2nd and 3rd (complete) degree heart block
- Hyperkalaemia.

In an advanced station, you may also be asked to comment on the initial management of the condition you have identified on the ECG, for example, a non-ST elevation myocardial infarction.

Further Reading

Macleod's Clinical Examination, Chapter 6, 'Cardiovascular System', especially the section on 'investigations in heart disease'.

Macleod's Clinical Diagnosis, Chapter 6, 'Chest Pain'; Chapter 25, 'Palpitations'.

Advanced Life Support Handbook, published by the Resuscitation Council UK, and widely available in most medical libraries.

Inserting an intravenous cannula

4.2

CANDIDATE INFORMATION

Background: You are a junior doctor in general medicine. You have been asked to cannulate Miss Thompson as she has been admitted with severe vomiting and diarrhoea and is not tolerating any oral fluids.

Task: Demonstrate how you would place an intravenous cannula in order to commence fluid replacement. Please perform the procedure on the manikin but address all communication to Miss Thompson as though you were performing it on her.

APPROACH TO THE STATION

This is a classic practical procedure station as it is one of the commonest skills needed by a junior doctor. Keep calm, clearly demonstrate aseptic non-touch technique (ANTT, see Table 4.2.1) and ensure safe disposal of sharps. Communication with the simulated patient is a must and you must counsel them as you would a real patient. Finally, be prepared to answer questions from the examiner regarding the risks of intravenous cannulation and sites to avoid (Table 4.2.2).

Table 4.2.1 Principles of aseptic non-touch technique	
Principle	**How to apply**
Always wash hands effectively	7-stage approach with hot water and soap. Dry thoroughly.
Maintaining an aseptic field	A tray should be used and cleaned with the appropriate wipe, as per local policy. Equipment should be removed from sterile packaging and placed in the tray with clean, gloved hands.
Never contaminate key parts	Key parts are those that, if contaminated, are most likely to lead to infection; in this procedure—the cannula (unsheathed) and connector ports.
Take appropriate infective precautions	Wash your hands and wear clean (non-sterile) gloves and an apron. One pair of gloves should be worn when preparing all your equipment, then discard these, re-sanitise hands and put on clean gloves immediately prior to the actual procedure.

4

Risk	Advice
Failure of procedure	Patients should be warned that intravenous cannulation is not always straightforward and that the procedure may fail.
Extravasation of vein	Fluid may extravasate into the surrounding tissue. The cannula must be removed and swelling allowed to resolve. This complication can occur at any time. Certain medications (highly irritant) are more likely to cause problems and it also tends to occur more frequently with smaller veins.
Haematoma	May occur at the site during a failed cannulation attempt or on removal of a cannula. Pressure should be placed over the site.
Infection - local phlebitis or bacteraemia	Local infection may occur or may involve introduction of bacteria into the systemic circulation. This can normally be avoided by good hand hygiene, thorough cleaning of the skin and ANTT. Most hospitals have local policies that involve daily checks of cannula sites and the removal of cannulas 72 h after insertion to further lower infection risks.
Embolism	Embolism of air or of a fragment of the catheter tip is very rare. The risk can be reduced by removing air bubbles from flushes and priming connectors. The risk of fragment embolism can be minimised by not re-threading a needle once removed.

Table 4.2.2 Risks of intravenous cannula insertion

PATIENT INFORMATION

Name: Miss Ann Thompson   **Age:** 32 years   **Sex:** Female

You have been suffering with severe diarrhoea and vomiting for 2 days and over the past 24 hours you haven't been able to tolerate anything orally. You haven't passed urine in over 12 hours. You are happy to have a cannula for intravenous fluids, though you would like to know the risks, and how long the cannula will be in place.

You will be laid on an examination couch, with a drape over your shoulder and the manikin arm for realism.

CLINICAL KNOWLEDGE AND EXPERTISE

Equipment
- Tray
- Sharps bin
- Cleaning wipes
- Gloves and apron
- Disposable tourniquet
- Cannula (of appropriate size)
- 2 × 5 ml 0.9% saline ampoules
- 2 × 5 ml syringe and 2 × green needle
- White syringe cap
- Connector
- Cannula dressing
- Gauze.

Procedure

1. Check you have all the necessary equipment (see Fig. 4.2.1). In an OSCE, a tray will often have been prepared. However, remember normally you must collect your equipment, wash your hands and apply gloves, and clean your tray with wipes (allow it to dry), before removing equipment from sterile packages and placing in the tray.
2. To prime a cannula connector, first open an ampoule of 0.9% saline. Draw up using a green needle (or drawing-up needle) and 5 ml syringe. Remove and dispose of the needle in a sharps bin. Apply the syringe to the port and flush through (about 1 ml). If the connector has multiple ports, each port needs to be flushed and clamped. Then remove the flush and place the connector in the tray.
3. Repeat the process as above to prepare a flush. However, after discarding the needle, place a sterile syringe cap onto the syringe and place in the tray.
4. Wash your hands again.
5. Introduce yourself and confirm the patient's identity.
6. Explain that you have been asked to place a cannula and tell them why. Obtain verbal consent and be prepared to answer questions about the possible risks of cannulation.
7. Ensure the patient is positioned comfortably and their arm or hand is resting on the bed or a pillow.
8. Apply a disposable tourniquet. Choose and palpate a vein (see Fig. 4.2.2).
9. Clean hands with alcohol gel and don clean gloves.
10. Clean the area with appropriate wipe or cleaning device (check local policy) and allow it to dry.
11. In the meantime, remove the sheaf from the cannula and fold down the wings.
12. Warn the patient to expect a sharp scratch. Use one hand to place some traction on the skin, avoid touching the cleaned area, and with the cannula in your other hand, insert into the skin at an angle of about 30°, with the bevel upwards. If the cannula has entered a vein, there will be a flashback of blood into the barrel of the cannula.
13. Keep the needle still and slide the cannula into the vein, over the needle.
14. Remove the tourniquet.
15. Put pressure on the vein immediately above the cannula site to reduce bleeding and remove the needle. You can place some sterile gauze below the cannula before you remove the needle, in case any blood drips from the cannula.
16. Dispose of the needle in the sharps bin.
17. Remove the cap from the connector and screw onto the cannula end.
18. Secure the cannula by applying the strips provided with the dressing. Ensure the site of cannula entry can be visualised.

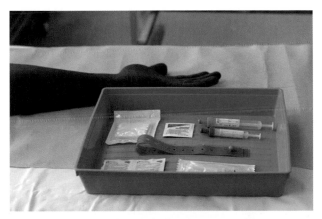

Figure 4.2.1 Example of manikin used for cannulation and venepuncture

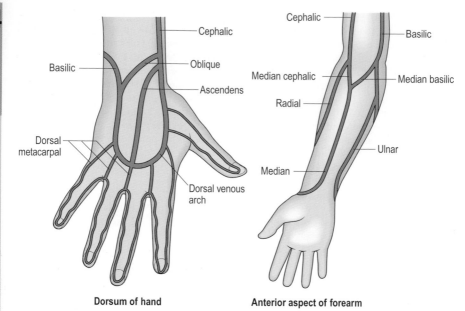

Dorsum of hand   **Anterior aspect of forearm**

Figure 4.2.2 Veins of the hand and forearm

19. Clean the port of the connector with a cleaning wipe and allow to dry. Open the clamp and flush the cannula. Ensure the patient does not feel any discomfort as the cannula is flushed.
20. Apply the rest of the dressing. If the dressing contains a date sticker, complete and apply.
21. Thank the patient.
22. Remove any equipment. Dispose of waste in a clinical waste bin and clean the tray.
23. Wash your hands.
24. Document procedure in the patient notes or on a relevant chart (as per local policy).

⚠ WARNING

- Remember never to place a cannula in a limb affected by the following: lymphoedema or lymph node surgery, arteriovenous fistula, fracture.
- Avoid placing a cannula in a limb that is weak (e.g., affected by a stroke) when possible.
- Avoid placing a cannula close to an existing wound and never in an area with a current skin infection.

✓	How to excel in this station		
Action	**Reason**		**How**
Communicate.	Builds rapport and produces a calm and reassuring environment for the procedure.		Introduce yourself and check consent prior to starting. Talk through the steps as you are performing them.
Demonstrate ANTT.	Minimise infection risk.		Refer to the principles of ANTT in Table 4.2.1. If unsure of the practicalities of the procedure while maintaining ANTT, approach an infection control nurse as they regularly run training sessions

Common errors in this station		
Common error	**Remedy**	**Reason**
Failure to ask consent.	Briefly ensure consent prior to beginning.	Explain why you have been asked to perform the procedure, warn that it will be briefly painful and check they are happy to proceed. Learn the risks of the procedure (Table 4.2.2), in case asked.
Causing undue pain or distress.	Warn the patient prior to starting that the procedure will be briefly painful. Warn immediately prior to needle insertion.	Part of informed consent is that it helps to prepare the patient for what they should expect. It minimises the shock of the procedure and limits possible distress.

STATION VARIATIONS

4

◯ Basic

- Venepuncture is a similar but simpler procedure than intravenous cannulation as it does not involve using a flush/connector or applying a dressing. There are different venepuncture systems available and you should become familiar and competent with the system that is used locally.
- The principles of ANTT should be adhered to and equipment prepared in the same manner.
- Communication skills are still important in this station, and again consent should be taken.

Further Reading

Association of Safe Aseptic Practice, international guidance available at http://www.antt.org.uk.

Royal College of Nursing, 'Peripheral Venous Cannulation in Children and Young People', free workbook available at http://www.rcn.org.uk.

Arterial blood gas sampling

4.3

CANDIDATE INFORMATION

Background: You are a junior doctor in Accident & Emergency and have been asked to take a radial arterial blood gas sample from Jack Shanahan, who has presented with shortness of breath.

Task: Demonstrate how you would take an arterial blood gas sample by performing the procedure on the manikin—address all communication to Mr Shanahan as though you were performing it on him.

APPROACH TO THE STATION

This is a common procedure for junior medical staff. This station details arterial blood sampling from the radial artery — this is the most appropriate initial site. Keep calm, clearly demonstrate aseptic non-touch technique (see Table 4.2.1 in Station 4.2 for further information) and ensure safe disposal of sharps. The setup normally involves a simulated patient and a manikin to perform the procedure on (possibly draped so it looks like their arm). Communication with the simulated patient is essential and you must counsel them as you would a real patient. This procedure is frequently extended to include interpretation of arterial blood gas results — there are other stations in this book that cover this skill in detail (Stations 7.3 and 7.5).

PATIENT INFORMATION

Name: Mr Jack Shanahan **Age:** 52 years **Sex:** Male

You have been suffering with increasing shortness of breath for 3 days, but it has got much worse over the past 24 hours. You have not had an arterial blood gas sample taken before and are unclear why the procedure is being done as you have already had some bloods taken.

You will be laid on an examination couch, with a drape over your shoulder together with a manikin arm for realism.

CLINICAL KNOWLEDGE AND EXPERTISE

Equipment
- Tray
- Sharps bin

- Cleaning wipes
- Gloves and apron
- Heparinised syringe
- Syringe cap (usually supplied with syringe)
- 22G needle (may be supplied with syringe)
- Gauze.

Procedure

1. Check you have all the necessary equipment. In an OSCE station, a tray may have been pre-prepared. Normally you must collect your equipment, wash your hands and apply gloves, and clean your tray with wipes (allow to dry), before removing equipment from sterile packages and placing in the tray.
2. Often an arterial blood gas syringe comes in a pre-prepared pack with a needle and syringe cap to place over the syringe after discarding the needle. Sometimes you will need a separate needle. The syringe will either contain liquid heparin or may be coated with dry heparin.
3. Wash your hands again.
4. Introduce yourself and confirm the patient's identity.
5. Explain that you have been asked to take an arterial blood sample and explain why. Obtain verbal consent and answer questions about possible risks (Table 4.3.1).
6. Ensure the patient is positioned comfortably and their arm or hand is resting on the bed or a pillow, with the wrist well extended.
7. Palpate the radial artery with three fingers so that you have an idea of the patient's local anatomy and the passage of the artery.
8. Clean hands with alcohol gel and put on clean gloves.
9. Clean the area with appropriate wipe or cleaning device (check local hospital policy) and allow to dry for at least 30 seconds.
10. In the meantime, remove the sheath and attach the needle onto the syringe hub. If the syringe contains liquid heparin, you need to squirt this out onto a piece of gauze. If the syringe contains dry heparin, it is provided ready to use with the syringe already partly withdrawn to allow an appropriate amount of blood for analysis (usually 1–2 ml).

4

Table 4.3.1 Risks of arterial blood gas sampling	
Risk	**Advice**
Failure of procedure	Patients should be warned that arterial blood gas sampling is not always straightforward and that the procedure may fail.
Pain	Arterial is more painful than venous blood sampling due to the structures surrounding the usual site of sampling (most commonly the radial artery). It is particularly painful to hit the periosteum with the tip of the needle—the artery is relatively superficial so only advance the needle very slowly.
Haematoma and bruising	Haematoma is relatively common after arterial blood sampling due to the high pressure causing increased leakage of blood into the surrounding tissues following puncture. This can be minimised by pressing firmly over the puncture site with a clean gauze swab for at least 2 min (you may be able to ask the patient to do this after demonstrating firm pressure).
Vasospasm of artery	Arteries are prone to spasm once punctured. This is usually a transient phenomenon and the artery returns to normal very soon after. However, it may be more difficult to take further samples from the same site.
Ischaemia of distal structures	This is very rare and much more likely to occur following insertion of an arterial line than after arterial sampling. However, if there is increasing pain and pallor of distal structures with difficulty palpating the pulse, then senior support should be summoned immediately.

4

11. Warn the patient to expect a sharp scratch. Place two or three fingers of your non-dominant hand onto the radial artery which you palpated before. With the needle in your dominant hand, place the needle at the skin just distal to your fingers (do not put the needle too close to your fingers or in between your fingers as this increases the risk of a needle-stick injury). Puncture the skin with the needle at an angle of 90° to the skin.
12. Advance the needle very slowly until bright red blood flushes into the syringe.
13. Keep the needle still while the syringe fills – there should be no need to draw back as it should fill on its own due to the arterial pressure. You should only need 1–2 ml of blood to be able to analyse.
14. With your non-dominant hand, get some clean gauze ready while you remove the needle.
15. Put firm pressure on the puncture site immediately after removing the needle. After demonstrating firm pressure, you may be able to ask the patient to provide pressure while you finish the procedure.
16. Carefully remove the needle from the syringe and dispose of the needle in the sharps bin.
17. Place the cap on the syringe and try to expel any air at the top of the syringe. Do not shake the sample. Put the syringe carefully back in your tray.
18. Check the patient's puncture site and apply a dressing if necessary.
19. Thank the patient.
20. Remove any equipment. Dispose of waste in a clinical waste bin.
21. Wash your hands.
22. Put on clean gloves and apply a patient label (if available) to the blood gas syringe and arrange for it be analysed or take it to the analyser yourself.
23. Document the procedure in the patient notes or on a relevant chart (as per local policy).

⚠ WARNING

- Arterial blood sampling is painful even when performed proficiently. If a patient requires repeated analysis of arterial blood gas samples, consider whether they could have capillary sampling or monitoring of venous bicarbonate instead. If not, they should be considered for admission to a clinical area that allows insertion of an arterial line.
- If any distal structures blanch or appear pale or dusky or are disproportionately painful after arterial blood sampling, consider the possibility of arterial damage or severe vasospasm and seek senior help immediately.

	How to excel in this station		
Action	**Reason**	**How**	
Communicate.	Build rapport and produce a calm and reassuring environment for the procedure.	Introduce yourself and check consent prior to starting. Talk through the steps as you are performing them and answer questions appropriately.	
Minimise bleeding and pain.	Use your knowledge of the local anatomy to avoid over-advancing the needle or missing the artery.	Advance your needle slowly and remember that the artery is relatively superficial. Apply firm pressure after removing the needle.	

Common errors in this station		
Common error	**Remedy**	**Reason**
Failure to explain procedure.	Explain why this test, as well as other blood tests, is required (e.g., it allows you to find out the amount of oxygen in the blood).	Explain why you have been asked to perform the procedure, warn that it will be briefly painful and check they are happy to proceed. Learn the risks of the procedure (Table 4.3.1), in case asked.
Causing undue pain or distress.	Warn the patient prior to starting that the procedure will be briefly painful. Warn immediately prior to needle insertion.	Part of informed consent helps to prepare the patient for what they should expect. Minimise the shock of the procedure and limit possible distress.

STATION VARIATIONS

4

O Advanced

- This station is very commonly combined with interpretation of an arterial blood gas result and possibly some relevant patient management questions. Refer to Chapter 7 for stations containing arterial blood gas interpretation.

Further Reading

See Stations 7.3 and 7.5 for further information on arterial blood gas interpretation.

Capillary blood glucose measurement
4.4

CANDIDATE INFORMATION

Background: You are a junior doctor in general practice and have seen a patient who has symptoms of increased urinary frequency. You have decided to check a random blood glucose measurement.

Task: Demonstrate how you would perform a blood glucose test with a capillary sample. Discuss the result with the patient and suggest a management plan. You are not required to take any further history.

APPROACH TO THE STATION

In this station, the practical procedure is not of primary importance. Performing glucose monitoring is simple (Fig. 4.4.1) and the expectation is that it will be performed competently. However, all glucometers are slightly different, so make sure you are familiar with the equipment in your skills lab. Performing well in this station relies on good communication with the patient and appreciating the implications of different results. You would also be expected to know a reasonable next step of management (Tables 4.4.1 and 4.4.2). For example, if the patient was found to be normoglycaemic, other explanations for urinary frequency should be explored, such as prostatic symptoms or hypercalcaemia.

When you are informed of a blood glucose measurement it is important to establish whether the patient has been fasting (for at least 8 hours), in order to interpret the results correctly. It is also important to note that a diagnosis of diabetes should never be made solely using a bedside glucometer and that abnormal results should be confirmed with a venous glucose sample. Be aware that glucose levels may be transiently higher during periods of inter-current illness or secondary to trauma and surgery. If identified in these circumstances, the levels should be monitored but normally resolve spontaneously. Other causes of hypo- and hyperglycaemia are listed in Table 4.4.3.

Figure 4.4.1 Performing a capillary blood glucose test

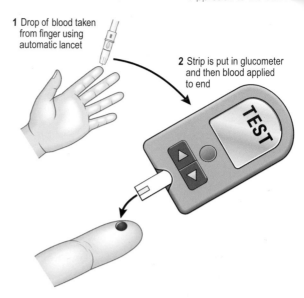

1 Drop of blood taken from finger using automatic lancet

2 Strip is put in glucometer and then blood applied to end

Table 4.4.1 American Diabetes Association (2005) diagnostic threshold for diabetes[a]

	Normoglycaemia	Impaired fasting glucose	Impaired glucose tolerance	Diabetes
Random	—	—	—	>11.1 mmol/l[b]
Fasting	<5.6 mmol/l	5.6–6.9 mmol/l	—	>7.0 mmol/l
2 h post 75-g glucose load[c]	<7.8 mmol/l	—	7.8–11.1 mmol/l	>11.1 mmol/l

[a]Please note that the ADA criteria differ from the World Health Organization (WHO) criteria (2002).
[b]If asymptomatic, the blood glucose should be repeated on a different day, preferably whilst fasted.
[c]An oral glucose tolerance test (OGTT) requires a minimum 8 h fast followed by a measurement prior to the test. The patient then ingests 75 g of glucose within 5 min and a further glucose measurement is taken 120 min post-ingestion. The diagnosis of impaired glucose tolerance can only be made if an oral glucose tolerance test is performed (WHO). Note that the ADA preferentially suggest performance of a fasting glucose, and if this is between 5.6-6.9 mmol/l, describing the patient as having an impaired fasting glucose or 'pre-diabetes', as opposed to performing OGTTs.

Table 4.4.2 Response to blood glucose measurements

Fasting glucose measurement (mmol/l)	Action required
<5.6	Normal blood glucose measurement. No further action required. Further explore the differential diagnosis for symptoms.
5.6–6.9	Suggests impaired fasting glucose. Recommend dietary and lifestyle advice and agree on a time frame for follow-up. Screen for associated problems (hypertension, hypercholesterolaemia).
>7.0	Suggests diabetes (if no intercurrent illness). Repeat a venous lab sample for confirmation. Discuss management plan, which may include lifestyle modifications ± medical therapy. Screen for associated problems (hypertension, hypercholesterolaemia)

Table 4.4.3 Causes of hypoglycaemia and hyperglycaemia

Causes of hypoglycaemia (all rare except with diabetic treatment)	Causes of hyperglycaemia
• Insulin (exogenous or endogenous) • Oral diabetic medications • Inborn error of metabolism • Alcohol abuse • Some medications and poisons • Prolonged starvation • Sepsis	• Diabetes mellitus (type 1 and type 2) • Some medications (notably steroids) • Critical illness including myocardial infarction and stroke • Sepsis • Dysfunction of thyroid, adrenal or pituitary glands • Disorders of the pancreas • Intracranial disease (inc. tumours, infection)

PATIENT INFORMATION

Name: Mr Harry Preston **Age:** 66 years **Sex:** Male

Recently you have noticed that you need to pass urine more frequently. You are waking in the night 3 or 4 times to go to the toilet. You are not sure if you are drinking more than usual. You have come to the GP to get some answers.

You consent to the procedure and are cooperative with it. Regarding the results of the test, you are not interested in science; you just want to know what is wrong with you.

CLINICAL KNOWLEDGE AND EXPERTISE

Equipment
- Tray
- Cleaning wipes
- Glucometer
- Glucometer strips
- Finger prick lancet
- Cotton wool
- Gloves.

Procedure (see Fig. 4.4.1)
1. Introduce yourself and briefly explain what you are about to do and gain consent.
2. Confirm the patient's identity.
3. Wash your hands and ask the patient to also wash their hands. Apply gloves.
4. Check the expiry date of the glucometer strips and when the glucometer was last calibrated. Then insert a new test strip into the glucometer.
5. Select one of the patient's fingers and clean with a cleaning wipe.
6. Warn the patient, and then use a lancet to prick the patient's finger.
7. Dispose of the lancet in a sharps bin.
8. Squeeze the finger gently till a drop of blood forms. Wipe away the first drop with a piece of cotton wool. Touch the glucometer strip to the edge of the next drop of blood to allow it to take it up.
9. Hold cotton wool to the finger (you can ask the patient to do this); a plaster is not normally necessary.
10. The glucometer will automatically show a result on the screen once it is ready.
11. Thank the patient and clear away any equipment.
12. Document the result in the patient's notes.

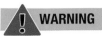

WARNING

- A high blood glucose in an unwell patient should prompt immediate investigation. Diabetic ketoacidosis (DKA) is potentially life-threatening and diagnosis is based on a triad of hyperglycaemia, ketonuria and acidosis. DKA may be the initial presentation of type 1 diabetes or occur in patients with known diabetes. It requires urgent care, including intravenous insulin and intravenous fluids (see Station 7.5).
- A blood glucose level of <4.0 mmol/l is defined as hypoglycaemia, and without treatment patients may lose consciousness or have seizures. A conscious patient can take oral glucose; an unconscious patient will require IM glucagon or IV dextrose.

How to excel in this station

Action	Reason	How
Know the diagnostic criteria.	Demonstrates knowledge of the subject as well as the procedure.	Consult the guidance on diagnostic criteria. Remember that the ADA and WHO criteria are slightly different.
Recognise emergencies.	It is critical to recognise emergency situations and initiate required management.	Check local policies on the management of DKA and hypoglycaemia.

4

Common errors in this station

Common error	Remedy	Reason
Lack of differential diagnosis.	Remember the differential diagnosis of hypoglycaemia and hyperglycaemia.	The ability to suggest alternative diagnoses can mark you out as an excellent candidate. It is important not to assume a diagnosis of diabetes—bear in mind other possibilities.

STATION VARIATIONS

Intermediate

- This station could be combined with writing an insulin prescription (see Station 6.4 for further information).
- The patient information may be that of a known diabetic who needs their regular insulin prescribing, or a correction dose of short-acting insulin prescribing for high levels.
- Be familiar with the insulin prescription forms used in your local hospital trust.

Further Reading

Station 5.4, 'Explaining a new diagnosis of type 2 diabetes'
Station 6.4, 'Prescribing insulin'
Station 7.5, 'Acute management of a diabetic emergency'
American Diabetes Association, http://www.diabetes.org.
Diabetes UK. http://www.diabetes.org.uk.
WHO guidance, 2006. Definition and Diagnosis of Diabetes Mellitus and Intermediate Hyperglycaemia. Available at, http://whqlibdoc.who.int/publications/2006/9241594934_eng.pdf.
Joint British Diabetes Societies Inpatient Care Group, 2010 guidance, 'The Management of DKA in Adults'. Available at http://www.bsped.org.uk/clinical/docs/dkamanagementofdkainadultsmarch20101.pdf.

Urinary catheter insertion

4.5

CANDIDATE INFORMATION

Background: You are a junior doctor in general medicine and have been asked to catheterise Mr Stewart to help monitor his urine output.

Task: Demonstrate how you would place a urethral catheter using the manikin (Figs. 4.5.1 and 4.5.2). Address all communication to the simulated patient.

APPROACH TO THE STATION

This is a practical procedure that involves using a sterile field and pack. Your sterile technique needs to be perfect and, if you make a mistake, it is best to admit it and ask to start with a fresh pack. You will be performing the procedure on a manikin, but address all communication to the simulated patient. You need to take consent prior to commencing. Make sure you are aware of the potential complications and the contraindications (Table 4.5.1).

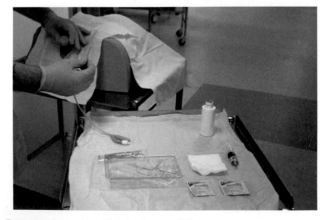

Figure 4.5.1 Example of a male catheterisation manikin

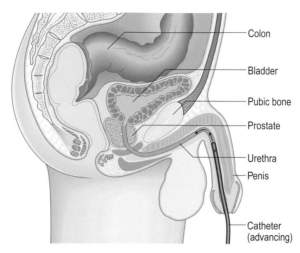

Figure 4.5.2 Male catheter insertion (From Douglas G., et al., *Macleod's Clinical Examination*, 13/e (Churchill Livingstone, 2013) with permission.)

4

Table 4.5.1 Important points regarding catheterisation	
Indications	Urinary retention Monitoring of urine output, for example in acute kidney injury Incontinence (if skin integrity is at risk) After surgery or in severe illness To give intravesical chemotherapy For investigation, e.g., micturating cystourethrogram
Contraindications	Suspected urethral injury History of false passages or strictures
Complications	Bleeding (transient haematuria) Pain Infection Stricture or creation of a false passage
Causes of lack of urine draining on insertion	Blocked catheter—try to flush it with saline Empty bladder (e.g., acute kidney injury) Catheter incorrectly placed

PATIENT INFORMATION

Name: Mr James Stewart   **Age:** 74 years   **Sex:** Male

You are unwell with pneumonia and a catheter needs to be placed in order to monitor your urinary output. You are happy to consent to the procedure and are cooperative with it.

4 CLINICAL KNOWLEDGE AND EXPERTISE

Equipment
- Silver procedure trolley
- Cleaning wipes
- Sterile dressing pack including towel, drape, gauze, gallipot and sterile gloves
- Cleaning solution, e.g., chlorhexidine
- Lignocaine lubricating gel
- Male catheter (containing syringe for inflating balloon)
- Catheter bag.

Procedure
1. Ensure you have all the equipment and clean the silver trolley.
2. Open the sterile dressing pack, then open onto it the catheter (in its plastic wrapper) and syringe, the syringe of lignocaine lubricating jelly and the catheter bag, without contaminating them. Pour the cleaning solution into the gallipot.
3. Introduce yourself to the patient, confirm their identity and gain verbal consent.
4. Put on an apron. Scrub your hands, then dry on a sterile towel from the dressing pack. Apply sterile gloves.
5. Explain that you would position the patient lying on the bed comfortably with his legs slightly separated, genital area exposed and an absorbent pad on the bed in case of any spillages. Explain that you would maintain the patient's privacy and dignity by ensuring the curtains are drawn and minimising risk of interruptions.
6. Explain that you need to begin the procedure and that you are first going to clean the area. Hold the penis with a piece of gauze, with your non-dominant hand. Clean the penis thoroughly, making sure you retract the foreskin and clean around the meatus of the urethra.
7. Make a hole in the drape and place around the penis.
8. Still holding the penis with a piece of sterile gauze, inject some lubricating jelly into the urethra. Explain that you would normally leave this for 3–5 minutes to numb the area.
9. Explain that you are now about to introduce the catheter. Tear open the plastic wrapper containing the catheter in to expose the tip. Try not to touch this and gently advance the catheter into the urethra, discarding the plastic wrapper as you proceed. Advance until only the Y-shaped section remains visible. Urine should be draining through the catheter.
10. Inflate the balloon with the prefilled syringe, ensuring the patient does not feel any pain; inflating the balloon is painless if within the bladder, but it is very painful if it is in the urethra (i.e., if the catheter is not advanced far enough) and can be potentially dangerous.
11. Gently withdraw the catheter until slight resistance is felt and then replace the foreskin. Attach the bag to the end of the catheter.
12. Inform the patient you have finished and clean away your equipment and help the patient in re-dressing if necessary.
13. Record the procedure in the patient's notes; include the residual volume and whether a sample was sent for culture.

NB: Some packs do not include a pre-filled syringe and you may need to include a syringe of sterile water in your equipment. The catheter wrapper will have the balloon volume written on it.

WARNING

- Never use a female catheter for a male patient — the catheters are shorter and this could lead to the balloon being inflated in the urethra, potentially causing serious damage.

✔ How to excel in this station

Action	Reason	How
Perfect sterile technique.	Minimise risk of infection to the patient.	Indwelling catheters can lead to infections and to minimise the risks it is important to have perfect sterile technique.

✖ Common errors in this station

Common error	Remedy	Reason
Inadequate communication.	Engage with the patient, confirm consent and then keep up a commentary, warning of discomfort as appropriate.	It is sometimes difficult, when performing a procedure on a model, to talk to the simulated patient, but this is a critical skill as you could fail on poor communication.
Failure to maintain privacy and dignity.	Close the curtains and preferably hang a 'do-not-disturb' sign. Offer a chaperone. Only expose the patient for the minimum time. After the procedure, help the patient to clean/dress or seek nursing assistance for them.	Respect for your patient and their feelings during this intimate procedure is paramount. You must demonstrate that you intend to put the patient at ease, and minimise any embarrassment or distress.

4

STATION VARIATION

⬤ Basic

- The procedure for female catheterisation is essentially the same, but on a female anatomical model. In clinical practice doctors are less frequently asked to catheterise females, as many nursing staff are trained to perform this skill.

Further Reading

Macleod's Clinical Examination, Chapter 9, 'The Renal System', for further information regarding conditions requiring urethral catheterisation.

Speculum examination

4.6

CANDIDATE INFORMATION

Background: You are a junior doctor working in a general practice. You have been asked to review a patient by the practice nurse. She performed a cervical smear yesterday on Mrs Sandra Ball and noticed a small lump on the cervix, and she wants your opinion to determine whether a referral to gynaecology is indicated.

Task: Please perform a speculum examination on this patient.

APPROACH TO THE STATION

This station asks you to carry out a practical procedure, with all the relevant history already given. In an OSCE this would be performed using a manikin, but it is still important to behave as you would do normally when examining a patient: consenting prior to the examination and offering a chaperone, talking through the procedure, checking for discomfort throughout and ensuring the patient is adequately covered at the end. Although this may feel artificial, demonstrating these skills will form a significant part of your mark so they should not be omitted.

It is important to be aware of the different equipment that may be used so that it does not appear to the examiner (or the patient) that you are performing the procedure for the first time. Speculums come in a variety of sizes and lengths and can be metal or plastic (Fig. 4.6.1); metal speculums are cold so you should offer to warm them under the hot tap prior to use for patient comfort. Choice of speculum size may

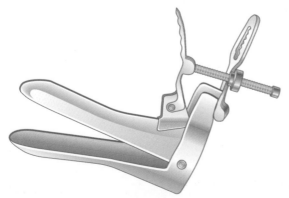

Figure 4.6.1 Bivalve speculum (From Douglas G., et al., *Macleod's Clinical Examination*, 13/e (Churchill Livingstone, 2013) with permission.)

dependent upon patient size, whether they are post-partum and patient preference and comfort.

PATIENT INFORMATION

Name: Mrs Sandra Ball   **Age:** 42 years   **Sex:** Female

You are asymptomatic and normally fit and well. You are up-to-date with your cervical smear tests and have a regular menstrual cycle with no intermenstrual or post-coital bleeding. You have no abnormal vaginal discharge. You have been married for 10 years and are not at risk of sexually transmitted infection. You have three young children, all of whom were normal vaginal deliveries and your husband has had a vasectomy. You don't take any regular medication or have known allergies.

4

Once you have familiarised yourself with the procedure, it is important to practise with a colleague or senior observing you on several occasions to check technique. This could be either done within the clinic setting, e.g., colposcopy clinic, or using a manikin in your skills centre. It is important to review the normal appearance of a healthy cervix in nulliparous and parous women so that you can more easily identify abnormalities (Table 4.6.1).

CLINICAL KNOWLEDGE AND EXPERTISE

Equipment
- Sterile pack, with sterile gloves
- Lubricant (jelly or warm water)
- Speculum (size used is dependent on body habitus and previous history).

Procedure
1. Ensure you have all the equipment and clean the silver trolley.
2. Open the sterile dressing pack and open onto it the speculum and lubricant.
3. Introduce yourself, confirm the patient's identity, obtain consent and offer a chaperone. Allow the patient to undress below the waist and offer a blanket or towel to cover them. Ask the patient to lie supine on the bed with knees drawn up and legs dropped apart to a comfortable position; explain to the patient what is going to happen before proceeding.
4. Wash your hands and apply gloves.

Table 4.6.1 Abnormalities of the cervix

- Cervical erosion/ectopy (extrusion of the columnar epithelium through the os (common when on combined oral contraceptive pill))
- Cervical polyps (grey/white and on surface of cervix)
- Endocervical polyps (cherry red and pedunculated on a stalk)
- Nabothian cysts (a mucus-filled cyst on the surface of the cervix)
- Cervicitis (inflammation with contact bleeding that can indicate chlamydial or gonorrhoeal infection)
- Cervical malignancy (an irregular vascular area)
- Cervical fibroids
- Cervical endometriosis (blue black spots on surface of cervix)

4

5. Expose the introitus by separating the labia with the forefinger and thumb of your left hand commenting on any discharge, inflammation, atrophy or ulceration.
6. Apply lubricant jelly to the tip of the speculum and then gently insert the speculum with blades closed and handles positioned next to the patient's left leg.
7. Once fully inserted, rotate the speculum 90° so the handles are positioned upwards and gently open out the blades to visualise the cervix.
8. Secure the speculum by tightening the screw in the handle (or twisting the plastic lock 90° in some plastic speculums).
9. Look for any abnormalities of the cervix and vaginal walls and comment on shape of the cervical os.
10. Offer to take swabs if any evidence of abnormal discharge and a cervical smear test if appropriate (only if due).
11. If you are struggling to visualise the cervix, withdraw the speculum slightly, close the blades then angle the blades more anteriorly or posteriorly and slightly deeper before re-opening.
12. Withdraw the speculum to just clear of the cervix before loosening the speculum screw and closing the blades, continue to slowly withdraw the speculum whilst rotating the handles back to their original position.
13. Offer tissues and privacy so the patient can dress.

⚠ WARNING

• The size of the speculum used depends on the body habitus of the patient and their previous history (for example, whether they have had previous vaginal deliveries). Bear in mind that the use of a larger speculum may be uncomfortable or painful for the patient.

How to excel in this station

Action	Reason	How
Ensuring a patient-centred approach.	This is a very intimate, and sometimes embarrassing, examination for women and care should be taken throughout to avoid harm or distress.	Make sure that the patient has consented prior to starting and talk through the different stages allowing the patient the opportunity to stop if it is too painful, or take a short break.
Maintain privacy and dignity throughout.	As mentioned above, this is paramount given the nature of this intimate female examination.	Ensure that curtains are fully pulled around. Offer the patient either a blanket or towel to cover themselves so that they don't feel fully exposed. Cover on completion, offer tissues afterwards and give opportunity to dress in private.

✗ Common errors in this station

Common error	Remedy	Reason
Forgetting to treat the manikin as a patient.	Try to visualise a real patient underneath the cover and talk normally as you would do when explaining a procedure.	It can feel an artificial situation having to perform an intimate procedure without the opportunity to first take a history and build up rapport, and even more so when the station involves a manikin only.

Common errors in this station—cont'd

Common error	Remedy	Reason
Lack of explanation.	Ensure that there is discussion around the procedure before and during the examination so the patient remains fully aware of what to expect.	In order to ensure that the patient is fully consented, they must be made aware of what the procedure involves, even if they have had it done before; this should avoid surprise or distress during the examination.

STATION VARIATIONS

○ Intermediate

4

- Most manikins used for this procedure have a removable cervix, so a normal cervix may be replaced with an abnormal one to provide more of a challenge when describing findings to the examiner or patient, and in considering differential diagnoses.

Further Reading

Macleod's Clinical Examination, Section 10, 'The Reproductive System: The Gynaecological Examination: The Physical Examination'.

Patient.co.uk, 'Uterine Cervix and Common Cervical Abnormalities'. http://www.patient.co.uk/doctor/uterine-cervix-and-common-cervical-abnormalities.

Fastbleep.com, 'Bimanual/Speculum Examination'. http://www.fastbleep.com/medical-notes/o-g-and-paeds/17/37/380.

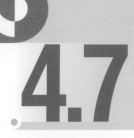

Suturing a wound

4.7

CANDIDATE INFORMATION

Background: You are a junior doctor in the Emergency Department where a patient has presented with a wound on her anterior thigh, made by accidently walking into a broken piece of glass.

Task: Discuss the requirement for sutures with the patient and then demonstrate this on the equipment provided.

APPROACH TO THE STATION

There are several components to this station, which incorporates a fairly complex skill. These are:
- Patient consent and explanation (brief);
- Understanding of the assessment of wounds and their basic management (Table 4.7.1);
- Aseptic non-touch technique (ANTT), universal precautions, and safe disposal of sharps;
- Ability to suture; and
- Follow-up and after-care as appropriate.

This station can be difficult to complete in the allotted time, so you must be aware of this and not take too long in any one area. See the chapter introduction for more details about managing your time in practical procedure stations and Station 4.2 for an overview of ANTT. Due to the time restriction, this station will normally involve an uncomplicated, superficial wound; however, make sure you are aware of how to assess a wound prior to closure (Table 4.7.1).

Table 4.7.1 Assessing a wound
- Is the wound clean? What implement made the wound? Antibiotics may be indicated for certain contaminated wounds.
- Could there be a foreign body in the wound (e.g., a piece of glass or other material)?
- Has haemostasis been achieved?
- Can the wound edges be easily opposed?
- Does the wound involve any other structures (e.g., tendons, nerves, joints)? Could it penetrate body cavities or deep tissues?

PATIENT INFORMATION

Name: Ms Maria Grabowski   **Age:** 25 years   **Sex:** Female

You have a fairly deep gash on your thigh made by a piece of glass. It has stopped bleeding now. You have never had any stitches before and want to know if they will hurt and if they will scar.

CLINICAL KNOWLEDGE AND EXPERTISE

Equipment (Fig. 4.7.1)

- Silver trolley
- Sterile dressing set
- Sterile gloves (may be included in dressing set)
- Suture
- Irrigation solution (usually sterile normal saline)
- Suture holders, forceps, scissors or stitch cutter (may be together in a 'suture set')
- Dressing
- Sharps bin
- Local anaesthetic (lignocaine 1%), syringe, drawing-up needle and narrow gauge injecting needle. Due to time constraints and limitations of simulated equipment you are not likely to be expected to demonstrate anaesthetising the wound; however, you may be asked to talk through it.

4

Procedure

1. Introduce yourself and briefly explain what you are about to do and gain consent. Answer any questions (see above). Check the patient has been immunised against tetanus.
2. Confirm the patient's identity.
3. Set up your sterile field by opening the equipment using ANTT. Put some saline into the galley pot in your dressing pack. Clean your hands thoroughly and put on sterile gloves.
4. Clean the wound using sterile gauze and the irrigation solution, taking care not to touch the wound with your gloves until after it has been cleaned.

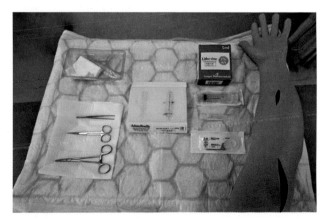

Figure 4.7.1 Suture equipment and simulated skin

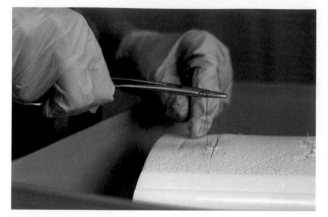

Figure 4.7.2 Instrument tie

5. Examine the wound. State that you would want to ensure that haemostasis had been achieved, that the wound edges were opposable, and that the wound did not involve any other structures such as joints, nerves, tendons, etc. You should also ask about a possible foreign body in the wound (answer in an OSCE will be 'no').
6. Explain that you would draw up some local anaesthetic and inject it subdermally along the wound edges. Explain what you are doing as you go along. Local anaesthetic should work quickly but it is prudent to check the skin is anaesthetised sufficiently by checking with the patient.
7. Place the suture in the suture holder and hold in your dominant hand. Take the forceps in your other hand. Gently hold the skin at the wound edge with the forceps and put the suture through the skin near the wound edge. Unclasp your suture holder and pick up the other end of the suture to pull through to the other side.
8. Repeat step 7 on the other side of the wound (this time moving from inside the wound edge to outside) and then take the threads and do an instrument tie (Fig. 4.7.2).
9. Perform another suture (steps 7 and 8) approximately 1 cm further along the wound. The examiner will usually ask you to stop after completing two sutures.
10. Carefully dispose of sharps in the sharps bin provided.
11. Explain that the sutures can be removed at the patient's GP surgery in 7–10 days. The wound should be kept dry and it is helpful to provide a spare dressing in case the other gets wet. Tell the patient to go to the GP or return to A&E if the wound edge starts looking inflamed or if the wound starts discharging.

You may be asked about the advantages and disadvantages of other types of wound closure — refer to Table 4.7.2 for further information.

Table 4.7.2 Mechanisms of wound closure		
Wound closure	**Advantages**	**Disadvantages**
Sutures	Good for wounds on areas with lots of movement, and wounds that are still bleeding slightly.	May scar. Requires patient compliance (difficult with needle phobic patients and children). Skin may be too delicate (e.g., pre-tibial).

Table 4.7.2 Mechanisms of wound closure—cont'd

Wound closure	Advantages	Disadvantages
Steri-strips	Usually a good cosmetic result. Easy to apply. Good for small/complicated/uneven wounds and delicate skin (e.g., face).	May not stay on if good haemostasis has not been achieved. Cannot be applied to areas that undergo lots of movement.
Staples	Quick to apply so good for larger wounds, e.g., abdominal, large scalp wounds.	Can be uncomfortable and unsightly. Not as good cosmetic result.
Wound glue	Excellent for small wounds on delicate skin areas and wounds within hair. Good cosmetic result.	Requires good haemostasis. Wound's edges must oppose well. Only suitable for small wounds.

 WARNING

- If a wound is directly overlying a joint, if you suspect nerve or tendon involvement or (sometimes) if it is on the face, then you should not attempt to suture it and should ask for involvement from specialists (such as plastic surgery or orthopaedic surgery).
- Bear in mind the mechanism of injury and if there is anything of concern about all injuries. Could this be a presentation of domestic violence, child abuse, elder abuse or abuse of a vulnerable adult?

How to excel in this station

Action	Reason	How
Good patient communication.	Do not overlook the consent and explanation elements to the station.	View the patient holistically—is there anything else they want to discuss?
Recognise complexities.	It is reassuring to the examiner that you would confirm that the wound is suitable for the suggested treatment.	Discuss the wound management details outlined above and confirm that you would speak to a senior doctor or discuss with other specialists if concerned.

Common errors in this station

Common error	Remedy	Reason
Perfect suture technique but poor rapport.	Practise the skill and remember that there are several elements to the station.	It is more important that you are able to communicate effectively and perform ANTT with safe sharps disposal than that your suture technique is perfect.
Running out of time.	Pace yourself. You can talk about wound management as you set up.	You cannot get a really high score unless you manage to cover all the elements that the station is examining.

STATION VARIATIONS

○ Basic

- This station may be combined with the process of drawing up a solution for injection (for example, local anaesthetic). This station would examine the demonstration of ANTT technique and safe disposal of sharps.

4

4

○ Intermediate

- You may be asked to focus on taking detailed consent for this procedure, rather than actually performing it as a practical skill (see Station 5.2 for more details on taking informed consent).
- Make sure you are aware of the risks of the procedure and advice regarding ongoing wound care and scarring.

Further Reading

If you are struggling to find opportunities to suture and practise instrument ties in your clinical placements there are several resources on the Internet, including videos on YouTube (search for 'interrupted sutures' and 'suturing — instrument ties').

Adult basic life support

4.8

Background: You are a junior doctor in general surgery. You are walking along a quiet hospital corridor near ward B4 and see an adult lying on the floor further down the corridor. There is a wall-mounted phone on the corridor.

Task: Demonstrate how you would manage this situation.

APPROACH TO THE STATION

It is essential that all medical students and junior doctors can perform good quality adult basic life support when required. You should be able to perform the following procedure confidently and are likely to be marked harshly if you cannot manage at least a competent demonstration. Some institutions use this station as a standalone certification or 'must-pass' station and students/doctors must reach the passing level in this or will have to retake on a separate occasion.

The UK Resuscitation Council basic life support algorithm was modified in 2010 to place more emphasis on effective chest compressions – see the notes below and Further Reading section.

This station is almost always performed with an examiner and a resuscitation manikin. Remember that many manikins have sensors to monitor the efficacy of chest compressions and rescue breaths. It is often helpful to the examiner to give them a running commentary of your actions. Ability to perform basic life support may also be assessed as part of a more complex station such as those in Chapter 7.

CLINICAL KNOWLEDGE AND EXPERTISE

Equipment
- BLS manikin
- Telephone (to demonstrate calling for help).

Procedure
1. SAFE approach
   a. Shout for help.
   b. Approach with care.
   c. Free from danger.
   d. Evaluate patient (call to patient loudly and shake their shoulder), then proceed with assessment.

4

2. Position yourself to the side of the patient and perform a head tilt, chin lift procedure with the first two fingers of your right hand under the patient's chin (see Fig. 4.8.1). Use your other hand to palpate the carotid artery (Fig. 4.8.2). Put your head near to the patient's mouth and nose and tilt your head so that you are looking down at the patient's chest.

3. Look, listen and feel for a carotid pulse and any signs of breathing — breath on your cheek, gurgling noises or other breath sounds and chest movement. Do this for 10 seconds. It is helpful to the examiner if you count aloud.

4. If there are no signs of life after 10 seconds (informed by the examiner), call the cardiac arrest team on the nearby phone, giving your location, and return to the victim immediately. (If another person is available, ask them to call the team while you start chest compressions.) Immediately return to the patient.

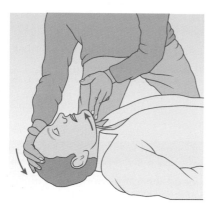

Head tilt chin lift
Palm of hand on forehead. Index and middle fingers under chin. Lift gently.

Figure 4.8.1 Head tilt chin lift

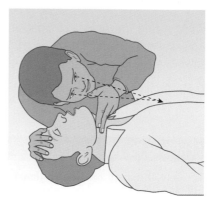

Simultaneous pulse and breathing check
1. Maintain head tilt whilst checking carotid pulse.
2. Look, listen and feel for breathing, pulse, chest movement or signs of life for 10 seconds.

Figure 4.8.2 Head tilt chin lift and simultaneous pulse check

5. Perform 30 chest compressions (Fig. 4.8.3). Place the heel of your hand in the centre of the victim's chest with the heel of your other hand on top, approximately over the lower half of the patient's sternum. There is no need to measure the exact position, just commence compressions without delay. Keep your shoulders over the victim's chest and keep your arms straight with the elbows locked.

6. Ensure your chest compressions are at a rate of approximately 100–120/min with a depth of 5–6 cm or approximately a third of the depth of the victim's chest.

7. After the 30 chest compressions, give two rescue breaths by performing a head tilt, chin lift manoeuvre, opening the victim's mouth, taking a deep breath and applying your mouth around the patient's to form a seal and blowing into the victim's mouth. Look for rise and fall of the chest following the breaths. If after the first breath there is no rise and fall, re-check the mouth for obstruction, re-position the patient and have one further attempt. Do not attempt more than two breaths before returning to chest compressions.

8. If help arrives without a defibrillator, clearly ask the helper to fetch an automated external defibrillator (AED) or a cardiac arrest trolley from the nearest clinical area (in this situation) and immediately return to you. Continue chest compressions and rescue breaths at a rate of 30:2 until their return.

Figure 4.8.3 Performing chest compressions

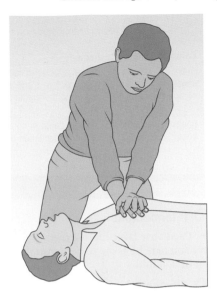

4

9. When the helper returns, ask them to take over chest compressions (you will be tiring by now) while you connect the defibrillator (if they have one) or perform rescue breaths. Demonstrate the procedure if necessary (though this is unlikely to be tested in a BLS station), and ensure that your helper is already in position to take over chest compressions as soon as you stop.

10. Continue at a rate of 30 chest compressions to two rescue breaths until further help arrives or someone brings a cardiac defibrillator. Do not stop to check the victim or discontinue CPR unless the victim starts to show signs of regaining consciousness, such as coughing, opening their eyes, speaking, or moving purposefully and starts to breathe normally.

⚠ WARNING

- Basic life support is an essential skill for all medical students and junior doctors, and a good knowledge of the procedure and fluent performance is essential.
- Basic life support is the first link in the 'chain of survival'. The chain is only as strong as its weakest link. Poor quality basic life support increases the chance of a poor outcome.
- Remember that there is a different algorithm and procedure for performing infant and child Basic Life Support. Please see the UK Resuscitation Council website for more information.

✔ How to excel in this station

Action	Reason	How
Clear explanation.	The examiner cannot tell what you are thinking and may interrupt to ask.	Perform the procedure giving a clear and succinct commentary to the examiner.
Confident and fluent performance.	This is an essential skill for all medical undergraduates and practitioners.	Practise the procedure in a skills lab, and ask your colleagues or skills teachers to observe to ensure fluent performance and efficacious compressions.

4

Common errors in this station		
Common error	**Remedy**	**Reason**
Delay in instituting chest compressions.	Minimise delay in commencing chest compressions and restarting them after rescue breaths.	Delays in commencing and restarting compressions have been clearly shown to reduce the chances of a good outcome following cardiac arrest.
Poor quality chest compressions.	Practise depth of compressions with a resuscitation manikin.	Research shows that good quality chest compressions improve outcomes.

STATION VARIATIONS

○ Intermediate

- Paediatric basic life support.
- You may be asked to demonstrate how the procedure is modified for use in infants or children.

○ Advanced

- Advanced life support (ALS).
- A basic life support station may be extended to include some parts of advanced life support (for example, use of an AED) or some knowledge of the ALS algorithms. See the Further Reading section below for more information.

Further Reading

Resuscitation Council: Refer to the basic life support algorithm at http://www.resus. org.uk or it can be found in any of their resuscitation publications (such as the course manual for *Intermediate Life Support* or *Advanced Life Support*). These publications are normally available in medical school and hospital libraries. This site also offers information on the advanced life support algorithm and the initial treatment of many other emergency medical scenarios.

Death verification

4.9

CANDIDATE INFORMATION

Background: You are a junior doctor on nights at the hospital. The nursing staff have called you as an elderly patient, Mrs Doreen Hobson, has been found to have possibly died in her sleep. She was terminally ill with metastatic pancreatic cancer and 'not for resuscitation' and there are no suspicious circumstances.

Task: Please demonstrate how you would verify this patient's death.

APPROACH TO THE STATION

This station asks you to confirm death, although obviously within an OSCE this would be performed on a manikin rather than a deceased patient. There is no request to provide a death certificate so the emphasis should be on examining for signs of life, such as cardiac output, respiratory effort, response to painful and verbal stimuli and pupillary responsiveness, and recording your findings within the patient records. Although demonstrating your examination on a manikin in this instance, it is important to still show dignity and respect for the deceased person as well as the grieving family by maintaining a systematic professional approach and ensuring that the patient is adequately covered on completion of the examination.

Although there is no actual legal definition of death within the UK, it is the clinician who determines whether death has occurred using a thorough clinical assessment. Within the acute hospital setting, there may also be the additional support of ECG monitoring or invasive monitoring within intensive care, but this does not replace a clinical examination, no matter how confident you may be that the patient has died. As the background information states that this patient has a signed Do Not Resuscitate directive, no attempt should be made to perform CPR, although this would be appropriate in other cases even if the timing of death is not known and may have been some time previously.

Documentation of death verification is very important, and may well be part of the OSCE station. Candidates are likely to score poorly if this is missed out altogether or findings are not recorded accurately. See Box 4.9.1 for more information on what should be recorded in the notes.

4

| Box 4.9.1 | Documenting death verification in patient records |

- A record of the date and time you performed your examination
- A summary of your findings
- A record of whether the patient has a pacemaker fitted (dangerous if not removed prior to cremation)
- Your signature, name and designation

CLINICAL KNOWLEDGE AND EXPERTISE

1. Confirm the patient's identity using both medical records and a name tag that should be attached to the patient's wrist (even in instances when the patient is known to you).
2. Wash hands or apply alcohol hand-gel prior to beginning the examination and on completion.
3. Ensure privacy and dignity throughout, asking any relatives present to wait outside during verification.
4. Look externally for obvious signs of post-mortem, e.g., pallor of face and lips, rigor mortis (generalised muscle stiffening), lividity (red/purple discolouration of skin in gravity-dependent areas of the body, e.g., buttocks and back if lying supine), eyes open and staring with possible corneal clouding and relaxation of facial muscles, with sometimes drooping of jaw.
5. Assess pupillary reactivity using a pen-torch or light—in death pupils are fixed and dilated.
6. Look for signs of spontaneous movement or respiratory effort.
7. Palpate for the presence of a carotid or femoral pulse for at least 1 min.
8. Check there is no motor or withdrawal response, or facial grimace to painful stimuli, e.g., sternal rub or supraorbital pressure.
9. Listen for heart sounds (over the cardiac apex) and breath sounds for at least 2 minutes.
10. Check for corneal reflexes (blinking when touching edge of cornea lightly with cotton wool, see Fig. 4.9.1).
11. Check for the presence of a pacemaker (palpable superficially on the left anterior chest wall) and ensure it is documented in notes if present or absent.
12. Document your findings in the notes.

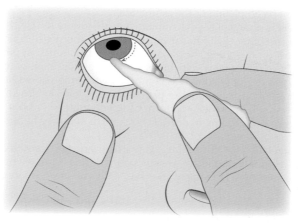

Figure 4.9.1 Testing corneal reflex (From Douglas G., et al., *Macleod's Clinical Examination*, 13/e (Churchill Livingstone, 2013) with permission.)

WARNING

- Remember that verification of death relies upon the combination of examination findings rather than any one in isolation and there can be certain clinical manifestations that may make it appear that the patient has died, e.g., severe hypoglycaemia, making a thorough assessment crucial.
- Always document in the medical notes whether the patient had a pacemaker fitted, as these must be removed prior to cremation.

How to excel in this station

Action	Reason	How
Demonstrate knowledge.	Show a thorough and consistent method to verification of death, using a step-by-step approach to avoid missing any key areas.	The excellent candidate should work through the examination systematically, explaining to the examiner as they go along what they are looking for and documenting clearly their findings in the patient record.
Show dignity and respect for the deceased patient.	Demonstrate professionalism and compassion throughout for not only the deceased patient but also their family.	Ask any family members to wait outside during the examination, if relevant, and ensure that the patient is covered up appropriately at the end of the examination, closing their eyelids if possible.

Common errors in this station

Common error	Remedy	Reason
Rushing through the verification stages.	Work through the examination slowly and systematically, as plenty of time is allowed for the completion of this station.	In order to accurately verify death, breath and heart sounds should be absent for at least 2 min, so rushing through this could mean potentially missing an alternative diagnosis.
Failing to adequately document examination finding on completion.	It is important to remember not only to document the findings relevant to certify death, but also date and time the notes entry with a legible signature.	It is a legal requirement to have a patient's death accurately verified with thorough documentation prior to the body being moved to a place of rest and the death certificate being issued.

STATION VARIATIONS

○ Intermediate

- To increase the complexity of the case, the candidate could be asked in addition to complete a death certificate for the patient (on the assumption that they have seen them in the preceding 14 days before their death).
- You would be offered either use of the medical records for guidance on past medical history that may be required or additional information regarding the patient's background at the beginning of the case.
- Make sure you are aware of how to accurately and appropriately complete a death certificate.

4 ○ **Advanced**

- To add complexity to the case, candidates may wish to consider how their examination may differ if the patient was on an intensive care unit being mechanically ventilated, i.e., what methods could be used to determine brain stem death.

Further Reading

Macleod's Clinical Examination, Chapter 18, 'Assessment for Anaesthesia And Sedation: Confirming Death'.

Patient.co.uk, 'Death (Recognition and Certification)', http://www.patient.co.uk/doctor/Death-(Recognition-and-Certification).htm.

Academy of Medical Royal Colleges, 2008. A Code of Practice for the Diagnosis and Confirmation of Death. available at http://www.bts.org.uk/Documents/A%20CODE%20OF%20PRACTICE%20FOR%20THE%20DIAGNOSIS%20AND%20CONFIRMATION%20OF%20DEATH.pdf.

Ethics, communication and explanation

5

Introduction to ethics, communication and explanation

5.0

Good communication skills are central to OSCEs, and are likely to be tested in the majority of stations. You will not be assessed as competent in performing a physical examination or practical procedure if you cannot explain to the patient the process and gain consent. The cases contained within this chapter give examples of common communication stations that focus on more challenging communication tasks, which require great sensitivity and empathy, as well as other crucial skills needed to become an effective communicator. Most of these stations utilise simulated patients, who may have been asked to behave in an aggressive or in a challenging way manner to test your ability to calm the situation and maintain a professional approach. Although this can be unnerving to begin with, the actors are trained to respond positively to good communication. Recognising and acknowledging the patient or relative's concerns or dissatisfaction early on can often allow the situation to be diffused and the consultation to progress.

Also tested within this chapter are attitudinal skills that often are intertwined with communication, including the ability to maintain an ethical approach and respect a patient's autonomy within decision making as well as demonstrating professional behaviour and values. Although it can be difficult to sit down and learn these techniques from a book (all communication skills require repeated practice using both patients and colleagues) it is important to have a good knowledge of the GMC's guidance (or similar), especially around topics such as consent and medico-legal issues. This information may often be tested towards the end of the OSCE by the examiner asking specific questions. In the event that you are unsure of how to proceed in a difficult ethical or medico-legal situation, you should acknowledge this and mention the need to discuss the case with senior team members, or with your medical indemnity body. Doing this does not automatically lead to a failure, as to recognise limitations in your knowledge or experience is an important demonstration of the professional attitude required to practise safely.

➡ KEY SKILLS

This list is not exhaustive and may appear simple and intuitive, but without a well-structured and communicated discussion or explanation, it can be difficult to engage a patient in a management plan or diffuse an emotionally charged situation.

- Use verbal and non-verbal communication to help the patient feel at ease.
- Ask the patient their opinions and thoughts to allow shared management decisions.
- Recognise and acknowledge their emotions and fears and allow time to express them using empathy.
- Avoid the use of medical jargon and check understanding throughout.
- Allow the patient or relative time to ask questions and offer follow-up if needed.
- Respect the need for autonomy, even if their viewpoint may be different from your own.

Explaining inhaler technique

5.1

CANDIDATE INFORMATION

Background: You are a junior doctor working in general practice. James Price is a 19-year-old student with a persistent nocturnal cough and wheeze whom you have been reviewing for a few weeks and he has been confirmed to have mild asthma on spirometry. You wish to start him on a Salbutamol inhaler, to use as required.

Task: Please explain to James how to use the inhaler and get him to demonstrate taking two puffs.

APPROACH TO THE STATION

This is a communication skills station, which requires you to discuss and demonstrate the technique to the patient in a series of simple steps that the patient can then repeat back to you. Getting the patient to repeat the technique ensures understanding and gives the patient the opportunity to practise within a safe environment, then ask any questions afterwards. This is known as the 'teach-back' method or 'closing the loop'.

You should initially perform the task in a step-wise fashion, first working through the demonstration in silence (pre-warn the patient that you are going to do this to avoid confusion) and then repeat whilst talking through each stage. Once this has been completed, ask the patient to demonstrate the technique, using the same steps, first by talking through the steps and then by demonstrating in silence themselves.

Allow the patient the opportunity to ask questions at the end of their demonstration so as not to distract them from following the steps and so that they have had a chance to see how they would use the inhaler in practice and establish any potential problems. Avoiding having more than four or five steps to any explanation makes it more likely that the patient will be able to retain and repeat the information back to you, and each step should be simple and discussed using language that is easy to understand.

Don't forget that, in order to teach a patient about using a device, you must also have confidence in your own ability to use it so make sure that you are familiar with several different devices and have had the opportunity to practise (with and without a spacer) before the exam.

PATIENT INFORMATION

Name: James Price   **Age:** 19 years   **Sex:** Male

Occupation: Student

Presenting symptom: Nocturnal cough and wheeze for last few months.

Opening statement: You believe that you can probably use an inhaler okay if given a chance as you've seen friends use them and it looks pretty straight forward.

Other symptoms (if asked): You do also experience mild wheeze on exertion and do have to catch your breath when playing sport sometimes as a result.

Past medical history: Hay fever during summer months only.

Drug history: Cetirizine 10 mg daily (during summer only).

Social history: You live with your parents. You are at 6th form college doing A Levels. You have never smoked.

If asked:

Ideas: You understand that you have a bit of asthma that is causing you to cough at night and that the inhaler should hopefully improve this.

Concerns: You are slightly concerned about the fact that you're not able to play football as well as you used to because you start to get a little wheezy when running around.

Expectations: You hope that the inhaler will help your night-time cough and mean that you can return to normal activity levels again.

5

CLINICAL KNOWLEDGE AND EXPERTISE

Inhaler technique is a common skill that requires teaching within primary and secondary care at the point of initiating or changing inhalers and should be checked regularly, ideally annually. If taught incorrectly or rushed, it can lead to a reduced beneficial effect, or an increased risk of potential side effects, such as oral thrush with steroid inhalers.

Written or verbal instructions on inhaler use are insufficient and it is important to use the opportunity at the point of initiation to demonstrate on a placebo device and allow the patient the chance to practise and ask questions after doing so.

Unfortunately, it has been demonstrated that health professionals themselves often struggle to perform inhaler technique correctly; in part this is as a result of the number of different inhaler devices available, and a lack of confidence may lead to reluctance to check inhaler technique with the patient.

The choice of a particular device, or whether to add in a spacer to improve drug delivery, depends upon acceptability and the patient's inhalation ability as well as dexterity in manipulating devices. Breath-activated devices may be considered in a patient who struggles to coordinate the inhaler with breathing in or who has problems with dexterity, which make holding the inhaler difficult, e.g., arthritis. The inspiratory flow rate required for each inhaler differs, and the patient's ability to take a full deep breath in can also affect inhaler choice. Aerosol (or metered dose inhaler, MDI) devices require a slow deep breath to allow the inhalant to make it to the lungs without sticking at the back of the throat, whereas some of the dry powder

5

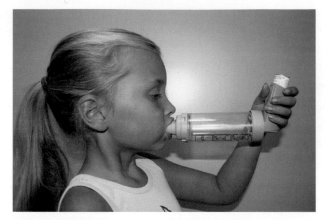

Figure 5.1.1 A child using an inhaler via a spacer (From Taussig LM et al., *Pediatric Respiratory Medicine*, 2/e (Mosby, 2008) with permission.)

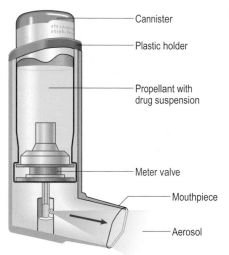

Cannister

Plastic holder

Propellant with drug suspension

Meter valve

Mouthpiece

Aerosol

Figure 5.1.2 Inside a metered-dose inhaler

inhalers require a more forceful inhalation in order to draw the particles of drug out of the inhaler, which may be difficult for certain patients, e.g., those with advanced COPD.

Although using a spacer greatly increases drug delivery, it can be difficult to achieve compliance if the patient does not understand the benefit of adding it, or if the device is too bulky and cumbersome to easily transport. It can be a good option for children (Fig. 5.1.1), or patients requiring a high dose of inhaled steroid, which is more likely to give localised side effects if used incorrectly. For the purpose of this station, we will be focusing on demonstrating the use of an aerosol (MDI) inhaler without a spacer (see Fig. 5.1.2).

Inhaler technique for using an aerosol device (MDI) without a spacer

1. Remove the inhaler cap, shake the inhaler, then hold it upright with your index finger placed on top of the inhaler.

2. Breathe out completely then place the mouthpiece between the lips and breathe in slowly and deeply whilst pressing firmly on the top of the inhaler canister at the same time.
3. Hold your breath for 10 seconds after breathing in deeply.
4. Breathe out normally and repeat the procedure after a few seconds before replacing the inhaler cap.

 WARNING

- Don't forget to check the patient's understanding of when to use the inhaler as it is being prescribed 'as required', as well as advising them to seek medical help if it is not working or no longer effective.
- Don't assume that the patient will be able to understand and follow your instructions on the first attempt; allow time for practising within the station.

✓ How to excel in this station		
Action	**Reason**	**How**
Discuss planned steps prior to starting.	The patient can feel pressurised and uncomfortable if suddenly asked to perform a task without warning and may freeze.	Talk the patient through the planned stages prior to starting so that they are aware that they will be expected to repeat the technique back to you later on, and reassure them that you are not testing their knowledge, more your ability to explain the technique to them.
Check understanding throughout.	The patient may be embarrassed or too shy to ask questions during or after the explanation but not understand what is expected of them and therefore not perform the task correctly.	Check for understanding throughout in a non-confrontational manner, e.g., 'Does that make sense?' or 'Please let me know if I'm not explaining this clearly enough to you.'

✗ Common errors in this station		
Common error	**Remedy**	**Reason**
Overcomplicated explanation.	Break down any explanation into bite-sized chunks that are easily reproducible and that the patient can learn in a step-wise fashion.	When explaining about new medication or devices, it can be easy to fall back on medical knowledge previously learnt from texts which can then lead to the overuse of medical terminology and jargon.
Focusing too much on history and running out of time.	All the salient points are included within the background information given, so, after a brief introduction and obtaining of consent, start the demonstration straight away.	The temptation can be to take a full history around asthma prior to starting the task. This is not necessary and will only cut into the allocated time for explaining and demonstrating the technique.

STATION VARIATIONS

● Basic

In a more basic station, you may be asked to check the inhaler technique of a patient who is already established on using an inhaler and has more experience. Remember, however, that the technique they have developed may not be completely correct, so this requires observation and advice on any errors.

5 ○ Advanced

In a more advanced station, the opportunity may be given to discuss different devices that may be suggested in different clinical circumstances and to offer a demonstration or discussion around the options and preferences with a patient, e.g., breath-activated device.

Further Reading

Rees, J., 2005. ABC of asthma: methods of delivering drugs. BMJ 331, 504.

Practice educator, 2011. How to teach inhaler technique. NursingTimes 107 (8), 16–17. Available at http://www.nursingtimes.net/Journals/2013/01/18/c/n/z/010211How-to-teach-inhaler-technique.pdf.

Obtaining consent for gastroscopy 5.2

CANDIDATE INFORMATION

Background: You are a junior doctor in a gastroenterology clinic. Mrs Freda Jones (57 years old) has been referred by her GP with indigestion, weight loss and iron deficiency anaemia. Clinical examination is unremarkable. You discuss her case with your consultant, who agrees that Mrs Jones requires an endoscopy to exclude an ulcer or a gastric cancer.

Task: Please explain the procedure to Mrs Jones and gain her informed consent for an oesophago-gastro-duodenoscopy (OGD).

APPROACH TO THE STATION

Gaining informed consent using shared decision making with patients is a key skill. You need to be satisfied that the patient understands the reason for the procedure including alternative options, the nature of the procedure and associated side effects or complications. If you have doubts that the patient is able to understand or weigh up the risks and benefits of the procedure, then you may need to formally assess their capacity.

PATIENT INFORMATION

Name: Mrs Freda Jones **Age:** 57 years **Sex:** Female

Occupation: Supermarket worker

Opening statement: You have been referred by your GP with the history as above. They have told you to expect that you will need a 'camera test' but you are not sure what this entails. When the doctor explains the test, you are reluctant to have it and if it has not been already discussed this, ask if you can be put to sleep.

Ideas, concerns and expectations: You are worried that you may have cancer as your uncle had stomach cancer and died 3 months after he had a gastroscopy. The doctor should explain the reasons for wanting to do the test and you should ask them directly if they think that you have cancer.

You are also worried about having to take a long time off work following the procedure and you can't afford this.

(Continued)

5

If the doctor answers all your questions to your satisfaction, then you will agree to have the procedure done. If not, you will say that you are not sure and want to think about it.

If asked: If the doctor asks, tell him/her you have been taking ibuprofen for arthritis in your hands.

CLINICAL KNOWLEDGE AND EXPERTISE

How to gain informed consent

You must be satisfied that a patient understands the need for a procedure, the potential results (including diagnosis of cancer), the technical aspects and the complications and side effects (including failure of a procedure, for example, if offering a surgical treatment).

You should explain who will carry out the procedure. It is best practice for the person performing the procedure to gain consent but for a straightforward and common procedure such as an OGD, a person who understands the procedure can gain consent on their behalf.

It is very important to check that the patient has understood the information. The best way to do this is to ask them to tell you what they have understood.

You must establish if the patient has any ideas about what the procedure entails and why they are having it, any concerns and what expectations they have of success/ failure. You should support the patient in making their decision by providing them with written information and reassure them that they may change their mind or seek further advice at any stage and that signing a written consent form does not invalidate this. If the person cannot decide, you should offer time to think and discuss with anyone. It is good practice to suggest a follow-up meeting to go through things again.

The differential diagnosis of iron deficiency anaemia

The history suggests an upper gastrointestinal cause for iron deficiency anaemia. The most common cause for this is aspirin or non-steroidal anti-inflammatory drug (NSAID) use, followed by benign gastric ulceration and then gastric cancer. Oesophagitis and coeliac disease are slightly less common.

Technical aspects of an OGD

The patient will need to be 'nil-by-mouth' for 4 hours pre-procedure. A small camera (approximately a thumb width in diameter) is inserted through the mouth and into the stomach. Many patients only have a local anaesthetic spray on the back of their throat, although some require sedation. Patents lie on their left side as the scope is passed into the mouth. If a lesion is seen, a small biopsy sample may be taken. An uncomplicated procedure takes about 5 minutes. Patients are usually able to drive or return to work immediately after the procedure. However, if sedation is given they will not be allowed to drive that day. Sore throat is a common side effect. Complications are rare (<1:1,000) but include aspiration of stomach contents causing pneumonia, bleeding and perforation.

 WARNING

- In this case it is important to outline the diagnostic value of OGD.
- The most likely diagnosis is a benign cause such as gastric irritation due to NSAID use or an ulcer. However, you should recognise the patient's concerns about cancer and discuss them.

✓ How to excel in this station

Action	Reason	How
Confidently explain the procedure to the patient.	This will reassure them you know what you are talking about!	Take time to explain, and use non-technical language as much as possible. Listen to any questions and answer these.
Check understanding of the proposed procedure.	Without this, you will not be getting informed consent.	Ask the patient to tell you what they understand or to summarise back to you what the procedure entails.
Acknowledge the patient's fears and anxieties.	It is important to gain the patient's trust and demonstrate that you are listening to them.	Offer some reassurance—for example, express sympathy about the death of their uncle but say that although one of the reasons for doing the test is to look for a cancer, other causes are more likely.

✗ Common errors in this station

Common error	Reason	Remedy
Not recognising that the patient is worried about cancer.	Failure to elicit ideas, concerns or expectations.	Avoid falsely reassuring them that cancer is not a possibility. Make sure that an appropriate balance is given as to the likely outcomes.
Using technical jargon.	When learning new medical terms, it can be easier to use these rather than 'translate' them back.	Use simple terms—e.g., 'camera test' rather than 'OGD' or 'inflammation of the stomach' rather than 'gastritis'.

5

STATION VARIATIONS

○ Basic

A basic station may just have you explaining a procedure to a patient rather than gaining informed consent.

○ Intermediate

Other intermediate stations could include taking consent for other common procedures so you should know about the technical aspects of these, including colonoscopy and lumbar puncture.

○ Advanced

An advanced station might be where the patient says that they do not want to have the procedure done. This would involve exploring reasons for not wanting the OGD, explaining potential consequences (responding calmly and appropriately even when the patient appears to be acting unreasonably) and offering them a follow-up appointment if they change their mind.

Further Reading

British Society of Gastroenterology, 'Guidelines for the Management of Iron Deficiency Anaemia'. Available from http://www.bsg.org.uk/clinical-guidelines/small-bowel-nutrition/guidelines-for-the-management-of-iron-deficiency-anaemia.html.

General Medical Council, 'Consent Guidance: Patients and Doctors Making Decisions Together'. Available from http://www.gmc-uk.org/guidance/ethical_guidance/consent_guidance_index.asp.

Macleod's Clinical Diagnosis, 'Gastrointestinal Haemorrhage', p. 148.

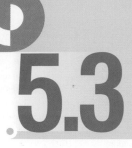

Driving and epilepsy

.5.3

CANDIDATE INFORMATION

Background: You are a junior doctor in a general medicine clinic. Darren Hill (34 years old) has a routine follow-up after being admitted 4 weeks ago with a collapse and the presumed diagnosis was a seizure. He was given advice not to drive on discharge. He has had an outpatient CT head and EEG, both of which were unremarkable.

Task: Discuss the patient's history, explain the results of the investigations and discuss driving advice.

APPROACH TO THE STATION

This station and variations are encountered frequently both in OSCEs and in clinical practice. In order to do well you need to be familiar with guidance from the GMC on your duties as a doctor, and on guidance regarding confidentiality (see Further Reading).

It is important to remember that this station needs to be conducted as a follow-up clinic appointment, and you should not dive straight in to the driving regulations. You need to hear the available history for yourself, and explain the test results. This station tests communication skills and a big part is to review the history and explain the uncertainty regarding the diagnosis.

PATIENT INFORMATION

Name: Darren Hill   **Age:** 34 years   **Sex:** Male

Occupation: Car salesman

Opening statement: You complain about the difficulty finding a parking space to the doctor. You had a collapse 4 weeks ago following several late nights and higher than usual alcohol intake. You cannot remember any details and it was not witnessed but you had wet yourself. You were very sleepy afterwards. Your girlfriend found you and called an ambulance. You have driven to the hospital today as you have had some follow-up tests (a brain scan and a brain-wave recording) and the people who did them said they looked OK, but that they would send the full reports. You think that is why you are here today. You recall that the doctors in hospital told you that they thought you'd had a fit and couldn't drive but assumed that was just until the tests were done.

If asked:

Further information: You normally drink moderate amounts of alcohol (about 10 pints a week), but had had a lot more in the days leading up to the collapse as you were away with friends. You had also had very little sleep for a few nights. The doctors in hospital said that they thought this is what might have triggered the fit so you have decided that as long as you avoid these situations you will be fine and can drive.

Concerns: Driving a nice-looking car is very important to your job. You did not tell your workmates that you could not drive following your hospital admission and instead said the car was being repaired. It would be embarrassing and frustrating not being able to drive in your line of work. Additionally, you are divorced and your 4-year-old son lives with your ex-wife almost an hour's drive away. Being unable to drive would make it much more difficult to see your son as you have him every other weekend and usually drop him at school on Monday morning. You are also worried that you might have epilepsy as the collapse that you had was quite frightening, and you do not want to have to take medication or be unable to drive in the long term.

5

CLINICAL KNOWLEDGE AND EXPERTISE

The history is highly suggestive of a generalised seizure. Alcohol and sleep deprivation are common triggers, but their avoidance does not mean no further fits will occur. It is always difficult to express diagnostic uncertainty, but you must not give false reassurance about the future likelihood of further seizures. In view of this, the licensing authority for England and Wales (DVLA) advise that any patient presenting with a probable isolated seizure should inform the DVLA and cannot drive for 6 months (usually 12 months seizure free where more than one seizure), provided that the consultant thinks it is unlikely the patient will have another seizure and the DVLA is satisfied that the patient is unlikely to be dangerous as a driver. Where there is uncertainty about the diagnosis, anti-convulsants would not normally be considered following a first seizure if the investigations were negative. All patients with possible epilepsy should have an assessment by a neurologist. You should discuss this with the patient.

Dealing with potential breaches of confidentiality

There are several circumstances as a doctor where you may have to breach doctor-patient confidentiality, such as in cases of communicable diseases, road traffic accidents or criminal acts. Below are some tips for this complex ethical situation:
- Ensure you are clear about the legal position – do you definitely need to disclose?
- Explain to the patient the reasons why they need to disclose information to the relevant authority or person.
- Remain polite and tactful; the primary goal is to get the patient to disclose.
- If the conversation is not going well, suggest a further appointment and offer the option to speak to a senior or help find a second opinion.
- It is good practice to discuss complex ethical cases with senior colleagues and with your medical defence organisation.
- Make clear, legible and contemporaneous medical notes.

5

- If you do decide that you need to breach confidentiality, inform the patient (and record this), disclose the minimum amount of information necessary and ensure you are speaking to an appropriate person.
- Write to the patient to tell them what information you have disclosed to a third party.

 WARNING

- Remember that there are also driving restrictions following stroke, myocardial infarction, percutaneous coronary intervention and many neurological conditions. If you're unsure about the advice, check the relevant licensing authority's website for more information.
- Anyone under investigation for potential epilepsy should be advised not to go swimming alone and to take showers rather than baths.

✓ How to excel in this station

Action	Reason	How
Communicate uncertainty.	Part of the task is to conduct a follow-up clinic appointment and explain the difficulty in excluding a diagnosis of epilepsy.	Use communication skills in history-taking, listening and summarising to recap the events preceding admission. Explain the residual diagnostic uncertainty.
Empathise.	Being unable to drive for a year would inconvenience many people, and having the additional worry about a major diagnosis is very stressful.	Approach the discussion in a non-confrontational manner. Try to get the patient to imagine the situation from the point of view of the general public. Highlight the risks to both himself and others if he was to continue to drive.
Understand what to do next.	You must demonstrate that you know the protocol to follow regarding a potential breach of confidentiality.	If the patient is very reluctant to accept the driving advice, it is good practice to suggest that he could speak to one of your seniors or seek a second opinion. Explain about the need for a specialist neurological review.

✗ Common errors in this station

Common error	Remedy	Reason
Not establishing a rapport.	This station will be made significantly easier if you can gain the patient's confidence and get him to disclose.	If you do not manage to keep the situation calm, then the patient may become increasingly hostile and you may lose control and not really know what the patient plans to do.
Not making the final position clear.	Be tactful and empathetic but ensure that you make your duty as a doctor clear—that you must inform the DVLA if he refuses to.	It is always best in situations of potential breach of confidentiality to persuade the patient to disclose the information to the other party themselves.

STATION VARIATIONS

O Basic

This station could be made less difficult with the patient having definite epilepsy (ongoing seizures) and readily accepting the advice.

O Advanced

The scenario could comprise a more hostile patient who continues to drive despite repeated advice not to, and who absolutely refuses to contact the licensing authorities.

Further Reading

General Medical Council, 2009. Confidentiality. GMC, London.

General Medical Council, 2009. Supplemental guidance—confidentiality: reporting concerns about patients to the DVLA or DVA. GMC, London.

Check the website of your relevant driving licensing authority to find out more information about driving restrictions following seizures and other diagnoses or treatment.

5

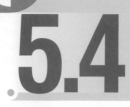

Explaining a new diagnosis of type 2 diabetes

5.4

CANDIDATE INFORMATION

Background: You are a junior doctor in general practice. Brian Williamson (58 years old) was found on annual blood-testing for hypertension to have a raised fasting glucose of 6.8 mmol/l, and subsequently 6.6 mmol/l. You arranged for him to have a Hba1c, which has confirmed the diagnosis of type 2 diabetes.

Task: Please explain the diagnosis of diabetes to Mr Williamson.

APPROACH TO THE STATION

Although designed primarily to test communication, you must have a good knowledge of diabetes and its management in order to be able to answer questions during the discussion and provide appropriate advice and support. Patients often have some degree of understanding of diabetes, especially when there is a strong family history. Therefore, it is important to establish their comprehension, as well as elicit any fixed beliefs about the condition, at the beginning in order to tailor any explanation accordingly.

There is often a fear or, at times, a sense of fatalism amongst patients diagnosed with a chronic disease that disability and premature death are unavoidable. In turn this affects motivation to engage with treatment and lifestyle modification. In the case of type 2 diabetes, which is closely linked with obesity, lifestyle changes can make a significant impact on both blood sugar and blood pressure control and alter the need to commence medication. Given this, it is important that discussion from the start should focus on health promotion and education and encourage the patient to take responsibility for management of their condition.

You should not overload the patient with information around diabetes all at once and time should be allowed for the patient to ask questions and digest explanations. Checking understanding and providing the patient with written information and an opportunity for a later discussion can give the patient time to consider the information and raise any additional concerns.

PATIENT INFORMATION

Name: Brian Williamson   **Age:** 58 years   **Sex:** Male

Occupation: HGV driver

Opening statement: You were quite shocked to find out that you are diabetic as you do not feel unwell. No one in your family has diabetes, so you don't understand why you have it and you're not sure what it will all mean, especially as you spend a lot of time away from home with work.

Other symptoms (if asked): No polydipsia or polyuria. You've gradually gained weight over the past 5 years and you know that you are significantly overweight (102 kg). You have an erratic diet because of your job and tend to grab snacks and eat pre-prepared foods when you can.

Past medical history: Hypertension for 10 years. High cholesterol (not on treatment).

Drugs history: Ramipril 2.5 mg od, Amlodipine 5 mg. No allergies.

Social history: You live with your wife and two teenage children. You smoke five cigarettes per day and drink 25 units of beer per week.

Family history: Your father had a heart attack aged 67. There is no family history of diabetes.

If asked:

Ideas: You have heard that you can get diabetes from eating too much sugar and you wonder if adding sugar to your tea has caused the condition.

5

Concerns: You are worried about the effect that having diabetes will have on your life and especially on your job as an HGV driver as you know someone who lost their licence after being diagnosed with diabetes.

Expectations: You hope that you won't be expected to take more tablets as you don't like taking tablets and you already have to take some for your high blood pressure.

CLINICAL KNOWLEDGE AND EXPERTISE

Diabetes is an escalating problem due to increasing obesity and can lead to macro- and microvascular complications affecting the heart, eyes, kidneys, feet, nerves and blood vessels, which highlights the need for close monitoring and strict glycaemic control. Type 2 diabetes differs from type 1 in that insulin resistance rather than deficiency predominates in the early stages and management is focused on reducing insulin resistance through weight loss, dietary modification and medications. New patients with diabetes should be encouraged to see a dietician and the emphasis of any medical input should be on education and promoting self-management. Hypertension and hypercholesterolaemia greatly increase the risk of complications of diabetes and management of these factors is just as important as achieving good glycaemic control, especially where there is already evidence of complications (Table 5.4.1).

Management of type 2 diabetes within general practice is focused on regular screening and early identification of individuals who are at risk of complications from diabetes. A holistic approach is required given the wide-ranging complications that can occur.

The majority of patients diagnosed with type 2 diabetes on routine screening do not require immediate intervention with treatment and patients should try modification of diet and lifestyle first and increase physical activity, although it may be necessary to start a statin (cholesterol-lowering medication) or anti-hypertensive if at high risk of cardiovascular complications.

5

Table 5.4.1 Complications of diabetes and their screening and management	
Complications of diabetes	**Screening/management options**
Cardiovascular disease/stroke	Encourage smoking cessation, treat hypercholesterolaemia, educate on lifestyle modification, dietary advice and physical activity. Strict blood pressure and glycaemic control is needed.
Nephropathy	Check urinary albumin:creatinine ratio. Strict blood pressure and glycaemic control is needed and consider ACE inhibitor.
Neuropathy	Set up annual foot screening to check sensation and circulation, podiatry input if patient is deemed to be at 'high risk'. Strict blood pressure and glycaemic control is needed.
Retinopathy	Organise annual retinopathy screening by accredited optician. Strict blood pressure and glycaemic control is needed.
Depression	Organise annual screening to include 2 depression screening questions: • During the past month, have you often been bothered by feeling down, depressed or hopeless? • During the past month, have you often been bothered by little interest or pleasure in doing things? Consider intervention if patient answers 'yes' to both.

Dietary and physical activity advice in diabetes

- Diet should include high-fibre, low-glycaemic-index sources of carbohydrate, e.g., wholemeal bread, porridge oats.
- Encourage low-fat dairy products and oily fish.
- Limit foods containing saturated fats and trans fatty acids.
- Discourage use of foods marketed specifically for people with diabetes.
- NICE recommend taking two and a half hours each week of moderate intensity physical activity, e.g., brisk walking or cycling on flat terrain, or one hour and 15 minutes of high intensity exercise, e.g., jogging or playing football.
- If overweight, gradually lose 5–10% of body weight/year, aiming towards a BMI (Body Mass Index) within the healthy range (18.5–24.5).

 WARNING

- Don't forget to include discussion around general health promotion and lifestyle modification rather than just focusing on diabetes; it is an equally important part of the management plan.
- Patients often have secondary complications of diabetes at the time of diagnosis, e.g., peripheral neuropathy, so don't forget to check for symptoms of these within the history.

How to excel in this station		
Action	**Reason**	**How**
Demonstrate knowledge.	Show a good understanding of type 2 diabetes and its possible complications, and initial management following diagnosis.	Provide the patient with 'bite-sized' chunks of information and summarise when appropriate, allowing the patient time to digest the information given and the opportunity to ask questions.

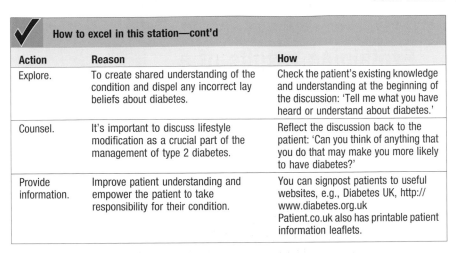

How to excel in this station—cont'd		
Action	**Reason**	**How**
Explore.	To create shared understanding of the condition and dispel any incorrect lay beliefs about diabetes.	Check the patient's existing knowledge and understanding at the beginning of the discussion: 'Tell me what you have heard or understand about diabetes.'
Counsel.	It's important to discuss lifestyle modification as a crucial part of the management of type 2 diabetes.	Reflect the discussion back to the patient: 'Can you think of anything that you do that may make you more likely to have diabetes?'
Provide information.	Improve patient understanding and empower the patient to take responsibility for their condition.	You can signpost patients to useful websites, e.g., Diabetes UK, http://www.diabetes.org.uk Patient.co.uk also has printable patient information leaflets.

5

Common errors in this station		
Common error	**Remedy**	**Reason**
Overloading patient with information.	Check understanding regularly and provide patient information leaflets to take away.	Attempting to show the examiner everything you know about diabetes may end up making the patient feel confused and overwhelmed.
Overuse of medical jargon.	Use lay terms throughout explanation and ask patient to relay information back to you to confirm he/she has understood.	It can be easy to fall into using medical terminology when explaining factual information. *Bad candidate*: 'We check you for a raised albumin:creatinine ratio, which can indicate nephropathy.' *Good candidate*: 'We check to see if your kidneys are leaking protein, which is a sign they are not working properly.'

STATION VARIATIONS

Basic

The case could be made more straightforward by simplifying the patient's past medical history so that they have no other comorbidities to discuss within the time.

Advanced

This case could be made more challenging by having the patient refuse to acknowledge the need for any lifestyle changes or the need for any new medication.

Further Reading

NICE clinical guideline CG66: type 2 diabetes; the management of type 2 diabetes, May 2008.
NICE quality standard 6: diabetes in adults, March 2011.

Explaining results of a cervical smear test

5.5

CANDIDATE INFORMATION

Background: You are a doctor in general practice. Mrs Gillian Brown (35 years) has attended after receiving notification that the results of her recent cervical smear test are abnormal and that she has been referred to the colposcopy clinic.

Cervical smear result: Mild dyskaryosis present. Human papilloma virus POSITIVE—Direct referral to colposcopy.

Task: Please explain to Mrs Brown the significance of her cervical smear result and discuss the process of colposcopy and the reasons behind the referral.

APPROACH TO THE STATION

This station reflects a common consultation within general practice and demonstrates the importance of good communication skills and background knowledge when counselling a patient. Although it is primarily examining communication, in order to do well you need to have an understanding of the classification of cervical smear results and the significance of different grades of cervical changes in relation to the risk of cancer.

Mrs Brown has a mildly abnormal cervical smear and has been referred because of the presence of the higher risk human papilloma virus (HPV) on testing. The likelihood is that this abnormal result will return to normal in future without needing any further treatment. Any abnormal result can understandably cause anxiety and an effective consultation should recognise this anxiety whilst avoiding false reassurance. The station requires you to offer a basic explanation of the smear result, without using overcomplicated medical jargon, and discuss colposcopy.

PATIENT INFORMATION

Name: Mrs Gillian Brown **Age:** 35 years **Sex:** Female

Occupation: Secretary

Opening statement: You had your smear test with the practice nurse 3 weeks ago. You have received your result through the post and were shocked to find that it was abnormal and that you need further investigation. Your smears have always been normal in the past, and you have always kept them up to date.

Other symptoms (if asked): No intermenstrual or post-coital bleeding.

Past medical history: You are normally well with no previous significant medical history. You have had two normal vaginal deliveries three and five years ago. You use condoms for contraception currently.

Drugs history: No regular medication or allergies.

Social history: You work as a secretary in an accounting firm. You live with your husband and two children. You are a non-smoker and drink socially only.

Family history: Nil significant.

If asked:

Ideas: You have recently seen that a celebrity on the television was diagnosed with cervical cancer and you are worried that this result could indicate a serious condition.

Concerns: You are worried about the possibility of cervical cancer and whether you may need treatment and what this could mean for your ability to have further children in future.

Expectations: You hope that the doctor will recognise your concerns and explain to you what your result means and what happens next at your clinic appointment.

5

CLINICAL KNOWLEDGE AND EXPERTISE

Before attempting to discuss any results, you need to establish the patient's prior knowledge, so that any explanation can be tailored to their level of understanding. For example, the explanation that you would give to a health professional would be very different from one to a patient with no medical knowledge, and failing to adapt explanation could lead to lack of comprehension or oversimplification that may be regarded as patronising.

You need to avoid relying upon medical terminology when explaining abnormal test results. A useful way to improve understanding is to use visual aids and there are a variety of online leaflets and resources that can be offered for the patient to take away.

The appearance of a cervical smear is described in terms of any abnormal (dyskaryotic) cells (Table 5.5.1). The histological diagnosis made at colposcopy after biopsy

Table 5.5.1 The classification of cervical smear results, dyskaryosis and CIN (cervical intraepithelial neoplasia)	
Normal smear result	No abnormal cells
Borderline smear result	Mild abnormality only (15–20% chance of needing further treatment), only significant if HPV positive.
Mild dyskaryosis	Mild abnormality, correlates with CIN 1. One-third thickness of the surface layer of the cervix is affected (15–20% chance of needing further treatment). Only significant if HPV positive.
Moderate dyskaryosis	Moderate abnormality, correlates with CIN 2. Two-thirds thickness of the surface layer affected.
Severe dyskaryosis	Severe abnormality, correlates with CIN 3. Full thickness of the surface layer affected—carcinoma-in-situ.

5

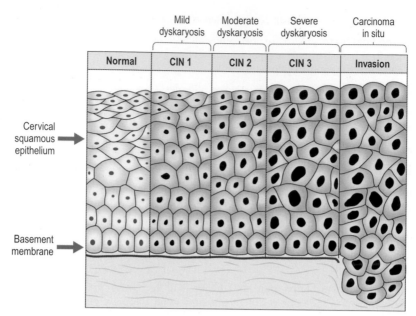

Fig. 5.5.1 Classification of cervical dysplasia

Table 5.5.2 The impact of testing for HPV in mildly dyskaryotic and borderline cervical smears	
Borderline smear result: HPV negative	Return to normal 3- or 5-yearly screening
Borderline smear result: HPV positive	Referral to colposcopy
Mild dyskaryosis: HPV negative	Return to normal 3- or 5-yearly screening
Mild dyskaryosis: HPV positive	Referral to colposcopy

classifies cervical changes into grades of intraepithelial neoplasia (CIN 1–3), depending upon the depth of abnormal cells (see Fig. 5.5.1). The addition of screening for 'higher risk' types of HPV (16 and 18) in mild or borderline cervical changes has altered the management of patients with mildly abnormal smear tests (see Table 5.5.2) and can lead to further anxiety. It is worth reassuring the patient that the majority of women are infected with HPV at some point (and may be asymptomatic for years) but that most viruses disappear without treatment and even 'high-risk' types rarely cause cervical cancer.

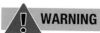 **WARNING**

- Acknowledge the patient's anxiety around the result and allow them time within the consultation to discuss their concerns rather than leading straight into the explanation around management.
- Avoid false reassurance when counselling around the referral as, although the changes are mild, she may still go on to require treatment at colposcopy.

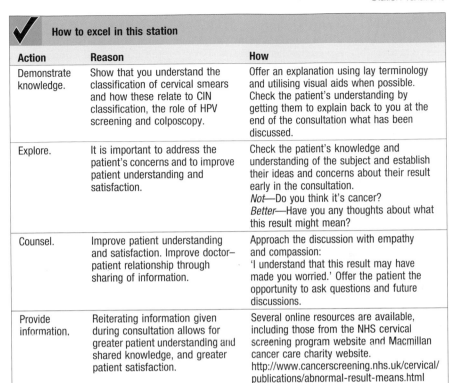

✓ How to excel in this station		
Action	**Reason**	**How**
Demonstrate knowledge.	Show that you understand the classification of cervical smears and how these relate to CIN classification, the role of HPV screening and colposcopy.	Offer an explanation using lay terminology and utilising visual aids when possible. Check the patient's understanding by getting them to explain back to you at the end of the consultation what has been discussed.
Explore.	It is important to address the patient's concerns and to improve patient understanding and satisfaction.	Check the patient's knowledge and understanding of the subject and establish their ideas and concerns about their result early in the consultation. *Not*—Do you think it's cancer? *Better*—Have you any thoughts about what this result might mean?
Counsel.	Improve patient understanding and satisfaction. Improve doctor–patient relationship through sharing of information.	Approach the discussion with empathy and compassion: 'I understand that this result may have made you worried.' Offer the patient the opportunity to ask questions and future discussions.
Provide information.	Reiterating information given during consultation allows for greater patient understanding and shared knowledge, and greater patient satisfaction.	Several online resources are available, including those from the NHS cervical screening program website and Macmillan cancer care charity website. http://www.cancerscreening.nhs.uk/cervical/publications/abnormal-result-means.html http://www.macmillan.org.uk/Cancerinformation/Testsscreening/Cervicalscreening/Abnormaltestresults.aspx

5

✗ Common errors in this station		
Common error	**Remedy**	**Reason**
Overuse of medical jargon.	Keep explanations simple and check understanding throughout.	Best candidates will use lay terms whenever possible. They will pause appropriately and allow time for the patient to digest information and ask questions, checking 'Does that make sense?'
Failure to acknowledge patient concerns.	Allow the patient the opportunity early in the consultation to express ideas and concerns.	Sometimes the rush to begin explanations can lead to patient's views being ignored and patients may be embarrassed or worried about admitting concerns

STATION VARIATIONS

⬤ Basic

You could change the patient's smear result to moderate dyskaryosis to minimise discussion around HPV testing and its significance for mild or borderline abnormal smear tests.

5

○ Advanced

You could add in further concerns from the patient about how she acquired HPV and whether this represents her husband being unfaithful in the context of it being a sexually transmitted infection. You could also discuss the implications that colposcopy may impact on the patient's ability to have more children, if this was a concern.

Further Reading

http://www.cancerscreening.nhs.uk/cervical/about-cervical-screening.html.

Jordan, J., et al., 2008. European guidelines for quality assurance in cervical cancer screening: recommendations for clinical management of abnormal cervical cytology, part 1. Cytopathology 19, 342–354.

Kelly, R.S., et al., 2011. HPV testing as a triage for borderline or mild dyskaryosis on cervical cytology: results from the sentinel sites study. Br. J. Canc. 105, 983–988. http://www.bjcancer.com, Published online 6 Sept 2011.

Kurtz, S.M., 2002. Doctor–patient communication: principles and practices. Can. J. Neurol. Sci. 29 (Suppl. 2), S23–S29.

Kurtz, S., Silverman, J., Benson, J., Draper, J., 2003. Marrying content and process in clinical method teaching: enhancing the Calgary–Cambridge guides. Acad. Med. 78 (8).

Discussing non-accidental injury (NAI) with a parent

5.6

CANDIDATE INFORMATION

Background: Jake Downes (2 years) has been referred by social services for a child protection medical examination after his nursery noticed a number of new bruises.

Task: You are the Paediatric trainee on-call and need to explain to Jake's mum (Wendy Downes) about the examination, why it needs to take place and gain consent. A consent form will be provided for you to complete with her. You do not need to progress on to the history or examination.

APPROACH TO THE STATION

Discussing potential non-accidental injury (NAI) with parents or carers can be stressful. However, by being open and honest and remembering a few tips, it can be made more bearable for both you and the family. In this case, a young boy has attended nursery where a number of bruises are noticed. This presentation is very common. Often, following a thorough examination, the bruises may be found to be consistent with a history of accidental injury. Unfortunately, NAI is much more common than most people realise and, in these cases, further action is taken by social services and possibly the police. Rarely, bruises may be due to a medical cause such as a clotting abnormality or idiopathic thrombocytopenia (ITP), and because of this, investigations, including a full blood count and coagulation studies, are often requested following a medical examination.

Child protection medical examinations (also called 'section 47 medicals' in the UK—1989 Children Act) can be requested by social services whenever a child is suspected to be suffering, or likely to suffer, significant harm. This may be due to physical injury, neglect or emotional abuse or a disclosure of abuse. Sexual abuse examinations are dealt with differently, and often referred to a regional centre for examination and interview. The purpose of a child protection medical is to elicit a history from the parents and child (if appropriate due to age and capacity), complete a thorough examination and determine whether further action needs to be taken to safeguard the child.

Most hospitals provide a specific proforma to record the details of the history and examination (look at one of these during your Paediatric attachment). It often consists of a consent form, demographics of the patient and family, sections for the history from social services, parents and the child and then a full medical history including past medical history, birth history, development and behavioural concerns, a record of all first degree family members and documentation of social circumstances and

5

concerns. Many of the questions can seem very personal; for example, it is necessary to ask about drug and alcohol abuse in the parents, domestic violence and mental health issues. A good approach is to show them the documentation before you begin and explain that you are completing a standard form, and have to ask all these questions, even if they seem irrelevant or intrusive.

PARENT INFORMATION

Name: Wendy Downes   **Age:** 24 years   **Sex:** Female

Opening statement: You have been visited by social services this morning and asked to attend A&E with Jake for a medical examination. You are initially very upset but will respond if things are explained appropriately to you, and will agree to the examination.

The candidate should not attempt to take any history from you until you have consented. If they do so — refuse politely and say you first want to know what this is about.

CLINICAL KNOWLEDGE AND EXPERTISE

Approach to discussing NAI
setting
- Choose a private and quiet area where you cannot be overheard.
- Explain you'll need a chaperone present for the history and examination.
- Minimise interruptions (get someone to cover your bleep).
- Be confident and clear about what information you need to give the patient and the next steps. Phone a senior doctor to ask advice prior to the conversation if necessary.

Initiating the session
- Introduce yourself and explain that you have been asked by social services to perform an examination, which involves taking a detailed history and thoroughly examining the child.

Giving information
- Explain this examination has been requested as there are some concerns that the child may have suffered harm and that you have to document clearly what has happened (the history) and the physical findings.
- Explain that following the history and examination, further investigations may be required (e.g., blood tests, a skeletal survey or CT head scan).
- You need to emphasise that the complete report will be shared with other agencies involved in safeguarding, most notably social services and the police, but also the GP, health visitor, etc.

Signing the consent form
- The consent form will state that the reason for, and nature of, the medical examination, as well as the need for information sharing, has been explained to the parent. It must be signed by you and the parent after you've fully informed them (Fig. 5.6.1).

CONSENT FORM

All children suffer injuries on occasions. These may occur in a variety of ways. Accidents are far more common but occasionally we may have to consider the possibility that an injury may have occurred in a non-accidental manner or that a child may have been subjected to some form of abuse.

CHILD'S NAME _____

DATE OF BIRTH _____

I have had the reason for a medical examination, further investigation and photographs explained to me by _____.

I understand that it may be necessary for information to be shared with the General Practioner, Social Services, and other agencies.

Signature of Parent/Carer/Social Worker
with parental responsibility _____

Signature of examining Doctor _____

Date _____

Figure 5.6.1 Example consent form

5

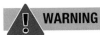 **WARNING**

- Remember that your safety is paramount. Try to always have another medical professional (nurse, junior doctor or health care assistant) in the room with you in case the situation becomes volatile or violent, and as a chaperone for your examination. Doctors have been accused of causing the marks they are being asked to examine, so it is important to have somebody else witnessing your examination and you should document their full name and job title in your report.

	How to excel in this station	
Action	**Reason**	**How**
Be honest.	Parents respond much better to honesty and problems often escalate if they feel they are being lied to.	Explain that you are performing the examination as there is a suspicion that the child may have suffered harm. However, explain that you will remain non-judgemental and are purely trying to document the facts. Explain that these examinations are performed nationwide in an effort to safeguard children and the examination has been requested as part of national guidance.
Be firm.	The examination is not really optional and although it is best to try to engage parents positively, do not allow yourself to be manipulated.	Although we get parents to sign a consent form, if they refuse the child will be admitted to a place of safety and a court order can be granted to perform the examination. If the parent leaves the hospital with the child, you cannot forcibly restrain them. However, the police should be called immediately as they can initiate a Police Protection Order (PPO) to admit the child to hospital (not requiring parental consent). If a parent is threatening to leave, try to persuade them to stay.

(*Continued*)

5

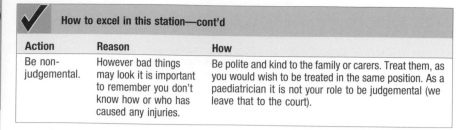

How to excel in this station—cont'd

Action	Reason	How
Be non-judgemental.	However bad things may look it is important to remember you don't know how or who has caused any injuries.	Be polite and kind to the family or carers. Treat them, as you would wish to be treated in the same position. As a paediatrician it is not your role to be judgemental (we leave that to the court).

Common errors in this station

Common error	Remedy	Reason
Focusing on a medical cause.	Explain that investigations may be necessary to exclude a rare medical reason for the bruising/fracture (as appropriate).	Do not focus on a medical cause or use it as a get-out clause to lessen the blow of performing the medical examination. Most cases turn out to be either a true accident or NAI, but are rarely due to clotting problems, etc.
Promising confidentiality.	Explain clearly that information from the report will be shared with relevant parties as part of the safeguarding process.	It is important to highlight that the report will be shared with the multiple agencies as appropriate to the case. You should emphasise that it will be only be seen by relevant parties.

STATION VARIATIONS

○ Advanced

Further communication challenges... The angry parent, the upset parent, etc.

This station could easily involve a 'challenging parent'. The simulated parent could either be very upset and difficult to deal with or angry and unreasonable. In these circumstances, stick to your central message that the examination is part of routine safeguarding measures due to various concerns. Whilst you appreciate they are upset/angry, the examination does need to be performed. Remember the points above as to where you stand if the parent leaves with the child or will not give consent. However, these discussions usually proceed more favourably if you can de-escalate and calm the situation down. Try to avoid using the threat of police and court orders as it does not tend to make parents calmer.

Further Reading

HM Government, 2013. Working Together to Safeguard Children. Available online at, http://www.workingtogetheronline.co.uk/documents/Working%20Together FINAL.pdf.

The whole document, though lengthy, is worth a look for an overview of all aspects of safeguarding policy.

Assessing a patient's capacity

5.7

CANDIDATE INFORMATION

Background: You are a junior doctor on the medical unit. Mr Thomas Anderson (78 years old) has come in with melaena. He has a past medical history of Alzheimer's disease, angina and chronic kidney disease. The consultant has noted that Mr Anderson has a significant anaemia and has requested a gastroscopy. You have been asked to discuss the procedure with Mr Anderson and gain informed consent. Mr Anderson's daughter has told the nursing staff that he is no more confused than normal, but is concerned he will not be able to understand the gastroscopy procedure.

Task: Please discuss the procedure with Mr Anderson and assess if he has the capacity to consent. After 10 minutes (with a 1 minute warning), the examiner will discuss your assessment and ask you questions.

APPROACH TO THE STATION

This station combines two elements. Firstly, you need to have the knowledge about how to consent someone for a gastroscopy—this is covered in station 5.2. You then need to be able to assess Mr Anderson's capacity to make a decision about the investigation. The assessment of mental capacity in the United Kingdom has been defined in a recent law and this is explained in more detail below. The principles of assessing an individual's ability to make decisions are applicable in all healthcare settings, but the legal framework may differ and you should be aware of local laws.

PATIENT INFORMATION

Name: Thomas Anderson   **Age:** 78 years   **Sex:** Male

Occupation: Retired shoemaker

Presenting symptoms: You have dementia. Your memory is poor as is your ability to retain and weigh up complex decisions. You have been admitted with black stools but cannot recall this. You know that you are in hospital but cannot understand why you are here. If asked, you will recall your date of birth but not your age.

The doctor should discuss your black stools and explain that you need to have a camera test ('gastroscopy') to look for the cause of bleeding. The doctor should explain what this involves. If they ask you whether you agree to have the

(Continued)

5

test done you should say yes. The doctor should then attempt to ensure that you understand the test and the potential implications. You *will not* be able to repeat what the doctor said, explain what the test involves or talk about potential complications. If they ask you to sign the form, then you should ask them what you are signing for.

For the examiner:

You should ask the following questions of the candidate:
1. Do you feel Mr Anderson has the mental capacity to consent to this procedure?
2. How did you arrive at this decision?
3. If Mr Anderson is considered to lack capacity, what should be done next?
4. How would you make a decision in someone's best interests?
5. If Mr Anderson required a blood transfusion, would this capacity assessment allow you to give it?

CLINICAL KNOWLEDGE AND EXPERTISE

This section refers to the Mental Capacity Act (2005) in the United Kingdom.

The Mental Capacity Act (2005) provides a legal framework for assessing individuals' abilities to make decisions. This ability to make decisions is what is referred to in the Act as capacity. There are five key principles:
1. Presumption of capacity until proven otherwise.
2. People must be given all practical support to make their decision (e.g. help with communication, vision, hearing).
3. People with capacity have the right to make unwise decisions.
4. Any decision made on behalf of a person lacking capacity must be in their best interests (see below).
5. Anything done on behalf of a person who lacks capacity should be the least restrictive option.

The assessment of capacity is *decision specific* (see Fig. 5.7.1). It means that, just because Mr Anderson may lack the capacity to consent to a gastroscopy, it does not mean that he lacks the capacity to consent to having a blood transfusion (and vice versa). Each decision must be assessed separately. The assessment of capacity is a two-step process:

> **1. Is there is an 'impairment of, or disturbance in, the functioning of the person's mind or brain?'**
>
> *Such as dementia, learning difficulties, mental health problems, delirium, unconsciousness*

> **2. Does the disturbance make the person unable to make a specific decision?**
>
> Are they able to:
> **Understand** the information relevant to the decision.
> **Retain** the information for long enough to make a decision.
> **Weigh** the information up to make the decision.
> **Communicate** that decision.

Figure 5.7.1 Assessing a patient's capacity

In this case you should attempt to take consent for gastroscopy as outlined in Station 5.2: You should determine:

- Does Mr Anderson *understand* what a gastroscopy is, why one is required, and what could happen if he declines to have the procedure?
- Can he *retain* the information long enough to make a decision?
- Can he *weigh up* the proposed benefits against the risks of the procedure?
- Can he *communicate* this decision to you?

The examiner will ask you questions about how you have made your decision and what you should do next. If you feel that Mr Anderson lacks capacity, then you should not complete the consent form. You should indicate that you would speak to your consultant who would have to make a decision in Mr Anderson's best interests about whether to proceed.

In order to make a decision in Mr Anderson's *best interests* the following should be considered:

- Whether he has a legally appointed power of attorney (health);
- His past and present wishes;
- Any beliefs and values that may influence his decision;
- The opinion of his family, friends and carers; and
- Whether he requires an independent mental capacity advocate (if he has no other representatives).

5

 WARNING

- Do not assume just because someone has dementia that they lack capacity for decisions.
- Indicate that you would carefully record your assessment in as much detail as possible.

✔ How to excel in this station

Action	Reason	How
Follow structured approach to assessment.	This shows that you understand the principles of the Mental Capacity Act and how to apply them.	E.g., 'I feel Mr Anderson lacks capacity to make this decision as he is unable to understand why he requires the procedure, is unable to retain the information for long enough to make a decision, and is unable to weigh the information to come to a decision. Consequently, even though he is able to communicate a decision, he does not have capacity.'
Ask for family to be present.	It is important to show that you are giving Mr Anderson as much help as required to help him make a decision.	Say to examiner when questioned that ideally you would like Mr Anderson's family to be present to support him in making his decision.

✘ Common errors in this station

Common error	Reason	Remedy
Forgetting capacity is decision specific.	Capacity may differ depending on the complexity of the decisions required.	Say to examiner that you would need to assess Mr Anderson's capacity to consent to a blood transfusion separately.

STATION VARIATIONS

O Advanced

You could be asked to assess capacity in someone with a temporary lack of capacity (for example, a patient with a delirium). In this case you would follow the procedure above but then state that you may delay the decision until the person regains capacity, if clinically indicated.

Further Reading

UK Department of Justice, Office of the Public Guardian, 'Mental Capacity Act', available online at http://www.justice.gov.uk/protecting-the-vulnerable/mental-capacity-act.

Nicholson, T., et al., 2008. Assessing mental capacity: the mental capacity act. BMJ 336, 322.

Discussing starting an SSRI

.5.8

CANDIDATE INFORMATION

Background: You are a doctor in general practice. Michael Barratt (18 years) is a student and has recently joined the surgery, but has been an infrequent attender at his previous GP. He complains of a 3-month history of feeling low in mood and is keen to discuss starting fluoxetine today.

Task: Take a history from Mr Barratt, then discuss management options with him, with particular focus on the prescribing of an SSRI.

APPROACH TO THE STATION

Consultations focused around mental health are extremely common in general practice, with 1 in 3 consultations having a mental health component, and around 90% of mental health problems are managed within primary care. You need to demonstrate skills in building the doctor–patient relationship, maintaining rapport using verbal and non-verbal communication and negotiating an appropriate management plan, taking into account the patient's perceived need. You must be able to discuss risks, benefits and side effects of SSRIs and have a good understanding of their use in depression.

PATIENT INFORMATION

Name: Mr Michael Barratt **Age:** 18 years **Sex:** Male

Occupation: Undergraduate student in politics

Opening statement: You have been feeling down for the past few months; friends and family have mentioned that you are 'not yourself' and your university marks are beginning to drop, whereas you were previously doing well. Your girlfriend has asked you to come in to talk about 'getting help'.

Other symptoms (if asked): No thoughts of self-harm or suicidal ideation. For a couple of months now you have had interrupted sleep, your appetite has 'gone off' and you think you've lost about half a stone. You are not sure what has precipitated you feeling down; your course is challenging but until recently you were enjoying it and getting good results.

Past medical history: Tonsillectomy aged 12 for recurrent tonsillitis; otherwise, fit and well.

(Continued)

5

Drugs history: No regular medication or allergies.

Social history: You share a house with four students on your course. You are a non-smoker and are a keen rugby player, but have not felt like playing recently and have been dropped from the university team. You drink 12–16 units of beer on an average night out, but haven't been out recently and previously only drank one night per week.

Family history: Your paternal uncle has suffered from depression throughout his life and is currently stable on fluoxetine; he attempted suicide by hanging in his early 30s.

If asked:

Ideas: You wonder if you are suffering from depression like your uncle as your father has mentioned that he started to become unwell around your age.

Concerns: You are worried about the effect that your mood is having on your university marks and your relationship with your girlfriend. You are anxious that if you do not address the problem now it will worsen and you may think about harming yourself like your uncle did.

Expectations: You know that your uncle has been a lot better since he has been on the fluoxetine and you hope that the doctor will prescribe you this today.

CLINICAL KNOWLEDGE AND EXPERTISE

Before considering antidepressants, you should assess the severity of the depression, and therefore the appropriateness of prescribing, as well as undertake a risk assessment of self-harm or suicide, as an increased risk not only affects overall management but the quantity and type of antidepressant. Certain patients have a 'higher risk' of depression and the presence of chronic diseases such as diabetes, a family history of depression, or a history of previous depression, suicide attempts or substance misuse should trigger a comprehensive assessment.

Depression can be classified into mild, moderate and severe, with treatment differing according to severity (Table 5.8.1). Three screening questionnaires are regularly utilised to assist diagnosis in patients presenting with low mood, as well as assess the response to antidepressants once initiated: the Hospital Anxiety and Depression Score (HADS), the Patient Health Questionnaire 9 (PHQ-9; Fig. 5.8.1) and the Beck Depression Inventory II (BDI-II). Each is self-administered by the patient and provides a score, which, if over a given threshold, can indicate the need for antidepressants, although they should only be used alongside a thorough clinical assessment.

Table 5.8.1 The classification of depression and recommended treatment approaches	
Severity of depression as assessed by screening	**Recommended treatment approach**
Mild	Antidepressants are not routinely used for first-line therapy; consider psychological therapies or 'watchful waiting'.
Moderate	Antidepressant OR psychological therapy may be considered (this may be dependent upon local availability and patient preference).
Severe	Consider commencing antidepressant therapy immediately, in combination with psychological therapy. Consider involving secondary care if significant risk associated.

Patient Health Questionnaire (PHQ-9)

Over the last two weeks, how often have you been bothered by any of the following problems?

Little interest or pleasure in doing things?	Not at all ☐ Several days ☐ More than half the days ☐ Nearly every day ☐
Feeling down, depressed, or hopeless?	Not at all ☐ Several days ☐ More than half the days ☐ Nearly every day ☐
Trouble falling or staying asleep, or sleeping too much?	Not at all ☐ Several days ☐ More than half the days ☐ Nearly every day ☐
Feeling tired or having little energy?	Not at all ☐ Several days ☐ More than half the days ☐ Nearly every day ☐
Poor appetite or overeating?	Not at all ☐ Several days ☐ More than half the days ☐ Nearly every day ☐
Feeling bad about yourself - or that you are a failure or have let yourself or your family down?	Not at all ☐ Several days ☐ More than half the days ☐ Nearly every day ☐
Trouble concentrating on things, such as reading the newspaper or watching television?	Not at all ☐ Several days ☐ More than half the days ☐ Nearly every day ☐
Moving or speaking so slowly that other people could have noticed? Or the opposite - being so fidgety or restless that you have been moving around a lot more than usual?	Not at all ☐ Several days ☐ More than half the days ☐ Nearly every day ☐
Thoughts that you would be better off dead, or of hurting yourself in some way?	Not at all ☐ Several days ☐ More than half the days ☐ Nearly every day ☐

Total = ☐ /27 ☐

Depression Severity: 0–4 none, 5–9 mild, 10–14 moderate, 15–19 moderately severe, 20–27 severe.

Figure 5.8.1 Example of PHQ-9 questionnaire

Table 5.8.2 Risk factors for suicide		
Social characteristics	**History**	**Clinical/diagnostic features**
Male gender	Prior suicide attempt(s)	Hopelessness
Young age (<30 years)	Family history of suicide	Psychosis or severe depression
Advanced age	History of substance abuse	Anxiety, agitation, panic attacks
Single or living alone	Recently started on antidepressants	Concurrent physical illness

Although each questionnaire touches on self-harm and suicidal ideation, you must ask additional open and direct questions to assess the patient's risk (Table 5.8.2). A review of their social situation and 'protective factors' which may reduce their suicidal risk, such as a network of family and friends, should be undertaken as this can determine the need and urgency to involve secondary care services.

The choice of antidepressant is dependent on underlying medical conditions, interactions with other medications, suicide risk and previous response to therapy. Due to their relative safety in overdose and fewer side effects, SSRIs are used first line to treat moderate and severe depression or mild depression not responding to conventional treatment.

Points to remember about SSRI prescribing

- It takes 2–4 weeks to see any therapeutic benefit (can be earlier for sleep improvement).
- Common side effects are nausea and gastrointestinal upset when first taking.
- There is a risk of gastrointestinal haemorrhage and hyponatraemia (especially in elderly people).
- Anxiety, agitation and suicidal ideation can worsen the first few weeks of taking (especially in young people).
- Patient can develop withdrawal symptoms if abruptly stopped.
- Antidepressants need to be taken for at least 4 weeks before consideration is given to switching due to lack of efficacy.
- Aim to continue antidepressants for at least 6 months, once effective, before considering gradual withdrawal.

 WARNING

- Never forget to ask about thoughts of self-harm or suicidal ideation in a patient presenting with low mood.
- Check the patient's safety in terms of protective factors against suicide or self-harm; a good support network of family and friends reduces the risk, whereas someone who lives alone and is socially isolated would be of greater concern.

✓	How to excel in this station	
Action	**Reason**	**How**
Demonstrate knowledge.	Show that you are able to diagnose and differentiate between different severities of depression and assess risk of self-harm.	Make use of a depression assessment questionnaire, e.g., PHQ-9, to assist diagnosis and assess severity. Ask direct questions about suicidal ideation:

Action	Reason	How
		'Have you ever thought about hurting or harming yourself?'
Explore.	Discuss the patient's expectations around the use of antidepressants.	Explore their understanding of antidepressants and what they hope will happen when taking them—are they aware that they are not effective straight away? Do they know that they may initially feel worse when taking?
Explain.	Patient-centred shared management plan.	Discuss risks and benefits of SSRIs and allow the opportunity for questions. Explain method of action using layman's terminology: 'Increase the amount of happy hormones in the brain.'
Provide information.	There is better adherence to medication when the patient fully understands possible side effects associated with antidepressants and how long they must take SSRIs in order for benefit to be evident.	Offer information leaflet, e.g. examples available on Patient.co.uk: http://www.patient.co.uk/health/ssriantidepressants Signpost patient to local voluntary counselling organisations or self-referral to university counselling services.

5

✖ Common errors in this station

Common error	Remedy	Reason
Formulaic symptom list.	Use of open questions; allow the patient to 'tell their story'.	Over-reliance on lists of questions and symptoms can lead to a regimented and cold, non-empathetic consultation. Allow time and pauses appropriately and explore patient's, ideas, concerns and expectations.
'The patient is always right'— giving the prescription without question.	Shared negotiation around the use of antidepressants and the risks and benefits of doing so.	Just because the patient has an expectation of antidepressants, it doesn't mean that this is necessarily the only or best option for the patient. *Good candidate*: 'Tell me what you understand about how antidepressants work.' 'Do you know of any problems with antidepressants?'

STATION VARIATIONS

O Basic

You could remove the expectation and prior knowledge of antidepressants from the history so that the explanation is more focused on discussing the available options for the patient and weighing up the risks and benefits of each.

5

O Advanced

You can make the case more advanced by changing the patient's age to 16 to provide a more challenging discussion around the use of SSRIs in children and adolescents, or increase the complexity by adding thoughts of self-harm and suicidal ideation.

Consider how your approach would alter if the patient was expressing active thoughts of suicidal ideation:

- Would you consider involving secondary care or the community mental health 'crisis team'?
- Would you prescribe antidepressants? If so, would it affect the quantity you prescribed?
- What level of follow-up would you arrange for the patient?
- How would you assess their safety in the community?

Further Reading

NICE clinical guideline 90: 'The Treatment and Management of Depression in Adults', available at http://www.nice.org.uk/guidance/CG90.

Clinical Knowledge Summaries with clinical scenarios, http://cks.nice.org.uk/depression.

http://www.bnf.org, chapter on prescribing antidepressants.

Example of PHQ-9 questionnaire is available at http://www.patient.co.uk/doctor/patient-health-questionnaire-phq-9.

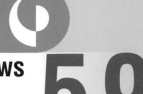

Breaking bad news

5.9

CANDIDATE INFORMATION

Background: You are a junior doctor completing a Medical rotation. Nick Thorpe (21 years) has presented with a few days history of easy bruising and a few weeks of fatigue. His initial blood tests have demonstrated a very high white cell count and the haematologist has phoned you to say that they can see blast cells and the presumptive diagnosis is Acute Lymphoblastic Leukaemia (ALL).

Task: Inform Nick of the results of his blood tests and explain he needs to remain in hospital for further investigation and initiation of treatment once a definitive diagnosis is made.

APPROACH TO THE STATION

Example scenarios of breaking bad news include informing a patient of a new and serious diagnosis, explaining an unpleasant treatment, or explaining to relatives about a death. The ability to break bad news in a sensitive and empathetic manner impacts on how well patients can cope with a new diagnosis and, when discussing death, can help relatives in the grieving process. Patients and relatives will often remember if news has been broken in a rushed or insensitive manner and this can impact upon the doctor–patient relationship, or compliance with treatment. It is important to get the setting right before you begin your conversation and then to follow a logical approach which can be applied to any scenario (e.g., SPIKES model). In this station, do not worry if you do not know much about ALL; the important thing is the way in which you break the news and not to overload the patient with information about chemotherapy regimens or statistics.

Nick Thorpe is a young man who presented with symptoms of easy bruising and generalised fatigue. The history is short and therefore he probably will not be expecting such a serious diagnosis; it is important to try to establish what his worries and concerns are at the outset.

PATIENT INFORMATION

Name: Mr Nick Thorpe   **Age:** 21 years   **Sex:** Male

Opening statement: You have been feeling more tired than usual over the past few weeks and in the past few days have noticed a number of bruises and you are not sure how you have got them. A few people have commented that you look quite pale. You have had some blood tests and are wondering what they show.

(Continued)

5

If asked:

Ideas: You wonder if there is a problem with how your blood is clotting but you haven't really given it much thought.

Concerns: You are concerned that it could be something serious, though you are not sure what. When leukaemia is mentioned, you are worried, as a kid at your school had it and seemed to need treatment for years and was really ill.

Expectations: You want to know what is wrong and are keen to be kept informed on what happens next.

CLINICAL KNOWLEDGE AND EXPERTISE

ALL is characterised by uncontrolled lymphoblast production. It has a peak incidence in children aged 2–5 years, but is seen up until the age of 25 years and there is a smaller peak in the elderly population. Although treatment can be lengthy, invasive and difficult, outcomes are good in young patients and there is a 5-year-survival rate of almost 95%.

ALL presents with symptoms of fatigue, recurrent infection, easy bruising or unexplained bleeding. It may also present with weight loss, fever, swollen lymph nodes and bone pain. The history is often short and symptoms present over a few days to weeks. The presence of a very high or low number of white cells, often with an anaemia and thrombocytopenia is suggestive, and the diagnosis is very likely if blast cells are seen on a blood film. However, a bone marrow biopsy is required for a definitive diagnosis. Chemotherapy is the mainstay of treatment for ALL and may last 2 years or more. Side effects include hair loss, fatigue, vomiting, and weight and appetite changes, depending on the exact regimen of drugs used.

The SPIKES model is set out below.

Setting
- A private and quiet room is most appropriate.
- Establish whether the patient would like a partner or family member present for discussions.
- Minimise interruptions (get someone to cover your bleep).
- Read up on the patient's admission so you can relate the news to their experience: 'Nick, I know you've come in with easy bruising...'.
- Be confident and clear about what information you need to give the patient and the next steps from here; phone a senior doctor to ask advice prior to the conversation if necessary.

Perception
- Introduce yourself and summarise the situation so far.
- Check the patient's ideas and concerns, and their expectations of this discussion.
- Find out what the patient has already been told or knows.

Invitation
- Try to obtain an invitation from the patient regarding the news. Patients may volunteer this by asking for their results or information themselves; however, if they don't, ask them directly, for example 'Is it ok if I talk to you about your results now?'

Knowledge and information
- Give a 'warning shot'; for example 'I'm afraid it is more serious than we had hoped...' or 'I'm afraid it isn't good news'.
- Give basic information in short sections.

- Check the patient's understanding as you proceed and be prepared to repeat important points.
- Be honest and direct and avoid euphemisms and long-winded descriptions.
- Try not to give too much information or overwhelm the patient.
- Avoid medical terms and jargon.

Emotions and empathy

- Try to recognise the patient's emotions (tearfulness, silence, shock, disbelief, anger or sadness).
- Acknowledge these emotions by naming them: 'I can see that you are sad/angry etc.', and tell them that you understand why they have that emotion, for example 'and that is natural given the news' or 'I know this isn't the news you were hoping for'.
- Act empathetically; for example, use active listening techniques, offer a tissue, make eye contact or move closer if appropriate.
- If the patient does not clearly express their emotions, you may need to explore further before making an empathic response, for example 'What is it that frightens you?' or 'You said you were worried about the future. In what way does it worry you?'

Strategy and summary

5

- Identify a plan for what will happen next and a time frame. If appropriate, discuss the future prognosis.
- Highlight support services and written information.
- If the patient or relatives are going home, ensure follow-up is given. In cases of death, this can include offering a debrief session with the consultant and team, and an appointment with the hospital bereavement service to collect the death certificate, etc.
- Offer to speak to relatives.
- Summarise the discussion and check the patient's understanding and any final questions.

! WARNING

- Be prepared that patients and their relatives may respond to bad news in a variety of ways. They may be upset or emotional, appear numb and shocked, or be angry and distressed. Occasionally parents or relatives can become confrontational when given bad news, so bear in mind your safety.
- It is good practice to have a nurse present during the conversation who can remain with the patient/family after you have left, for ongoing support. They also act as added support for you during the conversation.

 How to excel in this station

Action	Reason	How
Structured approach.	This will keep your discussion on track and prevent you from forgetting important points, such as giving a warning shot and arranging further support and follow-up.	Learning a structured approach (for example, SPIKES) as a framework for giving bad news that can be adapted to almost any situation.

(Continued)

5

✓ How to excel in this station—cont'd

Action	Reason	How
Sensitive approach.	This is the most important thing to do as it demonstrates you care, and can be empathetic towards patients.	Be aware of non-verbal cues. Pause regularly to allow the patient to take on board the information and ask questions. Respond to the patient's feelings with empathy and concern.
Remember ICE.	This is a helpful way to establish a baseline before you begin the discussion and then introduce the diagnosis.	Specifically ask about the patient's ideas and concerns at the start. It may be appropriate to ask them again, 'What are you most worried about?' after you have broken the news of the diagnosis. Clarifying expectations after you have broken the news is a useful way of offering support to the patient.

✗ Common errors in this station

Common error	Remedy	Reason
Giving false hope.	Be realistic and honest about the news you are giving, and avoid giving false hope, for example 'it'll be ok'. It may be better to make general comments such as 'we'll do everything we can' or 'we'll support you through this'.	Feel free to make hopeful comments where appropriate, for example 'survival for this condition is very good'. However, avoid making sweeping statements or giving false hope, as patient and relatives may cling onto those comments and then be upset later that they were misled.
Overwhelming with information.	Give basic information in short points initially. Only go on to give further information if the patient specifically asks for it.	This station is not designed to test your knowledge of the condition or management; it is to assess your communication skills, so focus on those. Patients often go into shock when they receive bad news, and often find it difficult to absorb any information you are giving them, so keep points to a minimum and repeat anything important.

STATION VARIATIONS

○ Basic

Breaking the news that an amputation is necessary

Another example scenario might be that you are asked to see a patient with type 2 diabetes with severe leg ulcers and the vascular surgeons have decided they require a below-knee amputation. Breaking the news in this scenario should be performed in the same way; the patient may be aware of the seriousness of the leg condition, but news of plans for amputation can still be potentially devastating. In this scenario, it is important to give a realistic message of hope, for example 'it is still possible to have a very active life following an amputation', and to focus on the quality of life aspects.

Further Reading

Baile, W.F., et al., 2000. SPIKES—a six-step protocol for delivering bad news: application to the patient with cancer. The Oncologist 5 (4), 302–311.Available online at, http://theoncologist.alphamedpress.org/content/5/4/302.full.

Breaking Bad News... Regional Guidelines. Developed from Partnerships in Caring, Department of Health, Social Services and Public Safety, February 2003. Available online at http://dhsspsni.gov.uk/breaking_bad_news.pdf.

5

Discussing a 'do not resuscitate' decision

5.10

CANDIDATE INFORMATION

Background: You are a junior doctor on the medical unit and are looking after Albert Roberts (90 years old), who was admitted following a collapse at home. He has a history of ischaemic heart disease, chronic obstructive pulmonary disease and prostate cancer with multiple bony metastases. He is very unwell and is hypotensive, tachycardic and unconscious. His chest radiograph shows consolidation of the right lung consistent with pneumonia. He has been treated with intravenous antibiotics and fluids, but is deteriorating and his oxygen saturations are dropping despite maximal therapy.

Task: The consultant has reviewed him and stated that he should be for ward level care only and not for cardiopulmonary resuscitation (CPR). She has asked you to discuss this with the patient's son, Mr Richard Roberts, who has now arrived.

APPROACH TO THE STATION

This station is a variant on the breaking bad news station (station 5.9). You should follow the principles of the SPIKES model as detailed in that station. In this case the patient is clearly not able to make decisions for himself, so the decision should be made in his best interests. In UK law if there is a legally appointed lasting deputy, then their views must also be sought (see station 5.7).

PATIENT INFORMATION

Name: Mr Richard Roberts (son)   **Age:** 55 years   **Sex:** Male

Opening statement: You have just arrived at the hospital following a phone call from the nurses. They have told you that your father is very unwell with pneumonia and you should come as soon as possible. When you arrive, the nurses take you to see your father and you realise that he looks very unwell. His eyes are closed and he is not able to talk to you. The nurses then tell you that the doctor would like to speak to you.

Ideas: You know that your father is very unwell and you have never seen him like this. You are very worried that he will die. Your father has not been a well man for the past year—he has been deteriorating since he was told that his prostate cancer had spread. He is now only able to walk a few steps, having been going to the shops by himself a year ago. Your father has often told you that he has 'had enough' and this was very upsetting for you. You had never discussed resuscitation with him but you are sure that he would not want to be resuscitated.

Concerns: You are worried that the doctors will ask you to make this decision as you do not want him to die. You assume that if CPR was offered it would be successful but he would probably be in a worse state than before. You are also worried that by agreeing to a 'not for CPR' decision your father will not have any further treatment and simply be left to die.

Expectations: You feel that your father will die and want him to be as comfortable as possible. You anticipate that the doctors will want to discuss resuscitation with you and if your concerns above are discussed, then you will agree that he would not want to be resuscitated.

5

CLINICAL KNOWLEDGE AND EXPERTISE

Cardiopulmonary resuscitation (CPR) involves both basic and advanced life support measures. This includes chest compressions, artificial ventilation, defibrillation (if the patient has a 'shockable rhythm' such as ventricular fibrillation or tachycardia) and the use of drugs to attempt to restart the heart. If resuscitation is successful most patients will need a period of treatment on an intensive care unit. Patients who have CPR are at risk of hypoxic brain injuries and rib fractures. The decision about whether to perform CPR needs to consider the likelihood of a good outcome versus the potential harm caused to the patient.

'Do not resuscitate' (DNR) (sometimes called 'do not attempt resuscitation' (DNAR) or 'allow natural death') orders are commonly used in hospitals and community settings. Such decisions should consider:

1) What is the likely outcome in terms of survival and disability?
2) What are the patient's wishes (either from discussion or by advanced care plan/ directive)?
3) If the patient is unable to discuss his/her wishes—what do the family/carers feel the patient's wishes would be?
4) The legal and ethical frameworks in the country you work in (e.g., in the UK the GMC guidance and the Mental Capacity Act).

There are two factors to consider when discussing outcome following a cardiac arrest—survival and level of disability afterwards.

Survival

The chance of surviving an out-of-hospital cardiac arrest is very low. This depends on the type of arrest—only 2% of people who have a 'non-shockable' rhythm cardiac arrest will survive. Around 20% of patients who have a cardiac arrest in hospital survive and are discharged. However, these statistics vary, depending on the reason for the arrest. If a cardiac arrest occurs following a predictable deterioration in the patient's health, then they are much less likely to survive than if the cardiac arrest is sudden and unexpected. This is because 'shockable' rhythms are usually due to sudden cardiac events that can be reversed. If a cardiac arrest occurs due to prolonged physiological stress with multiple organ dysfunction the chances of recovery are much lower. The

5

likelihood of success also depends on the baseline functional status of the patient—a younger person with no pre-morbid health conditions is more likely to survive than an older person with multiple chronic health problems.

Level of disability

These factors are also important in determining the likely level of disability following cardiac arrest. Patients who have a sudden cardiac arrest with a shockable rhythm are more likely to return to their normal functional status afterwards if they survive than those with prolonged physiological decline or who have a poor pre-event baseline function. Within this second group, a person is likely to have a significantly worse quality of life if they survive to discharge.

Communicating about CPR

It is good practice to communicate with patients and their relatives about CPR decisions. This is a variation on breaking bad news so the principles discussed in 5.9 also apply. You should use the SPIKES model to explore the patient's or family's ideas, concerns and expectations about CPR, including likely outcomes and potential harm. In most cases conflict about CPR decisions arises due to lack of understanding or communication about these factors. Whilst patients can refuse CPR they are not able to demand it if the medical team feel that it would be futile. If you are not able to allay these concerns, and there is still conflict about the decision, then it is good practice to involve the most senior member of your team, who may then seek a second opinion.

The SPIKES model

- *Setting*—This is set up in an OSCE, but you should introduce yourself, check whom you are speaking to and ask whether there is anyone else he would like to be present.
- *Perception*—The start is key. You should use open questions, such as 'Have you spoken to any of the staff and what have you been told so far?' After listening to the response you can consider asking how he feels his father is currently. If you want to establish further background information you could ask a similarly open question, such as 'How has your father been recently?' It is likely that Mr Roberts will tell you how unwell his father has been and may include some cues about prognosis. You could also ask, 'Is there anything that you are concerned/worried about that you would like to ask me?'
- *Invitation*—If Mr Roberts mentions prognosis, you should pick up on this cue and ask 'Would you like me to talk about what the treatment options are?' If there are no cues you may need to ask more directly, 'You have told me how unwell you think your father is and I wanted to talk to you about his treatment—is that OK?'
- *Knowledge and information*—You should outline how unwell his father is despite being treated with antibiotics and intravenous fluids. You should then ask whether his father had ever discussed with him what he would want in this situation. If it has never been explicitly discussed, ask his son what he feels his father would want. If resuscitation is mentioned, then you can explore Mr Roberts' perception of CPR. If he says that he wants his father resuscitated, you should explain that the medical team do not feel that if CPR was attempted it would be successful, and that it would be your medical opinion that it should not be attempted. If you feel that he requires more information on CPR, briefly outline what CPR involves, including potential benefits and side-effects and the likely outcome. Explain that it is the medical team's opinion that if Mr Roberts were to deteriorate to the point where his heart stopped or he stopped breathing, then CPR is very unlikely to be successful and you would propose it is not attempted.
- *Emotions and empathy*—You should respond appropriately to Mr Roberts by displaying active listening techniques and acknowledging any emotions.

- *Strategy and summary* — Finish by summarising the discussion and the outcome (either that the patient is not for CPR or that you will seek a second opinion if there is disagreement). You should close by checking his understanding of what has been discussed and asking whether he would like any further information.

⚠ WARNING

- All DNA-CPR decisions should be discussed with the most senior doctor available.
- A DNA-CPR order does not mean that treatment will be withheld. A further discussion about ceiling of care or withdrawal of treatment should also be held if appropriate.

5

✓ How to excel in this station

Action	Reason	How
Explore perception.	It is often easier to explore patient's/ relative's perceptions of the situation first; this helps build rapport and helps you to judge how to approach a sensitive discussion.	Ask open questions and let Mr Roberts explain his perception of events and his concerns before attempting to discuss the resuscitation decision.
Display empathy.	This is a distressing situation for any relative.	Actively listen and respond to cues from Mr Roberts. Acknowledge that this is a difficult situation for him and that you realise he is finding the discussion upsetting.

✗ Common errors in this station

Common error	Remedy	Reason
Asking relative to make decision.	Explain that this is primarily a medical decision but that you want to take on board the views of the patient and family to help guide you.	It can be very difficult for family if they feel they are being asked to make a 'life or death' decision.

STATION VARIATIONS

⦿ Intermediate

Discuss a resuscitation decision with a (simulated) patient. The same principles would apply, but you also need to consider if the patient would like anyone else with them for support.

⦿ Advanced

The scenario may be one where the patient or relatives demand CPR when it is the medical team's opinion that this treatment would be futile — if this is the case, then you should conclude the session by recognising their concerns and agreeing to seek a second opinion.

5

Further Reading

Baile, W.F., et al., 2000. SPIKES—a six-step protocol for delivering bad news: application to the patient with cancer. The Oncologist 5 (4), 302–311. Available online at, http://theoncologist.alphamedpress.org/content/5/4/302.full.

General Medical Council, 'Treatment and Care towards the End-of-Life'. Available at http://www.gmc-uk.org/guidance/ethical_guidance/end_of_life_care.asp.

American Medical Association, 'Do Not Resuscitate Orders'. Available at http://www.ama-assn.org.

Speaking to a dissatisfied relative

5.11

CANDIDATE INFORMATION

Background: You are a junior doctor on the Medical Assessment Unit. Mohammad Abbas (63 years) was admitted with increasing breathlessness and was diagnosed with a chest infection that your consultant wanted antibiotics prescribed for. He advised co-amoxiclav on the ward round but you did not get a chance to prescribe it before you left, so you handed it over to the on-call team. Co-amoxiclav was then administered overnight. The allergies box on the drug chart had been left blank by the admitting doctor.

Mr Abbas had a known penicillin allergy and had a moderate to severe reaction with severe rash and some face and tongue swelling and wheeze. He was treated and moved to the High Dependency Unit, but is now stable. His son arrives on the ward and asks to speak to someone. You are the only member of the team available. Mr Abbas has already given permission for the medical team to discuss his care with his son, and you recognise his son from when he visited previously.

Task: Please see Mr Abbas' son and speak to him about the error.

APPROACH TO THE STATION

Dealing with dissatisfied patients and relatives is a difficult aspect of medical care, but one which it is essential to perform well. In this scenario, a drug error has resulted from a combination of factors, resulting in harm. There were multiple personnel involved (medical staff, nursing staff, and pharmacists) and it is crucial not to blame one individual (for example, the doctor who wrote the prescription) as there has been a series of systems errors. In this example, the junior doctor clerking the patient, the consultant who asked for the drug to be prescribed, the doctor who handed the task over (you), the doctor who prescribed the drug, the ward pharmacist and the nursing staff all bear some responsibility for this error.

PATIENT INFORMATION

Name: Syed Abbas (son) **Age:** 30 years **Sex:** Male

Occupation: Solicitor

Opening statement: I've just been to see my Dad and he told me he was prescribed penicillin. This is appalling! What happened?

(Continued)

5

If asked: You have permission from your father to speak to the medical team about his care.

Ideas: You want to know how this happened and who is responsible.

Concerns: You are very concerned about your father and his ongoing care. You are unsure whether he can be safely treated here. Your wife is also due to give birth in the hospital and you are wondering if she should go elsewhere as well. You are considering making a formal complaint.

Expectations: You want to hear an apology, you would like an offer to speak to senior personnel about the error, and you want to know that a thorough investigation will take place of how the error occurred.

CLINICAL KNOWLEDGE AND EXPERTISE

Dealing with complaints and dissatisfied patients or relatives requires a slightly different approach to breaking bad news. However, it is useful to remember some aspects from the SPIKES model as it is important to ensure an appropriate setting, perform the introductions, as well as check what the patient's relative already understands about what has happened. The information states that you have permission from the patient to discuss his care with his son, but if you are in any doubt you should check. You should also maintain a calm and empathetic approach; it is understandable for the patient's relative to be angry and concerned.

In this case you are not a senior team-member and you may feel that this station places you a little out of your depth. However, sometimes senior team-members are unavailable, for example, when in clinic. Do not feel that you are solely responsible for 'fixing' this problem; you just need to make a good start. It is good practice for a member of the nursing team to accompany you.

The best approach is to offer an unreserved apology on behalf of the team as soon as possible. You may know a good deal about how serious untoward incidents (SUIs) are dealt with, and it might help to explain some of this to the patient's son. Avoid becoming defensive or confrontational. It is understandable that the patient's relative may want to make a formal complaint following a serious medical error; you should direct him towards services that will help him to do this.

Remember that the best way to diffuse upset and anger is to remain calm and empathetic. You may need to reiterate the apology several times. Do not be drawn into apportioning blame; explain that there were several systems errors and that the detailed analysis of the incident will look into exactly what went wrong and how the error occurred.

Try to cover the following points in your discussion:
- Ensure an appropriate setting, introduce yourself (and your role) and check the identity of the person. Explain that there is no one more senior to speak to currently, but that they will be available later.
- Double-check with the patient's son that the patient is happy for you to speak to him about the case.
- Review his understanding of the events.
- Apologise for the error on behalf of the team. Empathise with the patient's relative about his concern/anger/upset. You may need to repeat this and allow the patient's son time to talk or to digest this.
- Assure the patient's relative that this incident will be looked into in great detail. Explain that an incident form has already been completed (make sure it has been beforehand) and that a full and detailed analysis will be done. Admit that there have

been mistakes and that one outcome of the investigation will be about avoiding this happening in future.

- Do not blame individuals. Explain that no single individual was at fault, but there were a number of (systems) errors that contributed to the incident.
- Reiterate the offer to speak to more senior team-members. Offer to help them arrange this by ringing the consultant's secretary. It may also be helpful for one of the senior nursing staff or the ward manager to speak to the patient's son on behalf of the nursing staff.
- You can also suggest that the patient's son speaks to an independent advocate if one is available. In the UK, the Patient Advice and Liaison Service (PALS) offers this service. They can also instruct the family on how to make a formal complaint if their concerns are not dealt with satisfactorily.
- Sum up the conversation by reiterating the apology and summarising the action points, e.g., making an appointment for the patient's relative to speak to the consultant/senior nurse and/or contact PALS.

⚠ WARNING

- Sometimes the care provided falls below the standard expected and it is understandable for patients and their relatives to be upset and angry. However, it is not acceptable for them to behave in a violent or aggressive manner towards any staff. If you feel threatened, remove yourself from the situation immediately and call security.

5

 How to excel in this station

Action	Reason	How
Apologise.	The GMC states that 'You must respond promptly, fully and honestly to complaints and apologise when appropriate.'	Harm has occurred. Offer an honest, sincere and unreserved apology on behalf of the team.
Remain calm and empathetic.	The best way to deal with upset, frustration or anger is to remain calm yourself.	Remember to allow natural pauses and plenty of time for the patient's relative to talk and ask questions. Do not take the complaint personally. Consider what your own response would be in a similar situation.
Suggest action points.	The patient's relative will want to know what steps are being taken to address the error.	Offer the opportunity to speak to senior medical and nursing staff. State that the incident will be fully investigated. Suggest that he should contact an advocacy service such as PALS.

✗ Common errors in this station

Common error	Remedy	Reason
Becoming defensive or confrontational.	Stay calm and empathioo. It is understandable that the patient's son may want to make a formal complaint or even pursue litigation—you might want to take similar action if you were in his position.	If you become defensive or confrontational the situation may escalate. Remember that they are complaining about the situation, not about you personally. We need to be honest and open about mistakes, as well as putting systems in place to learn from them. The patient's relative may want to make a complaint but is

(Continued)

5

Common error	Remedy	Reason
		less likely to do so if their concerns are dealt with in an honest, open and empathetic manner.
Blaming absent team-members.	The patient's son may ask who is responsible. Try to explain that there were many system errors at fault, rather than one individual being responsible.	It is clear in this case that several individuals made errors or oversights which together resulted in harm, and blaming one person is unfair on your colleagues.

✕ Common errors in this station—cont'd

STATION VARIATIONS

○ Intermediate

A patient has had a pleural aspiration performed but unfortunately the samples have been damaged on the way to the laboratory. Explain to the patient that the samples have been lost and that the procedure will need to be repeated.

Further Reading

- The Medical Protection Society has issued guidance for doctors on how to handle complaints, entitled 'Handling Complaints', which is available to download for free as a PDF via their website http://www.medicalprotection.org.uk
- There are several resources on the National Patient Safety Agency website http://www.npsa.nhs.uk, including information on how medical errors should be dealt with, as well as links to a publication about reducing medication errors entitled 'Safety in Doses'.

A colleague who drinks too much

5.12

CANDIDATE INFORMATION

Background: You have recently started work in a general practice with three partners and two other GPs. You have become concerned that the senior partner, Dr McCormick, is drinking excessively as you have noticed him smelling of alcohol on a couple of occasions and found a bottle of whisky hidden in his bottom drawer when you went to borrow a thermometer.

Task: You approach Dr McCormick at the end of surgery; please discuss your concerns about his drinking.

APPROACH TO THE STATION

This is a classic ethical dilemma made more difficult because you are the new GP and the doctor involved is the senior partner. The discussion involves a fellow health professional as a colleague rather than a patient and your approach should reflect this, focusing not only on the effect of excess alcohol, but also the impact on practising safely as a doctor. Ultimately, your duty of care is to patients and if you have ongoing concerns about your colleague's fitness to practise you have an obligation to take these further though it is prudent to warn your colleague if you are planning to do this.

PATIENT INFORMATION

Name: Dr Paul McCormick   **Age:** 52 years   **Sex:** Male

Occupation: Senior partner in GP surgery

Opening statement: You admit that you may have been drinking a little more recently since your wife died, but you do not think that it is an issue in the surgery and don't feel that it has any impact on your patients or your ability to practise. You are embarrassed that the bottle of whisky has been found in your drawer but did not plan on drinking any of it in surgery (or lie and say that it was a present from a patient that you had forgotten to take home).

You ask the doctor approaching you not to tell anyone about your drinking.

Further information (if asked): Your wife died 10 months ago of a haemorrhagic stroke. Your only son lives in Australia and you are finding that you are drinking alone most evenings when you return home. Initially you were drinking a bottle of

(Continued)

5

wine per night but now you have started drinking spirits as well and you occasion-ally have a shot of whisky in the morning as an 'eye-opener' to get you ready for the day if you're feeling a bit shaky.

Concerns (if asked): You are worried that you may be reported to the GMC and suspended from practice now another GP has found out about your drinking. (If the discussion is going well, you may express relief that you have been able to confide in someone about your problems.)

You also require your car to drive to and from work and on home visits and are concerned that your colleague may report you to the DVLA and losing your licence would have a devastating effect on your ability to work.

CLINICAL KNOWLEDGE AND EXPERTISE

The General Medical Council (GMC) 'Good Medical Practice' guidance is clear that 'the safety of patients must come first' and doctors are obliged to 'protect patients from risk of harm posed by another colleague's conduct, performance or health'. This means that a failure to act upon concerns is unacceptable and you risk being investigated by the GMC yourself if it becomes evident that you were aware of the issue, but did not act. Although it would be appropriate to report your concerns to the Practice Manager, it is often better to be open and approach a colleague directly and honestly voice concerns. You can speak to your defence union for additional advice and support prior to doing so.

- Ensure that any discussions are in a private environment and try to avoid possible interruptions.
- Express concerns open and honestly — be frank and direct.
- Ask them if they have noticed a problem with their current behaviour or thought about seeking help.
- Explain your concerns about the impact of their behaviour on patient safety.
- Stress their duty of care to seek help.
- Highlight that you may have to raise concerns with others.
- Offer to support them in seeking help if wished.
- *Don't* offer false reassurances of confidentiality if asked.

⚠ WARNING

- Remember that patient safety should come above loyalty to a colleague.
- Speak to your defence union early if you are unsure how to proceed.

How to excel in this station

Action	Reason	How
Demonstrate knowledge.	Show awareness of the guidance in the GMC's 'Good Medical Practice' on concerns around a colleague's fitness to practise.	Discuss the responsibilities of a doctor when unwell in terms of seeking help, and what responsibilities you personally have to highlight any concerns.

✓ How to excel in this station—cont'd

Action	Reason	How
Explore.	Allow the doctor time to identify the problem themselves rather than dictate to them in a patronising way what should happen.	Approach the discussion in a non-confrontational manner, exploring what they think the proper procedure should be or how they would advise others in a similar position.
Counsel.	Demonstrate empathy and understanding within a non-judgemental approach.	Remember that, as this involves talking with another health professional, it should be a discussion between experts with less emphasis on health promotion and education.
Provide information.	Support the onward progression towards recognition of the extent of the problem and recovery.	Signpost to voluntary organisations that are tailored to confidentially supporting doctors with dependency issues, e.g., the British Doctors and Dentists Group or the Sick Doctor's Trust.

✗ Common errors in this station

Common error	Remedy	Reason
Turning it into a consultation.	Ensure a discussion between colleagues, rather than a consultation with a patient.	The temptation is to use the same approach as in a consultation with a patient. However, by doing so, you may come across as condescending to someone with a wealth of medical knowledge and experience.
False promises of confidentiality.	Remain open and honest throughout the discussion and don't falsely reassure.	Confidentiality cannot be guaranteed with concerns around patient safety so better to be honest at the time rather than reassure and end up breaking promises.

5

STATION VARIATIONS

○ Basic

You could reduce the conflict within the interview by removing the underlined statement from Dr McCormick requesting that his drinking levels be hidden from others.

○ Advanced

The role of Dr McCormick could be played with a greater level of confrontation for a more challenging consultation, with him attempting to pressurise the candidate into not disclosing his drinking or raising concerns with others.

Further Reading

General Medical Council, 2013. Good Medical Practice. GMC, London.
General Medical Council, 2012. Raising and Acting on Concerns for Patient Safety. GMC, London.

Prescribing and handover

Introduction to prescribing and handover 6.0

Prescribing and handover are very important skills in patient safety. As a result many schools now have specific training on these so that newly qualified doctors are better equipped to start practising medicine safely.

Prescribing skills of newly qualified doctors have been highlighted as a concern in the United Kingdom and this has led to the introduction of a national prescribing skills assessment. Remember though that is still possible to have OSCE stations on prescribing. It is important to know how you will be expected to prescribe in your exam — many universities have developed a standardised student prescription chart. You should familiarise yourself with the chart that will be used in your exam. It is important to write clearly on a prescription chart — in some cases this will mean completing charts in block capitals. If you make a mistake, then the safest way is to rewrite the prescription rather than altering a chart.

Handover is recognised as a very important skill and is increasingly being taught and tested. The best way to learn about handover is to use a structured approach (such as SBAR) and practise this whenever you see a patient. Think about how you would hand the patient over or present to a senior colleague. You should also watch experienced doctors hand over and see how they convey important information in a concise and accurate fashion. Simulation training is an ideal place to practise handover skills safely. You could use any of the acute management scenarios in Chapter 7 to practise your handover skills in this setting.

KEY SKILLS

- Be able to write a clear, legible and safe prescription.
- Be able to take a structured medication history including allergies and adverse reactions (this is described in station 6.1).
- Know how to prescribe medications that are high risk such as insulin, anticoagulants and analgesics.
- Be able to give and receive a concise structured handover using a tool such as SBAR.
- Be aware of how to escalate patient safety concerns.

Prescribing antibiotics

6.1

CANDIDATE INFORMATION

Background: You are the junior doctor on the medical admissions unit. You have assessed Mr Davis (60 years old) who has been admitted with an infective exacerbation of chronic obstructive pulmonary disease (COPD). He has a past medical history of COPD, type 2 diabetes and chronic kidney disease (CKD). You decide that he needs some oral antibiotics, steroids and some nebulised salbutamol and explain this to him. He hands you a list of his usual prescriptions.

Task: Prescribe his usual medications and add antibiotics and nebulised salbutamol. The examiner will play the role of Mr Davis; you can ask him any questions that you need to.

For the purposes of this station you *do not* need to explain the prescription to the patient.

A hospital antibiotic policy and a prescription chart have been provided.

The patient's medication list is as follows:

Mr C Davis. Date of birth 12/10/1953. Hospital ID 155423 Gliclazide 40 mg bd (8 am and 5 pm), Ramipril 5 mg, Amlodipine 10 mg, Simvastatin 40 mg at night, Salbutamol inhaler 2 puffs when required, Beclomethasone inhaler 2 puffs bd.

The hospital formulary states: Infective exacerbation of COPD: Non-severe—oral amoxicillin 500 mg tds for 7 days. 5 days of oral prednisolone (30 mg).

If penicillin allergic: oral clarithromycin 500 mg bd for 7 days (omit statins whilst on clarithromycin).

APPROACH TO THE STATION

Prescribing medication is an important skill and likely to be tested in OSCEs. This is because medication errors are common, especially at transitions in patients' care (such as on admission or discharge). You should provide a safe and clear prescription within the allocated time. Station 6.2 describes the key points in taking a medication history and you should follow this structure. In this case it is acceptable to check with the patient that the drugs on the supplied repeat prescription are still current. It is vitally important to check drug allergies especially when prescribing antibiotics.

In this case the patient has CKD and this should alert you to possible issues. Familiarise yourself with a formulary so you know where to look for possible drug interactions or restrictions (British National Formulary (BNF) in the UK).

Although prescription charts vary between hospitals most will have common themes. Familiarise yourself with the chart that is likely to be used in your OSCE. We would suggest using one of these when practising this station.

PATIENT INFORMATION

Name: Mr C Davis   **Age:** 60 years   **Sex:** Male   **Occupation:** Chef
- Confirm that you are Mr Davis.
- Confirm that the medications on the repeat prescription list are correct.
- State that you do not take any other medications or non-prescribed medicines.

Only if asked: Say that you are allergic to penicillin and that you had lip swelling with this previously.

CLINICAL KNOWLEDGE AND EXPERTISE

6

To write a safe and clear prescription you need to:
- Include patient identification — full name, date of birth and a third identifier (usually a patient identification number).
- Include any allergies or adverse reactions (with consequences) on a prescription chart.
- Write clearly and legibly the following information about each medication:
  - Name of medication, dose, route of administration, date of prescription, indication, name and signature of the prescribing clinician.
  - In the case of the antibiotic prescription a stop date should be provided (in this case 7 days).

An example of a completed drug chart is shown in Fig. 6.1.1.

In this case the important actions are:
1) Transcribing the previously prescribed medications.
2) Recognising that the patient has had a severe allergic reaction to penicillin previously, documenting this on the chart and then prescribing an alternative antibiotic as per the formulary.
3) Changing the salbutamol inhaler to a regular nebulised delivery at the appropriate dose (2.5 mg qds).
4) Recognising the interaction between the antibiotic and the simvastatin and omitting it accordingly.

⚠ WARNING

- Allergies to medications are vitally important and should be recorded on the prescription chart.
- Renal failure, liver disease and pregnancy are special considerations when prescribing new medications. If you are unsure, then you must check before prescribing.
- You should consider drug interactions when prescribing, particularly with medications such as warfarin.

6

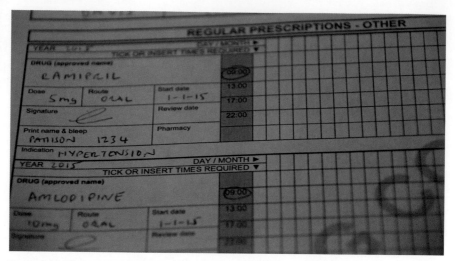

Figure 6.1.1 Example of a completed prescription on a hospital drug chart

✓ How to excel in this station

Action	Reason	How
Stop date on antibiotics.	This will avoid overtreating with antibiotics. Good antibiotics stewardship is essential in reducing complications of treatment.	State on the chart the intended duration of the antibiotic course.
Add a caution about renal failure.	Many medication doses must be reduced in renal impairment and some are contraindicated.	Write 'renal impairment' in cautions box and add a dated eGFR.

✗ Common errors in this station

Common error	Remedy	Reason
Not documenting allergy.	Write the drug the patient is allergic to and the reaction they had with it—in this case 'Penicillin: causes lip swelling'.	Not documenting the allergy could have catastrophic consequences. Documenting the reaction helps to gauge the seriousness of the allergy/adverse reaction.
Assuming medication list is accurate.	Always look for a second source of information to confirm medication list.	Medication list may be out of date and not all patients will be able to recall their medication and doses correctly, potentially leading to prescribing errors.

STATION VARIATIONS

Advanced
Indicate that the patient is on warfarin therapy and will require close monitoring of INR due to drug interactions. Another advanced skill may be to calculate a drug dose (such as a dose of the antiobiotic gentamicin that is prescribed according to the weight of the patient).

Further Reading
General Medical Council, 'Good Practice in Prescribing and Managing Medicines and Devices (2013)', http://www.gmc-uk.org/guidance/ethical_guidance/14316.asp.
Maxwell, K.S., Wilkinson, K., 2007. Writing Safe and Effective Prescriptions in a Hospital. J R Coll Physicians Edinb 37, 348–351.

6

Medication review

6.2

CANDIDATE INFORMATION

Background: You are a doctor in general/family practice and Mr Calder has come for a medication review. He normally sees Dr Khan, but she is away. Mr Calder has hypertension (30 years), hypercholesterolaemia (2 years) and previous smoking. The records show that his blood pressure is well controlled but cholesterol has remained high (last reading 7.5 mmol/l). Dr Khan has asked the patient to come in to discuss the cholesterol result and changing to a more potent statin (atorvastatin 40 mg).

Task: Please perform a medication review and discuss the change of medication with the patient.

APPROACH TO THE STATION

Firstly, check the patient's understanding of why they have come. Remember the task is to perform a medication review and then to discuss the blood test result and agree on a shared treatment decision. In a review you should check the patient's understanding of why they are taking the medications, if they are adherent to this and any side effects. You should also discuss any concerns that patients have about taking their medication.

PATIENT INFORMATION

Name: Mr Calder   **Age:** 60 years   **Sex:** Male   **Occupation:** Office manager

You have been asked back to the surgery to discuss your cholesterol test. You should tell the doctor that you are taking: aspirin 75 mg one tablet daily, ramipril 5 mg daily (both taken for 2 years), simvastatin 40 mg daily.

You have had high cholesterol for 2 years and have high blood pressure. Initially you tried to treat your cholesterol with exercise and diet, but 3 months ago it remained high so your doctor suggested simvastatin. You weren't keen and 2 weeks after starting it you had some aching in your arms and legs. You read that this may be a side effect so stopped it. You haven't told your doctor, as you didn't want to admit this.

If the doctor asks directly, you will admit to not taking the simvastatin and tell them why reluctantly. You are worried because the muscle pains stopped you from exercising, which you feel is important in feeling healthier. You would be willing to try either the simvastatin at a lower dose or another medication if the doctor suggests this.

You should also mention that you are worried that your regular doctor will be upset when they find out you have not been taking your medication.

CLINICAL KNOWLEDGE AND EXPERTISE

The purpose of the station is to test both clinical knowledge about medications and communication skills. Firstly, it checks whether the candidate can take a medication history and discuss medicine adherence. Then the candidate should discuss the patient's concerns in terms of side effects and understanding. Finally, the candidate should agree on a shared decision about the next steps.

You need to be able to take a structured medication history, which should include:
- Regular or recently prescribed or discontinued medicines
- Name, strength, dose, frequency, indications, side effects
- Adherence with regimes
- Non-prescribed medication, over-the-counter medications, herbal remedies
- Known medication allergies
- Previous adverse drug reactions
- Patient's understanding and expectations.

You also need to know the common side effects of regularly prescribed drugs. The cardiovascular drugs discussed in this case are among the most commonly prescribed medications in the world (Table 6.2.1).

Non-adherence, with medication, is very common, with studies quoting adherence rates of only 30–50% after 1 year in patients with chronic diseases. These patients have worse clinical outcomes and there are cost implications for healthcare systems. The World Health Organization (WHO) defines five common causes of non-adherence, several of which could apply in this case (see Table 6.2.2 and Further Reading).

6

Table 6.2.1 Common side effects of cardiovascular drugs	
Drug	**Some common side effects**
Statins	Muscle aches, GI disturbance, sleep disturbance
ACE inhibitors	Hypotension, cough, renal impairment, angioedema
β-blockers	Bradycardia, bronchospasm, sexual dysfunction
Calcium channel blockers	Ankle swelling, flushing, constipation, bradycardia
Aspirin	GI bleeding and upset, easy bruising

Table 6.2.2 Common reasons for non-adherence with medication (WHO)	
Health system	Poor quality provider–patient relationship; poor communication; lack of access to healthcare; lack of continuity of care
Condition	Asymptomatic chronic disease (lack of physical cues); mental health disorders (e.g., depression)
Patient	Physical impairments (e.g., vision problems or impaired dexterity); cognitive impairment; psychological/behavioural; younger age; non-white race
Therapy	Complexity of regimen; side effects
Socioeconomic	Low literacy; higher medication costs; poor social support

6

✓ **How to excel in this station**

Action	Reason	How
Elicit understanding.	This will ascertain whether patient knows proposed benefits of the medication.	Ask if they are clear why they have been prescribed the medication and what the intended benefits are.
Encourage openness.	This empowers patients to seek advice if they have problems with medication.	Suggest that if they are unsure about a side effect or reason for taking medication, or if they have any questions about their medication, they should discuss this with a pharmacist or doctor.
Agree a shared decision.	Shared decisions on treatment are more likely to be followed by patients.	Discuss the proposed treatment and come to an agreement about what to do. Offer a follow-up appointment to discuss further if required.

✗ **Common errors in this station**

Common error	Remedy	Reason
Undermining patient.	Show understanding for why they may have stopped taking the drug and acknowledge their concerns.	It is important to have a trusting doctor–patient relationship.
Not asking about adherence.	Be sure to ask patient if they are taking their medications and if they feel they have experienced any side effects from them.	Missing this key point may mean the consultation ends with the patient getting a prescription for a more potent statin which they are unlikely to take.

STATION VARIATIONS

○ Basic

A more basic station may just include taking a medication history and discussing concerns and concordance.

○ Intermediate

You could be asked to discuss prescribing a statin with the patient and counsel them about the likely benefits of the treatment and potential side effects. You might also consider the interactions or potential adverse effects of drug combinations, e.g., amlodipine and simvastatin. You should follow the model below when discussing new medication prescriptions with a patient:
• Name of medication
• Form (e.g., tablet, liquid, capsule)
• Dose
• How and when to take the medication
• Proposed length of treatment
• Benefits of medication
• Side effects of medication
• How long is it likely to take to work?
• What should they do if they have questions about medication?

You could consider the use of a patient decision aid to help patients understand the risk/benefit ratios of specific medications (see Further Reading).

Further Reading

WHO, 'Adherence to Long-Term Therapies: Evidence for Action', http://www.who.int/chp/knowledge/publications/adherence_report/en/.

Ho, P.M., et al., 2009. Medication Adherence: Its Importance in Cardiovascular Outcomes'. Circulation 119, 3028–3035 (open access).

NHS Patient Decision Aids http://sdm.rightcare.nhs.uk/pda/.

6

Prescribing postoperative fluids

6.3

CANDIDATE INFORMATION

Background: You are a junior doctor in a gynaecology unit. Mrs Jackson (58 years old) had an elective total abdominal hysterectomy yesterday to remove a uterine cancer. The operation was straightforward and there was minimal blood loss. The patient has not started to take any diet, and is being allowed sips of clear fluid only, but has managed to take very little as she is feeling nauseated (but has not vomited). Her observations are all normal. Other than her cancer, she has no other past medical history. She has been receiving postoperative intravenous fluids, but the last bag ran out 2 hours ago.

Task: Please prescribe some maintenance intravenous fluid for Mrs Jackson for the next 24 hours, and then put up a bag of intravenous fluids that you have prescribed at an appropriate rate. The giving set has only been used today and has been correctly primed with fluid already. A set of routine postoperative bloods has been performed today. The patient weighs 60 kg.

APPROACH TO THE STATION

This station is likely to be laid out with a desk and chair (usually next to the examiner) with fluid prescription charts available for you to complete (Fig. 6.3.1). A simulated patient will be seated with a cannula taped to their hand and a fully primed giving set attached to an empty bag of fluids. There will be a variety of different intravenous fluids available. The patient's blood tests for the day will be shown to you if you ask.

This station is testing your knowledge about intravenous fluid prescription for maintenance. The candidate information has explained why the patient cannot eat or drink, but states that her observations are normal, and that she has been receiving

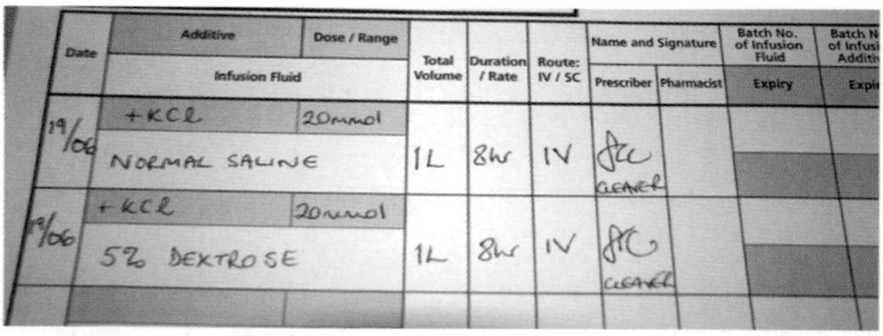

Date	Additive	Dose / Range	Total Volume	Duration / Rate	Route: IV / SC	Name and Signature		Batch No. of Infusion Fluid	Batch N of Infusi Additi
	Infusion Fluid					Prescriber	Pharmacist	Expiry	Expir
19/06	+KCL	20mmol							
	NORMAL SALINE		1L	8hr	IV	JC CLEARE			
9/06	+KCL	20mmol							
	5% DEXTROSE		1L	8hr	IV	JC CLEARE			

Figure 6.3.1 A completed fluid prescription chart

Figure 6.3.2 A fluid bag and giving set

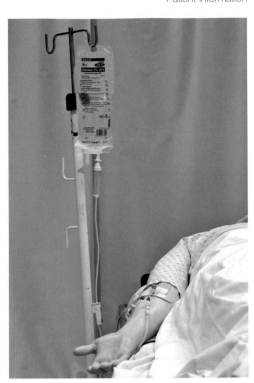

6

replacement fluid until recently, so no fluid resuscitation is required. To complete a fluid prescription correctly, you will need to know what the basic daily fluid and electrolyte requirements are for a 60-kg patient (this is explained below).

The second part of the task is to set up a bag of fluids and set the rate (see Fig. 6.3.2). This skill is being tested increasingly in OSCEs as administering intravenous fluids is a useful skill that is straightforward if you know how to do it, but very difficult if you have never done it before. If there is a simulated patient, it is important to remember to introduce yourself, check their identity and give a brief explanation of what you are doing and why.

PATIENT INFORMATION

Name: Mrs Loretta Jackson **Age:** 58 years **Sex:** Female **Occupation:** School secretary

You have had elective gynaecological surgery yesterday, which you have been told went well.

You are feeling fine and your pain is adequately controlled. You have been told you can't eat yet but can take sips of clear fluid. You feel slightly nauseated so you have been having fluids through a drip, but the last bag ran out a few hours ago.

You are in a hospital gown and you have a drip in the back of your hand.

6

Other information available to the candidate if requested:

Blood tests for Loretta Jackson		
Na+	136 mmol/l	(range: 135–145)
K+	3.5 mmol/l	(range: 3.5–5.4)
Urea	5.4 mmol/l	(range: 2.5–6.8)
Creatinine	67 μmol/l	(range: 49–90)
Hb	11.8 g/dl	(range:11.5–16)

CLINICAL KNOWLEDGE AND EXPERTISE

In order to correctly prescribe intravenous fluids you need to know what the indication is for prescribing fluids (e.g., maintenance, resuscitation, replacement of losses) and what the patient's daily fluid and electrolyte requirements are (Table 6.3.1). In this case, the station information is suggesting that the patient requires maintenance fluids only as she is unable to take sufficient volumes of oral fluids.

The patient's potassium level is at the bottom of the normal range, so you must add potassium to the fluids — 20 mmol would be inadequate; 40–60 mmol would be more appropriate (Table 6.3.2).

A 60-kg patient should not be prescribed more than 2 l of fluid a day for routine maintenance, whereas a 90-kg patient should be prescribed up to 3 l.

As the patient is nil by mouth, it is reasonable to administer some glucose-containing fluids—although bear in mind this does not constitute nutrition.

Table 6.3.1 Fluid and electrolyte requirements per kg

	Requirement per kg per day	Total required in this example (patient weight 60 kg)
Water	25–30 ml	1500–1800 ml
Sodium	1–2 mmol	60–120 mmol
Potassium	0.7–1 mmol	42–60 mmol

Table 6.3.2 Constitution of readily available intravenous fluids

	Na (mmol/l)	K (mmol/l)	Dextrose (g/l)	Other (mmol/l)
Normal saline (0.9% saline)	154	0—but is available with 20 or 40 mmol added	0	Chloride 154
Dextrose saline (0.18%saline/4% dextrose)	30	0—but is available with 20 or 40 mmol added	40	Chloride 30
Hartmann's solution (Ringer's lactate)*	131	5	0	Chloride 111, Ca 2, lactate 29
5% dextrose	0	0—but is available with 20 or 40 mmol added	50	—

*Other balanced isotonic intravenous crystalloids, such as Plasmalyte, are available. Check what is available in your hospital.

A reasonable fluid prescription could therefore consist of the following combinations:
- 1 l of Hartmann's solution plus 1 l of 5% dextrose with 40 mmol KCl added **OR**
- 1 l of 0.9% saline (normal saline) plus 1 l of 5% dextrose with 40–60 mmol KCl divided between the two bags **OR**
- 2 l of 0.18% saline/4% dextrose with 40–60 mmol KCl divided between the two bags.

The fluids could be administered over 6, 8 or 10 hours (the patient has had 2 hours without any fluid). Administering fluids over 12 hours is not advised as it does not take into account the frequent delays in administering fluids on a ward, and does not leave the patient with any 'drip-free' time.

Once you have completed the prescription you are asked to set up one of the prescribed bags. The method is outlined, but the easiest way to learn the technique is to perform it on the wards or in a skills suite.
- Select a bag and open the outer clear plastic wrapper (there should be no fluid leaking into the outer wrapper; if there is then discard the bag).
- Check the fluid against the prescription with another person to perform a second check — the examiner will offer. You also both need to check the expiry date and ensure there is no debris in the bag or fluid discolouration.
- Record the bag's lot number on the fluid prescription chart and sign — the second checker should also sign or initial in the space provided.
- Go to the patient. Introduce yourself and explain what you are doing.
- Ask to check the patient's wristband and that the prescription has the same name.
- Check the cannula — the dressing should have the date of insertion and there should be no swelling or erythema. State that you could check the cannula was still patent by flushing it with 5 ml of saline.
- Check that the giving set does not contain air bubbles and that the roller clamp is closed.
- If the fluid you have selected contains potassium, state that it would be administered via a pump as a safety measure (so that it cannot inadvertently be given too rapidly) — you will then be asked to continue to demonstrate the skill as if it were a non-potassium-containing fluid.
- Clean your hands and put on gloves and an apron.
- Unscrew the cap on the new bag and discard it — ensure you do not touch the port (key part) once the cap is removed. You can then hang the new bag from the drip stand — it will not leak.
- Take the empty bag off the stand and carefully take out the plastic 'skewer' part of the giving set (do not touch it as it is a key part) and screw it into the port of the new bag — you may find it easier to take the bag off the stand.
- With the bag hanging from the stand, gently squeeze the drip chamber of the giving set until it is approximately half full.
- Calculate a drip rate (see the formula below).
- Thank the patient.

Calculating a drip rate:

$$\frac{\text{Total volume of fluid in ml} \times \text{drop factor}}{\text{Time in minutes}} = \text{number of drops per minute}$$

The drop factor is available on the giving set but is usually 15, 20 or 60.

For example, to give a litre of fluid 10-hourly, using a standard giving set with a drop factor of 20, the calculation would be:

$$\frac{1000 \times 20}{600} = 40 \text{ drops per minute}$$

6

⚠ WARNING

- Electrolyte abnormalities can be life-threatening so it is crucial that you understand the basic daily fluid and electrolyte requirements.

✓ How to excel in this station

Action	Reason	How
Knowledge of basic requirements.	Difficult to tackle this question without knowledge of the daily requirements for fluid and electrolytes per kg per day.	Table 6.3.1 contains some brief information about calculating fluid and electrolyte requirements, but you can refer to the Further Reading section for more detailed information.
Obvious prior experience of procedure.	This station gives the game away if you have never put up a bag of intravenous fluid or calculated a drip rate.	On your ward placements, ask the nursing staff or junior doctors to show you how to administer IV fluids. Placements in anaesthesia or critical care will also provide good opportunities.

✗ Common errors in this station

Common error	Remedy	Reason
Incorrect interpretation of station.	Read the information carefully—it asks you to prescribe maintenance fluid only, not fluid for resuscitation.	Prescribing for resuscitation is a very different task to fluid prescribing for routine maintenance. Refer to the Further Reading section to find out more.
Poor rapport with patient.	Part of this station involves talking to the patient to introduce yourself, confirm their identity and explain what you are doing.	There are some easy marks on offer here if you remember to interact properly with the patient and perform routine safety checks such as checking the patient wristband and cannula site.

STATION VARIATIONS

○ Intermediate

You may have to demonstrate how to set up a bag of fluids for administration after inserting an intravenous cannula.

○ Advanced

An alternative setup is that you are asked to review an incorrect fluid prescription that has been completed by someone else. The prescription is likely to provide inadequate electrolyte replacement (for example, bags of 5% dextrose only) and may provide too much or too little fluid replacement.

Further Reading

The National Institute for Clinical Excellence (NICE) Guidance CG174—Intravenous fluid therapy in adults in hospital (December 2013) provides a detailed guide to fluid prescribing in different clinical circumstances in a hospital setting.

Prescribing insulin

6.4

CANDIDATE INFORMATION

Background: You are a junior doctor on a medical rotation. Mr McVitie has been admitted with pneumonia, but he is also known to have type 2 diabetes requiring insulin therapy.

Task: Please take a medication history from Mr McVitie about his insulin prescription and then prescribe his normal regime on the chart provided.

APPROACH TO THE STATION

This station is testing your familiarity with types of insulin, methods of administration and insulin regimens. You will also need to demonstrate that you recognise that insulin is dangerous if prescribed incorrectly, and ensure that it is prescribed safely. An examiner could also ask you more general information about insulin and diabetes; for example, familiarity of insulin-dosing regimens (Table 6.4.1), knowledge of insulin types (Table 6.4.2) and advice for patients regarding injecting.

Table 6.4.1 Types of insulin regimen		
Name	**Number of injections**	**Description**
Once daily	1	Suitable for type-2 diabetics who are also on oral medication. Patients take one dose a day of an intermediate insulin or long-acting analogue.
Twice daily	2	2 injections a day are normally given with breakfast and dinner. A mixed insulin that contains short and long-acting elements covers the glucose surge that occurs with breakfast and dinner and provides a background level for the rest of the day.
Basal-bolus regimen	4	A dose of short-acting or rapid-acting insulin is given with each meal (3x daily) and then a dose of long-acting or intermediate insulin is given at night. This covers the glucose peaks associated with meals but also provides background insulin to avoid high glucose levels between meals.

(Continued)

Table 6.4.1 Types of insulin regimen—cont'd

Name	Number of injections	Description
Continuous subcutaneous insulin infusions (CSII)	Continuous	Increasingly insulin pumps are being used to deliver a continuous infusion via a small subcutaneous cannula. Normally a low continuous dose is given of a rapid-acting insulin, and patients give a bolus with meals by touching a pump button. The cannula has to be changed every 3 days and the pump is about the size of a pager and can be worn on the patient's belt. This method allows better glycaemic control; however, the patient has to wear the device all the time and there can be risks of skin infections at the cannula site. Also, if the pump fails, the patients have no long-acting insulin so can develop hyperglycaemia very quickly.

Table 6.4.2 Types of human insulin*

Type	Speed	Examples	Effect
Human	Short-acting	Actrapid, Humulin S	Action within 30 mins. Peak of activity 60-90 mins. Duration – up to 10 hours. They ideally need to be given about 20 mins in advance of eating a meal and because of the longer effect they can cause hypoglycaemia after meals.
Human	Intermediate-acting	Humulin I, insulatard	Action within 2-4 hours. Peak of activity 4-10 hours. Duration – up to 18 hours.
Human	Premixed insulin	Humulin M2, Insuman Comb 15	Mixtures of short and intermediate-acting of various ratios. They must be given before meals so the short-acting component covers the prandial glucose surge, but the long-acting insulin will then act to reduce the glucose levels between meals as well.
Human analogue	Rapid-acting	Novarapid, Humalog	Action immediately. Peak of activity within an hour. Duration – up to 4 h. They can be given with a meal rather than 20 mins before and they have fewer issues with hypoglycaemias than short-acting. Often prescribed to be given with meals in basal bolus regimens to cover the prandial glucose surge.
Human analogue	Long-acting	Lantus, Levemir	Action within 2 h. Uniform activity (i.e., no peak). Duration – up to 24 h.
Human analogue	Premixed insulin analogues	Novomix 30, Humalog Mix 50	These combine rapid and long-acting in various ratios e.g., 30% rapid-acting and 70% long-acting.

*Most insulins are either human insulin (synthetically grown in a lab) or human analogues. The latter have been genetically modified to change the speed and duration of action and can be useful to achieve more steady glycaemic control; however, the cost is about twice that of human insulin. Animal insulin is now rarely used.

PATIENT INFORMATION

Name: James McVitie **Age:** 66 years **Sex:** Male

Background: You've had type 2 diabetes for the past 8 years and initially tried to control it with your diet but this was unsuccessful. You were on oral hypoglycaemic agents for a number of years but have required insulin over the past 18 months. You self-inject twice daily. You used to check your blood sugar fairly often but now only when you feel unwell. You use Novomix 30 insulin—20 units in the morning with breakfast and 10 in the evening with dinner.

CLINICAL KNOWLEDGE AND EXPERTISE

- Ask the patient to confirm their name and date of birth and then complete the insulin prescription chart—see Fig. 6.4.1 and below for how to do this safely.
- Ask the patient the type and dose of insulin used, remembering that patients may be on more than one type, and different amounts at different times of the day (Tables 6.4.1 and 6.4.2).
- Prescribe each type of insulin required at the appropriate times of the day.
- If the patient has a variable dose depending on carbohydrate counting, make this clear on the chart.
- Complete any additional sections of the chart; e.g., there is often an area to highlight whether a patient self-administers their insulin. There may also be an area to document how often they should have their glucose level checked. Make sure you are familiar with the charts used in your hospital.

To prescribe insulin safely:
- Always double check the patient details are correct.
- Write in clear and legible handwriting.
- Cross out errors with a single score and sign.
- Never abbreviate units to 'u'—always write out in full.
- Clearly document the route of administration.
- If in doubt, ask for advice.

6

Points to note about injecting insulin
- Injections are virtually painless and often given with a pen device that most patients can use to self-administer.
- Skin needs to be pinched prior to injection.
- Appropriate sites include abdomen, upper arms, thighs and buttocks.
- Injection sites should be rotated to avoid lipohypertrophy (which impedes absorption).
- A number of variables affect the rate of absorption of insulin; for example, exercise, local massage to the site and increased temperature all increase the rate of absorption.

6

INSULIN PRESCRIPTION CHART

NAME: ADDRESS: DOB:	PRE-ADMISSION DIABETES MEDICATION:
HOSPITAL NUMBER: WARD:	CHECKED:

When prescribing insulin never abbreviate units as "U" as this may be mistaken for a zero

REGULAR INSULIN PRESCRIPTION

Subcutaneous Insulin	Units	Date	Sig	Date and time given	Given by	Checked by
With breakfast						
With lunch						
With dinner						
Before bed						

Figure 6.4.1 Insulin prescription chart

⚠ WARNING

- Target blood glucose should be 4–7 mmol/l pre-meals and 4–10 mmol/l post-meals. Blood glucose levels below 4 mmol/l need urgent treatment to avoid the clinical complications of hypoglycaemia.
- Glucose levels above 10 are often tolerated more readily, but many patients are trained to give 'correction' doses of insulin if their blood sugar is above 12 or 15 to avoid diabetic ketoacidosis (DKA).

✓	**How to excel in this station**	

Action	Reason	How
Safe practice.	Insulin is a potentially lethal drug if administered incorrectly.	Demonstrate that you are aware of how insulin is prescribed safely, particularly writing legibly, crossing through and signing corrections and not abbreviating units to 'u'.
Background knowledge.	Impress the examiner with your knowledge and familiarity of diabetes and insulin management.	Attend diabetes clinic and talk to patients on the ward about their diabetic treatment. You will become used to the brand names of insulin. Ask clinicians about why a patient is on a certain regimen and how that impacts upon their diabetic control.

✗	**Common errors in this station**	

Common error	Remedy	Reason
Incorrect prescribing.	Carefully note the type and dose of insulin prescribed at each time of day. If the patient has a variable dose, make sure this is clearly documented.	The crux of the station relies on you carefully eliciting a patient's insulin regimen and then prescribing it carefully. Unfortunately, due to the often-complicated regimens (different types of insulin and different doses, at different times), errors are quite common in hospital, and can have catastrophic effects.

STATION VARIATIONS

○ Advanced

Calculating an insulin correction

You may be told a formula for correcting insulin doses and then asked to calculate this depending on a particular blood glucose level, and prescribe it.

For example, a patient may be correcting all blood glucose levels over 15 mmol/l with 1 unit of rapid-acting insulin for every 2 mmol/l of glucose over 10 mmol/l. If you were told that the patient had a blood glucose currently of 20 mmol/l, you would calculate that they are 10 mmol/l over 10 and therefore need 5 units of insulin correction.

There are no set formulae for correction doses. The formula a patient uses is normally decided upon by their diabetes team and may be changed over time once it is found what suits them best.

Further Reading

Station 5.4, Explaining a new diagnosis of type 2 diabetes.
Station 7.5, Acute management of diabetic emergency.

6

Prescribing analgesia

6.5

CANDIDATE INFORMATION

Background: You are a junior doctor in the Emergency Department. Ethel Miller (86 years old) has been brought in by her carer complaining of increasing right hip pain. She is known to have widespread osteoarthritis and takes paracetamol (1 g four times per day) but is now struggling to cope with the pain and is less mobile.

Task: Discuss with Mrs Miller the different options for additional pain relief, taking into account the side-effects and contraindications of the drug choices.

APPROACH TO THE STATION

You should use a step-wise approach to the prescribing of analgesia, utilising the World Health Organization's (WHO) pain relief ladder; taking into account that the patient is an older person, which can have implications for safety. You should consider the use of NSAIDs but, before prescribing any new medication, the risks should be assessed as well as whether any contraindications exist, and common or serious side effects should be discussed.

PATIENT INFORMATION

Ask a colleague to play the role of the patient. You may wish to consider practising how you would prescribe the chosen medication on a drug chart as this may be required as part of the examination.

Name: Mrs Ethel Miller   **Age:** 86 years   **Sex:** Female

Occupation: Retired cleaner

Presenting symptom: Right hip pain

Opening statement: You've come into hospital because you cannot cope with the pain in your hip any more. You have been told that you have bad arthritis but cannot have a hip replacement because it 'would not be safe at your age'. Your current painkillers are not helping and you want something different, in particular an anti-inflammatory.

Other symptoms (if asked): You have had no recent trauma or fall that has worsened the pain and there is no change in your pain to suggest any other underlying cause other than worsening osteoarthritis. You do not suffer from acid reflux or heartburn symptoms.

Past medical history: You have had high blood pressure for 25 years, which is well controlled. You had an operation for a repair of a perforated duodenal ulcer in your 30s following the birth of your second child.

Drug history: You are allergic to penicillin (it causes a rash). You take bendroflumethiazide 2.5 mg for your blood pressure as well as regular paracetamol (500 mg tablets, up to 8 daily).

Social history: You live alone in sheltered accommodation and have a carer who comes twice daily to help with meals. You are a non-smoker and drink a small sherry occasionally only.

If asked:

Ideas: You know that this pain is coming from 'wear and tear' in your hip, which you think is due to having a manual job for many years.

Concerns: You don't know how you will be able to continue coping at home if this pain worsens and you are struggling to wash and dress yourself now as a result.

Expectations: Your friend Doris takes diclofenac (an NSAID) and you wonder whether this would help your pain as you've heard that it's good for joint pain.

6

CLINICAL KNOWLEDGE AND EXPERTISE

The WHO's pain relief ladder was initially created to highlight management in patients with cancer, but is now widely used to manage pain, with non-opiate analgesia such as paracetamol and NSAIDs (if tolerated) forming the basis for all steps, with progression up through weak to stronger opiates (Fig. 6.5.1). The preferred approach is to use several different analgesics together in lower doses rather than one high dose analgesic, which has a higher risk of side effects.

Although this patient does not have any absolute contraindications to NSAIDs, there are several points within her background that suggest caution. The expectation is that you should discuss alternatives such as moving up the WHO's pain relief ladder, or introducing additional drug therapy to reduce the patient's risk with an NSAID (e.g., proton-pump inhibitor). You may add in a weak opiate such as codeine to her existing paracetamol (e.g., co-codamol), although you should explain the increased risk of side effects such as constipation, dry mouth and nausea, and warn about the risk of dependence and addiction.

You would not be expected to list all side effects of NSAIDs, but you need a good understanding of the most common or most serious, especially in older people and these should be discussed. Particular conditions preclude NSAIDs; these include:

- Hypersensitivity to aspirin or any other NSAID
- A history of cardiovascular disease
- Heart failure
- Active gastrointestinal bleeding or ulceration, recurrent GI bleeding and ulceration or prior haemorrhage or perforation relating to previous NSAID use
- Liver disease
- Renal impairment
- Pregnancy
- Taking oral anti-coagulants.

6

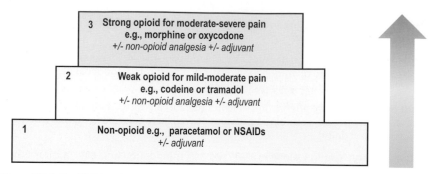

Figure 6.5.1 The WHO's pain relief ladder

Caution is also required when considering NSAIDs in patients with cardiovascular disease as they can increase the risk of thrombo-embolic events, and in mild to moderate renal impairment as there is a risk of precipitating renal failure. NSAIDs can also worsen hypertension as well as asthma (in approximately 20%), cause hepatic damage and exacerbate colitis and Crohn's disease. In older patients, to reduce the risk of GI haemorrhage with NSAIDs, it is worth considering prescribing gastro-protection, e.g., a proton-pump inhibitor such as omeprazole. NSAIDs associated with a lower risk of bleeding, e.g., ibuprofen and naproxen, are generally preferred and the aim should be to prescribe the lowest recommended dose possible to control symptoms for the shortest period possible.

 WARNING

- You must ensure there are no allergies or dangerous interactions with other medications.
- You must check that there are no contraindications within past medical history.

✓	How to excel in this station	
Action	**Reason**	**How**
Demonstrate knowledge.	Show that you are aware of the WHO's pain relief ladder and the process of increasing analgesia, and the risks and benefits of NSAIDs.	Discuss the options for pain relief after taking an appropriate past medical and drug history, making sure you establish whether there are any contraindications prior to prescribing.
Explain.	It is important to take into account the patient's preference and good communication.	Outline the risks and possible side effects of each medication proposed. Ask the patient whether they are aware of any problems with their preferred choice.
Counsel.	Reduce the risk of side effects and identify early any problems.	Advise on taking NSAIDs with meals 'to protect stomach' or consider using a PPI, e.g., omeprazole, and taking the lowest dose needed to control the pain.
Provide information.	Ensure a patient-centred approach, allowing informed choice.	Provide the patient with a drug information leaflet. These are available on the MHRA (Medicines and Healthcare Products Regulatory Agency) website http://www.mhra.gov.uk

Common error	Remedy	Reason
Over-paternalistic approach.	Establish the patient's ideas, concerns and expectations early within the consultation.	Poor candidates will decide on the analgesic choice without taking into account the patient's preference and expectation. Adherence relies upon a shared understanding of the benefits and risks with medication.
Missing possible interactions or contraindications.	Ensure a thorough drug and allergy history is taken. If you are unsure of a particular interaction it would be appropriate to ask to review the BNF.	It is impossible to know all side effects, interactions; doses and frequency of every drug, and time pressure within an exam situation can lead to information being omitted from the patient's background history that may be important.

Common errors in this station

STATION VARIATIONS

● Intermediate

6

Consider your approach to the station if the patient admitted that she was 'getting muddled' about when to take her painkillers and may therefore be taking more than prescribed on occasions when the pain was more severe. How would your management plan differ if this was the case and what could be offered to improve and monitor compliance with the medication?

Options you may wish to discuss could include:
- Only issuing analgesia on a weekly basis (via post-dated prescriptions) to monitor usage and reduce risk of overdose.
- Using a dossette box to help prompt the patient when and how often to take the analgesia.
- Using a slow-release buprenorphine or fentanyl patch (in severe pain only) that could be applied and removed by a relative or carer when due to ensure compliance (see station 3.18 Testing cognitive function).

Further Reading

British National Formulary, http://www.bnf.org.

General Medical Council, 'Good Practice in Prescribing and Managing Medicines and Devices (2013)', http://www.gmc-uk.org/guidance/ethical_guidance/14316.asp.

World Health Organization, 'WHO's Pain Relief Ladder', http://www.who.int/cancer/palliative/painladder/en/.

Handover of two patients

6.6

CANDIDATE INFORMATION

Background: You are a junior doctor on the medical ward. You are starting a long day shift on call for medicine in a large hospital. The junior doctor overnight does not normally work in the hospital and is in a rush to leave. There are some jobs to hand over from two of the patients admitted overnight.

Task: Please take a handover from the doctor finishing the night shift, and discuss with the examiner how you will prioritise the jobs.

APPROACH TO THE STATION

This station is challenging because the doctor giving the handover does not normally work at the hospital and is in a rush to leave. A doctor who is very reticent to give an adequate and safe handover can be very frustrating. However, it is of utmost importance that you are able to recognise the best way to take a structured handover, and how to best manage difficult colleagues. Remember that everyone responds well to politeness, courtesy and kindness and the doctor in this station is no different. The more polite you are, the more cooperative the night doctor will be. Be sympathetic to their personal concerns and recognise that they need to leave as soon as possible, but remember that a safe handover must take place to ensure patient safety.

PATIENT INFORMATION

You are the junior doctor covering the night shift.

You have covered the night shift as a locum but you are in a rush to leave as you need to get home for childcare before your partner needs to leave for work. Your young child has chickenpox and is not allowed in nursery so you will have to look after him today rather than going to sleep. You are very concerned that if you do not leave very soon you will get stuck in traffic. You are tired and you have not had a good shift as everything took you twice as long as it normally would because you have not worked in this hospital before.

There are two patients to hand over. (The other patients have already been reviewed and there are no outstanding jobs.) Do not volunteer any information unless asked. If the candidate is polite and asks you for information systematically then be cooperative and give the information you have been asked for. If the candidate is not structured then do not give the information in an ordered manner. Provided the candidate remains patient and courteous, then cooperate with handover and answer questions such as 'Is there anything else you need to tell me?' fully. Do not purposely mislead the candidate. If the candidate is rude to you, then refuse to give any further information and say you've had enough and you need to leave, and that the ward nurses will probably call them with the jobs.

Patient 1: Marjorie Jameson   **Age:** 72 years   **Sex:** Female

Ward 2B Hosp no: 03256118

Admitted with acute dyspnoea (probable pulmonary oedema). History of MI in the past and hypertension but no other medical history. Patient has been clerked but not yet reviewed by a senior doctor. There were widespread bilateral crackles on chest auscultation. You have prescribed a stat dose of furosemide 20 mg. Need to review chest radiograph, bloods and blood gas result.

Obs: Alert. Resp. rate 34/min, Sats 95% on 15 l oxygen. BP 98/67 mmHg, pulse 108/min, apyrexial.

Patient 2: Ashlie Cartwright   **Age:** 21 years   **Sex:** Female

Ward 3A Don't have hospital number.

Admitted following an intentional paracetamol overdose with alcohol. Has been seen and reviewed by a consultant but her paracetamol and salicylate levels were not back. The consultant has asked for N-acetyl-cysteine to be prescribed if the level is above the high-risk treatment line. Her GGT and ALT are slightly raised (you can't remember the result but the consultant is aware). Her clotting sample was underfilled and a repeat sample needs to be sent urgently.

Observations are normal.

6

CLINICAL KNOWLEDGE AND EXPERTISE

Ask questions in a structured manner. The first element is to ensure you have the correct patient. The best way of doing this is to have more than one patient identifier (such as date of birth and hospital number) as there can be more than one patient on a ward with the same surname. If more than one identifier is not available then just get as much information as you can, and remember to ask for the patient's location. The SBAR (situation, background, assessment, recommendation) structure is recommended for handover. Although the doctor in this scenario will not volunteer information in this format, you should ask for information according to this structure and the person giving handover should cooperate. This structure will help ensure that you do not miss anything out.

Table 6.6.1 gives some suggested questions for how to take handover according to an SBAR method.

In this station it is imperative that you take notes. You will not remember all the necessary information otherwise. It is also useful to summarise the information, and ensure you have not missed anything by asking something like 'Is there anything else I need to know?' at the end of the handover. Then briefly prioritise the jobs and explain to the examiner your next steps — this is a brief part of the station and you should leave no more than 2 mins. One of the patients is very unwell and needs an urgent medical review. However, the other patient has not had her paracetamol levels checked or a clotting sample taken — these are both imperative in order to find out if she needs treatment and whether she is developing liver damage, and a significant delay could affect her prognosis. If you think you need to get help from colleagues, then say so — one management possibility is to ask a senior colleague to urgently review the patient with probable pulmonary oedema while you deal with the urgent tasks for the other patient,

6

Table 6.6.1 SBAR method for communication	
Patient identity	Ask for the patient's full name, sex, age, date of birth, hospital number and location in the hospital.
Situation	For a new admission, ask for the presenting complaint. For an inpatient, ask what the current concern is.
Background	What is the relevant past medical history, or what has happened during this inpatient admission?
Assessment	Ask for a current set of observations and relevant clinical findings.
Recommendation	What needs to be done now? Are there any outstanding jobs? How urgent is it?

or ask if a phlebotomist or nursing colleague can take the bloods for you to check the result while you ensure the other patient is assessed.

 WARNING

- Poor or incomplete handover is a leading cause of serious medical errors. This station is testing your ability to communicate effectively with your colleagues and is fundamental to your role as a doctor.

✓ How to excel in this station

Action	Reason	How
Good rapport with colleague.	This will allow you to get the most information from your colleague.	Be polite and courteous and do not make dismissive remarks about the tasks handed over.
Structured approach.	Without a structure important information will be missed.	Ask about each patient in turn, ensuring you have patient identifiers then using the SBAR approach.

✗ Common errors in this station

Common error	Remedy	Reason
Running out of time.	You know there are two patients— allow about 4 mins for each patient with 2 mins to discuss management.	You cannot score highly if you do not manage to get a handover about both of the patients and have some time to summarise and discuss your next steps.

STATION VARIATIONS

Handover stations all demand a good understanding of clinical practice and consequently are all advanced level stations.

It is useful to refer to the other handover station in this chapter (station 6.7) for an idea of other styles of handover stations that you might encounter.

Further Reading

The World Health Organization (WHO) Collaborating Centre for Patient Safety Solutions have issued guidance on communication during handover: Communication during Patient Hand-overs, vol. 1 Solution 3, May 2007, available at/ http://www.who.int/patientsafety/solutions/patientsafety/PS-Solution3.pdf.

Referring a patient

6.7

CANDIDATE INFORMATION

Background: You are the junior doctor in the Emergency Department and have reviewed Michael Chan (52 years old), who has presented with shortness of breath. He has a past medical history of severe asthma and has been admitted to the intensive care unit on two occasions. His current medications include a salbutamol nebuliser 4 to 6 times daily, a steroid inhaler and a long-acting beta 2 agonist. His normal peak expiratory flow rate (PEFR) is 400 l/min.

He presented with shortness of breath with no cough. On examination you found him to be wheezy, unable to complete a full sentence. His respiratory rate was 32/min with saturations of 93% on air. His pulse is 110/min, blood pressure 140/90, temperature 36.8 °C. After giving him a combined salbutamol and ipratropium nebuliser, his peak expiratory flow rate is 180 l/min. His respiratory rate has improved to 28 and saturations to 95%. You feel that he requires hospital admission for further nebulisers and steroid treatment as his PEFR remains low.

Task: Speak to the on-call doctor for medicine and refer the patient using the information above. The examiner will then discuss the referral with you in the final 2 minutes.

APPROACH TO THE STATION

This station is similar to station 6.6 except you are handing the patient over rather than receiving the handover. You should follow the principles outlined for handover following a model such as SBAR (see station 6.6). The SBAR table has been adapted for use in this scenario in Table 6.7.1.

PATIENT INFORMATION

You are the on-call doctor for medicine. The candidate will speak to you about referring a patient with asthma who has presented with shortness of breath. You should listen to their handover and ask questions where appropriate.

(Continued)

6

You should then tell the junior doctor that you do not think that the patient needs to be admitted to hospital and that they should be discharged home on oral steroid treatment as they have improved with the nebulisers.

If they insist that the patient be admitted, you should tell them that you are too busy with unwell patients and again suggest they discharge the patient home. Finally you should say that you now have to see a very unwell patient.

CLINICAL KNOWLEDGE AND EXPERTISE

Classification and management of acute asthma attacks

The assessment of acute asthma is to decide whether the patient has a moderate, severe or life-threatening exacerbation. The stratification of this is covered in Table 6.7.2 (from recent UK guidance).

The history and examination point towards a non-infective, but severe, exacerbation of asthma due to an inability to complete sentences and PEFR between 33 and 50% predicted. Guidance suggests that these patients should be admitted until PEFR >75% predicted. His previous intensive care unit admissions also suggest that he is at risk of developing a severe asthma attack.

The treatment of acute severe asthma is as follows:
1. ABCDE assessment
2. Oxygen to maintain saturations >94%
3. β_2 agonist bronchodilators (such as nebulised salbutamol)
4. Steroid treatment—usually given orally if possible and continued for 5 days (e.g., prednisolone 40 mg)
5. Ipratropium bromide—usually added to nebulised salbutamol
6. Consider use of intravenous magnesium sulphate if no response to initial treatment.

Table 6.7.1	
Patient identity	Identify yourself. Give the patient's name, age.
Situation	Explain the presenting complaint—breathlessness on a background of asthma and that you think he has an acute severe attack of asthma.
Background	Explain that the patient has a previous history of intensive care admissions and asthma and that his usual PEFR is 400 l/min. He has no other relevant medical history. List his usual medication.
Assessment	Present his observations in an ABCDE format before and after the treatment that you have given.
Recommendation	Explain that as his symptoms have not fully resolved and his respiratory rate is still high and PEFR <50% predicted, he requires admission for further treatment and monitoring.

Table 6.7.2 Classification of severity of asthma	
Classification	Clinical features
Life threatening	Altered conscious level, exhaustion, arrhythmia, hypotension, cyanosis, silent chest, poor respiratory effort PEFR <33% best, oxygen saturations <92% PaO_2 < 8 kPa, 'normal' $PaCO_2$
Severe	One of the following: PEFR 33–50% best, respiratory rate >25/min, heart rate >110/min, inability to complete sentences
Moderate	PEFR >50% predicted, increasing symptoms, no features of acute asthma

Dealing with a difficult colleague and patient safety

As the scenario unfolds, you should recognise that the advice given to discharge is wrong and unsafe. It is your responsibility to ensure that the patient receives the correct treatment and that the potential risk to patient safety is addressed.

The acronym **PACE** has been used in the aviation industry to aid pilots to challenge each other. It describes a graded response to challenging a decision that you do not agree with and can be applied to this situation as well:

Probe for better understanding: In this situation ask the doctor why he thinks the patient is well enough to be discharged.

Alert to dangers: State that the patient has a severe exacerbation of asthma and that the guidelines suggest that he should be admitted for further observation.

Challenge current strategy: Say that you do not agree with his management plan, stating the reasons above.

Emergency warning of critical danger: Say that you do not feel the patient is well enough to be discharged and that you must discuss the situation with a senior colleague.

You should discuss both the correct management and the potential risk to patient safety. You should be satisfied that your senior will take steps to address the patient safety issue. As in all situations you should clearly document your actions and any discussions that have taken place.

 WARNING

6

- You MUST address and escalate patient safety risks appropriately whatever your stage of training.

✔ How to excel in this station		
Action	**Reason**	**How**
Use a structured approach to handover.	Using a structured approach minimises omissions and makes you appear slick.	Use the SBAR approach as demonstrated in 'Approach to the Station'. Practise using this when handing over other patients.
Highlight patient safety concerns.	Patient safety is always a major concern and examiners will want you to demonstrate how you would deal with this challenging situation.	Use the time to discuss your concerns with the examiner and suggest possibilities for dealing with them.

✘ Common errors in this station		
Common error	**Remedy**	**Reason**
Accepting the incorrect advice.	Read the acute asthma guidelines.	The guidelines clearly suggest this patient is unwell and should be admitted.
Becoming angry with the referrer.	You should politely but firmly challenge what you believe to be incorrect advice.	Although you may feel frustrated remember that you are a professional and that your primary duty is to the patient.

6 | STATION VARIATIONS

○ Basic

You may simply be asked to hand over a patient without the more complex patient safety element. You should practise this skill and get feedback on it, particularly in real life clinical situations or in simulated scenarios.

○ Intermediate

You could be asked to treat an unwell patient (such as any of the scenarios in Chapter 7) and then hand that patient over to another doctor or team. You can practise your hand-over by using the scenarios in that chapter.

Further Reading

General Medical Council, 'Good Medical Practice', Domain 2 Safety and quality (GMC, London, 2013). Available at http://www.gmc-uk.org/guidance/good_medical_practice/safety_quality.asp.

Scottish Intercollegiate Guidelines Network, 2012. British Guidelines on the Management of Asthma. Management of Acute Asthma, Chapter 6.

National Institute of Healthcare, Guidelines for the Diagnosis and Management of Asthma (US guidance), available at http://www.nhlbi.nih.gov.

Recognising and managing acutely unwell patients

Introduction to assessing acutely unwell patients

This chapter explores how to tackle stations involving acutely unwell patients. This increasingly common type of station can be conducted as a structured oral examination with an examiner asking you to describe your management (and possibly explain it to a simulated patient). More frequently, where facilities are available, you may be asked to act out your management in a simulated environment with a medical simulation manikin. In a simulated station you may also have a 'helper' (i.e., a person acting as a nurse whom you can issue instructions to), or your examiner may perform this role. If there is a 'helper' you must ensure that you give clear and concise instructions — they are likely to simulate performing the task so try to avoid giving a barrage of requests too quickly for them to complete.

KEY SKILLS

To attempt these stations it is helpful to know a little about the disease process and initial management of the various conditions. However, very little specialist knowledge is necessary to score well in these stations — the idea is to perform a rapid initial assessment and start urgent treatment, whilst ensuring that senior or specialist help is called. These stations share some common elements:

1. Using a systematic ABCDE approach to assess the patient;
2. Calling for assistance or senior help appropriately; and
3. Safe and appropriate initial management of the patient.

Other important themes for these stations include:

1. Establishing a rapport with the patient (and helpers if present);
2. Giving a running commentary so that the examiner can follow your train of thought and see that you are using a systematic approach; and
3. Remaining calm and systematic, giving clear concise instructions to helpers, or explaining your step-by-step management to the examiner.

It helps to practise these stations in larger groups (ideally 4 or more), so that you can act out the various roles (candidate, examiner, helper and patient) to enable better feedback on how you perform in this station type. You can use the practice mark-sheets provided online to get an idea of your performance. If you have any access to a simulation suite it is helpful to ask for extra training sessions or to sign up to them.

Acute management of chest pain

7.1

CANDIDATE INFORMATION

Background: You are the junior doctor in the Emergency Department and have been asked to see Mr Henry Jackson (64 years old). He has presented with a history of central chest pain and has a past medical history of type 2 diabetes, hypertension and ischaemic heart disease. He looks clammy and is in pain. He has been given 300 mg aspirin en route to the hospital.

Task: Please take a short history, examine him and initiate a management plan including pertinent investigations.

APPROACH TO THE STATION

This station would probably have a simulated patient with some key investigations to interpret. As with all of the acute management stations, a focused ABCDE assessment is a key skill. The differential diagnosis of chest pain is covered in station 2.1. In this case the history is suggestive of cardiac pain. You should ask a few quick questions to help with the diagnosis (station 2.1). If the person currently has chest pain, this must be managed as *acute coronary syndrome*. The most important investigation is an ECG—so you should ask for this as part of your ABCDE approach (Fig. 7.1.1), which detects the potential complications of acute coronary syndrome (Table 7.1.1). The management of acute coronary syndrome is constantly evolving, so be aware of the latest local and national guidance. Table 7.1.1 summarises the current approaches to management.

PATIENT INFORMATION

Name: Mr Henry Jackson   **Age:** 64 years   **Sex:** Male

You have had 40 minutes of central chest tightness. It is also present in your jaw and you feel breathless and nauseous. It is similar to your angina pain but is more severe and has persisted. You used your angina spray but it did not help.

Patient observations (given by the examiner):

Airway: Intact.

Breathing: Respiratory rate 32 breaths/min. Oxygen saturations 90% on air. Chest clear.

Circulation: Looks sweaty. Pulse 98/min. Blood pressure 160/90 mmHg. Capillary refill <2 s.

Disability: Glasgow coma scale 15/15.

Exposure: Coronary artery bypass graft (CABG) scar. Abdominal examination normal. No calf swelling.

Station will require
1) ECG showing acute ST elevation myocardial infarction (STEMI) (Fig. 7.1.1)
2) Oxygen mask
3) Chest radiograph showing acute pulmonary oedema (Fig. 7.1.2).

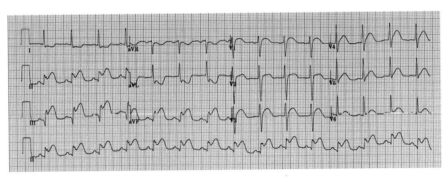

Figure 7.1.1 12-lead ECG showing inferior MI

Table 7.1.1 Potential complications of acute coronary syndrome

Complication	Detection	Management (on top of ACS management)
Acute pulmonary oedema	B—breathlessness, bilateral chest crepitations, hypoxia. Chest X-ray as below	Oxygen, intravenous diuretics, nitrates, opiates
Cardiogenic shock	C—hypotension, tachycardia, increased capilliary refill	250 ml fluid bolus; consider inotropic support
Arrhythmia	C—hypotension, tachy/bradycardia, ECG	Heart block—consider pacemaker Tachyarrhythmia—electrical or chemical cardioversion Cardiac arrest—as per advanced life support guidance

CLINICAL KNOWLEDGE AND EXPERTISE

The assessment and management of acute chest pain/coronary syndromes are covered in Figs. 7.1.3 and 7.1.4.

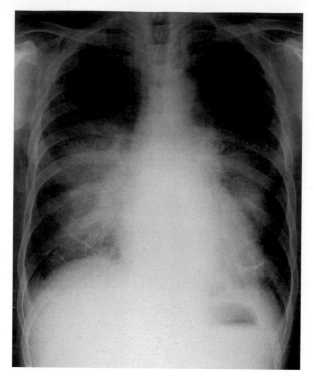

Figure 7.1.2 Chest X-ray showing pulmonary oedema

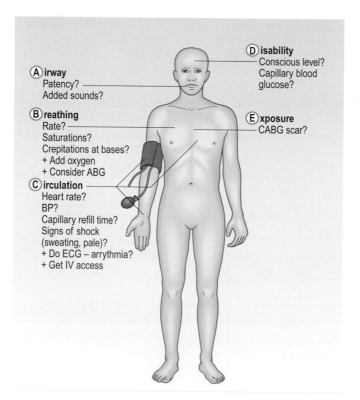

Ⓓisability
Conscious level?
Capillary blood
glucose?

Ⓐirway
Patency?
Added sounds?

Ⓔxposure
CABG scar?

Ⓑreathing
Rate?
Saturations?
Crepitations at bases?
+ Add oxygen
+ Consider ABG

Ⓒirculation
Heart rate?
BP?
Capillary refill time?
Signs of shock
(sweating, pale)?
+ Do ECG – arrythmia?
+ Get IV access

Figure 7.1.3 ABCDE approach in chest pain

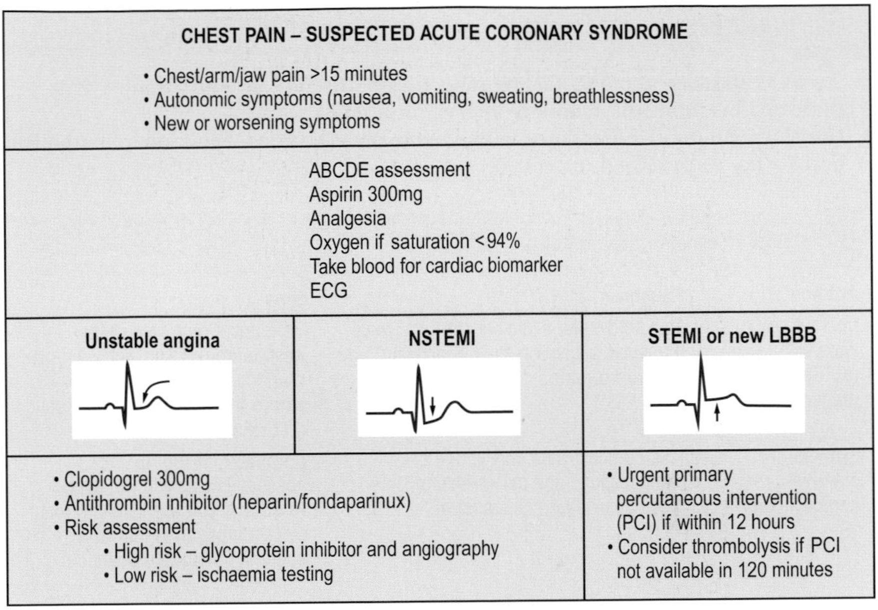

CHEST PAIN – SUSPECTED ACUTE CORONARY SYNDROME

- Chest/arm/jaw pain >15 minutes
- Autonomic symptoms (nausea, vomiting, sweating, breathlessness)
- New or worsening symptoms

ABCDE assessment
Aspirin 300mg
Analgesia
Oxygen if saturation <94%
Take blood for cardiac biomarker
ECG

Unstable angina	NSTEMI	STEMI or new LBBB

- Clopidogrel 300mg
- Antithrombin inhibitor (heparin/fondaparinux)
- Risk assessment
  - High risk – glycoprotein inhibitor and angiography
  - Low risk – ischaemia testing

- Urgent primary percutaneous intervention (PCI) if within 12 hours
- Consider thrombolysis if PCI not available in 120 minutes

Figure 7.1.4 Management of suspected acute coronary syndrome

7

ECG interpretation is a key skill and you should be able to recognise patterns of common abnormalities. However, it is important to look at the ECG in a structured manner to ensure that you do not miss anything. You can do this in the following way:

1. Calculate heart rate.
2. Determine heart rhythm.
3. Determine axis.
4. Examine the components of the ECG in order:
   a. P waves
   b. PR interval
   c. QRS complexes
   d. ST sections
   e. T waves.

The leads affected on the ECG show the area of the abnormality and the likely artery affected (Table 7.1.2).

Table 7.1.2 Area of abnormality and likely artery affected		
Inferior	II, III, AVF	Right coronary
Anterior	V1–V4	Left anterior descending
Lateral	I, V5–V6	Left circumflex
Posterior	ST depression V1–V3	Posterior descending

7

⚠ WARNING

- An ECG showing acute STEMI requires urgent discussion with a centre that performs percutaneous coronary intervention (PCI).
- Consider differential diagnoses with similar presentations—pulmonary embolism and aortic/oesophageal dissection.

✓ How to excel in this station

Action	Reason	How
Up-to-date knowledge of ACS management.	This shows the examiner that you have managed patients with ACS and that you keep up-to-date.	Read local guidance in the hospital/region you work in. Local management will depend on where the nearest interventional cardiology centre is.
Examine for potential complications.	This demonstrates knowledge of complications and awareness of how these can affect management.	Comment on the ABCDE assessment as you go along (e.g., that you are listening for basal crepitations that may suggest pulmonary oedema).

✗ Common errors in this station

Common error	Remedy	Reason
Running out of time.	Practise these sorts of scenarios with colleagues.	It is very tempting to treat this just as another history-taking station and to focus on that to the exclusion of the other parts. The key is a short, focused history.

STATION VARIATIONS

○ Basic

An easier station could simply involve a patient without pulmonary oedema or a simple ECG interpretation.

○ Advanced

If the ECG shows an acute STEMI you may be asked to discuss the patient with a cardiologist—you could do this using the SBAR handover approach shown in station 6.6.

Further Reading

Macleod's Clinical Diagnosis, Chapter 6, 'Chest Pain'.
American Heart Association guidelines, Part 10: 'Acute Coronary Syndromes' (2010).
NICE guidance 167, 'The Acute Management of Myocardial Infarction with ST—segment elevation' (2013).
NICE guidance 94. 'Unstable Angina and NSTEMI' (2010).

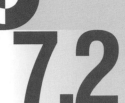

Acute management of breathlessness (1)

7.2

CANDIDATE INFORMATION

Background: You are the junior doctor covering general surgery and are asked to review a 53-year-old woman who underwent an elective (open) cholecystectomy 2 days ago. The nursing staff report that she has a respiratory rate of 28 breaths/min, oxygen saturation of 92%, and a temperature of 38.8 °C. She has no past medical history of note.

Task: Please review this patient.

APPROACH TO THE STATION

This station may be conducted as a structured oral with an examiner asking you to describe your management (and possibly explain it to a simulated patient). Alternatively, you may be asked to act out your management in a simulated environment with a manikin (Fig. 7.2.1; see station 7.0 for how to approach such stations). You may have a 'helper' taking part in the simulation (usually acting as a nurse whom you can issue

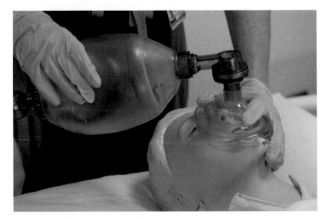

Figure 7.2.1 Simulation suite with manikin

7

instructions to), or your examiner may perform this role. If there is a helper you must ensure that you give clear and concise instructions and allow them time to perform the given task before asking them to do something else.

The key to the management of acutely unwell patients is to be systematic and to call for help from your seniors in managing unwell patients. The structured, systems-based ABCDE approach will help ensure that you don't miss anything and that you deal with adverse signs in order of urgency.

It is important to give a running commentary.

PATIENT INFORMATION

Name: Christine Barker   **Age:** 53 years   **Sex:** Female

You are breathless and hot. You still have some pain around the surgical site and a cough with green sputum. You were well prior to your operation.

Patient observations/clinical findings (given by the examiner):

Airway: Airway patent, talking but unable to complete sentences.

Breathing: Respiratory rate 28/min. Oxygen saturations 92% on air. Chest auscultation: left basal crepitations and reduced breath sounds at left base. Percussion: dull at left base but normal elsewhere. Bilateral chest expansion. ABGs not yet done but candidate should ask for them (will be told to wait for result). CXR has been done about 30 mins ago and will be shown to the candidate when they ask for a CXR.

Circulation: Pulse 122 bpm. Temperature 38.8 °C. BP 88/66. CRT <2 s, peripherally feels warm. The patient does not have a catheter but passed 240 ml of urine 2 h ago.

Disability: CGS 15/15, A on AVPU score. BM 6.2.

Exposure: Looks flushed. No rashes, calf swelling, etc.

CLINICAL KNOWLEDGE AND EXPERTISE

Table 7.2.1 gives a brief summary of the ABCDE approach. It is necessary to tailor your approach to the patient and respond to the physiological parameters you've been given. The idea of ABCDE is to not move on to the next element if you are not happy with the one you are on. It is acceptable, however, to institute some treatment for the abnormal parameters and to continue assessment while you wait for it to work. For example, if you find that the patient has a high respiratory rate, low oxygen saturation and wheeze, you could start oxygen and nebulisers and move on to assess circulation. You should explain that this is so the examiner knows that you have recognised the problem and are responding to it.

If you are stuck it can be helpful to reassess the patient starting from A.

This station includes interpretation of a chest X-ray (Fig. 7.2.2) — a quick reminder of how to present a chest X-ray:
- Confirm patient identity.
- Type of film — Antero-posterior (AP)/ postero-anterior (PA), erect, supine, etc. A mobile AP film is usually done if a patient is too unwell to attend the radiology department.
- Comment on the adequacy of the film (rotation, penetration and lung expansion), but if the X-ray shows an obvious abnormality it is more appropriate to state this first, then discuss adequacy at the end.

Table 7.2.1 General ABCDE approach

A	Airway	Do they have an airway?	If they are talking or groaning, yes; if noisy breathing or stridor, no; assess further.
B	Breathing	Are they breathing? Is the breathing normal?	Check for chest wall movements, respiratory rate, oxygen saturation, auscultate the chest, percuss if relevant. Give the patient oxygen. Ask for investigations as appropriate (CXR, ABG, etc.).
C	Circulation	Assess circulation.	Check pulse, blood pressure, capillary refill time, temperature, urine output (or ask for a catheter to be inserted if appropriate). Give the patient IV fluids if indicated. Ask for investigations (blood tests, lactate level, etc.).
D	Disability (+glucose)	What is the conscious level?	Calculate their AVPU or GCS. Ask for a capillary glucose (BM).
E	Exposure	Is there anything else to be aware of?	Expose the patient, looking for rashes, bleeding points, swelling, abdominal distension.

Figure 7.2.2 Lobar pneumonia (From Kumar, P & Clark M: Kumar & Clark's *Medical Management and Therapeutics* (Saunders 2011) with permission.)

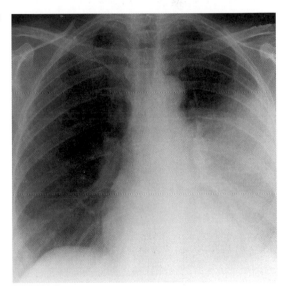

- 'The obvious abnormality is . . .' — Describe what you see, e.g., an area of consolidation in the left lower zone/a mass in the right upper zone/abnormal translucency on the left compared to the right, etc.
- 'This abnormality is in keeping with . . . infection (pneumonia)/a tumour/a pneumothorax.'
- If you cannot see an obvious abnormality, say so and proceed to your systematic structural description.
- Systematically comment on the other visible structures; check the lungs (including the apices), heart borders and heart size, mediastinum, bony structures (ribs, clavicles, scapulae, humeral heads), the diaphragm (including air under the diaphragm), the gastric bubble. It does not matter in what order you do this but make sure nothing is missed.

7

- Comment on any other visible structures/equipment (oxygen mask, ECG electrodes, sternal wiring, endotracheal tube, central line, nasogastric-tube, etc.). If you are unsure what it is, just describe it.

⚠ WARNING

- Pneumonia is serious and can carry a high mortality. Ask for input from seniors and the hospital critical care team, as appropriate. (Note that the CURB-65 pneumonia risk score is designed for community-acquired pneumonia and should not be used in this case.)
- Postoperative patients with poorly controlled pain are likely to deteriorate if their pain is not controlled due to an inability to cough and deep breathe. If there is severe pain, there may also be problems at the surgical site (for example, bleeding or anastamotic leak). Get advice from the hospital pain team, anaesthetist on call or surgical team as appropriate.

✓ How to excel in this station

Action	Reason	How
Clear, systematic management.	This demonstrates that you can methodically assess an unwell patient and begin emergency treatment.	Ask for senior support as soon as you recognise acute illness. Give your helper clear, calm instructions and talk through your assessment. Use the ABCDE approach.

✗ Common errors in this station

Common error	Remedy	Reason
Unstructured approach.	Become familiar with the ABCDE approach by talking through cases, practising in simulation suites or observing in acute clinical areas.	If your ABCDE approach becomes second nature, you can deal with cases of increasing complexity without overlooking things or getting flustered.
Inappropriate pace (too fast or too slow).	Practise stations like this in simulation suites or skills labs. Ask for feedback on how well you manage as a team-leader.	If your pace is too fast, both your helper and the examiner may get confused and instructions may be missed. If it is too slow, you appear hesitant and the patient may continue to deteriorate, making the station more stressful.

STATION VARIATIONS

⊙ Basic

Chest X-ray interpretation alone.

⊙ ⊙ Intermediate/Advanced

Discussion of appropriate prescribing of antibiotics or IV fluids in a patient with pneumonia.

Further Reading

Macleod's Clinical Diagnosis, Chapter 12, 'Dyspnoea'.
It is useful to read your hospital's management and antibiotic guidance for pneumonia as there are variations in local prescribing practice.

Acute management of breathlessness (2)

7.3

CANDIDATE INFORMATION

Background: You are the junior doctor on call and have been asked to see Mrs Mary Benjamin (53 years old). She has been admitted with breathlessness and has a history of chronic obstructive pulmonary disease (COPD) and hypertension. Her COPD is usually well controlled on regular inhaled steroids and long-acting tiotropium. She has been feeling unwell for 3 days and has become increasingly breathless despite using her inhaled salbutamol.

Task: Please assess and treat her for her breathlessness. A prescription chart is included for you to prescribe medication if required.

APPROACH TO THE STATION

With an acutely breathless patient, you may need to keep your history taking to a minimum as the patient may be too breathless to answer. Follow ABCDE and then request the appropriate investigations. When applying oxygen to a breathless patient it is important to know whether they have COPD as this will guide your initial oxygen prescription. Anticipate in this station that you will have to interpret investigations such as arterial blood gases and a chest X-ray and prescribe medication.

PATIENT INFORMATION

Name: Mary Benjamin   **Age:** 53 years   **Sex:** Female

You have COPD but it is normally well controlled and you can walk as far as you like. You have not been in hospital before with breathlessness. You have had courses of antibiotics and steroids from your general practitioner but only once or twice a year. You have been feeling breathless for 3 days with wheeze and a dry non-productive cough. You have been using your salbutamol inhaler more than usual but have become more breathless and are finding it difficult to talk. You do not have any allergies.

Patient observations:

Airway: Is intact.

Breathing: Respiratory rate 36 breaths/min. Oxygen saturations 84% on air. Chest sounds wheezy.

(Continued)

7

Circulation: Pulse 110/min regular. Blood pressure 130/70 mmHg. Capillary refill <2 s.

Disability: Glasgow coma scale 15/15.

Exposure: Looks sweaty. Abdominal examination normal. No calf swelling.

Station will require the following:
1. Blood gas result (shown below)
2. Normal ECG
3. Normal chest X-ray
4. Variety of oxygen masks (non-rebreathing mask and venture masks)
5. A nebuliser.

Blood gas result (on air)

pH 7.20 (7.35–7.45)

$PaCO_2$ 8.5 kPA

PaO_2 7.5 kPA

HCO_3 24 mmol/L (20–28)

Base excess 1.3 (+2 -2)

CLINICAL KNOWLEDGE AND EXPERTISE

An ABCDE assessment should be carried out and the following investigations requested:
- Arterial blood gas (ABG)
- CXR
- ECG
- Blood tests (FBC and U + E, consider D-Dimer if suspected PE depending on risk score).

These should help you to decide the cause of the breathlessness (Table 7.3.1). Table 7.3.2 summarises some of the key findings for some of the more common causes of breathlessness.

Oxygen prescription

Oxygen should be considered in all breathless patients. It may not be required if oxygenation is adequate (pulse oximeter saturation >94% or normal oxygenation on ABG).

If there is no concern about COPD give as much oxygen as required to get saturations >94% — this can be by either nasal cannulae, a controlled oxygen device, or a non-rebreathing mask (which can supply higher concentrations of inspired oxygen).

Table 7.3.1 Common differential diagnoses for acute breathlessness	
Airway	Foreign body, epiglottitis, trauma, anaphylaxis
Breathing	Asthma, COPD, pneumonia, pulmonary embolism (PE), pleural effusion, pneumothorax, mucus plugging, lobar collapse
Circulation	Pulmonary oedema, acute coronary syndrome, cardiac tamponade, aortic dissection, arrhythmia
Others	Sepsis and metabolic acidosis

Table 7.3.2 Key findings for the common causes of acute breathlessness

Condition	Clinical features	CXR	ECG	ABG
COPD	Smoking history, wheezing	Hyperinflation	Normal or right heart strain	Type 1 or type 2 respiratory failure
Pneumonia	Productive cough, lung, unilateral crepitations, signs of sepsis	Consolidation	Normal or tachycardia	Usually type 1 respiratory failure (see station 7.2)
Pulmonary oedema	History of heart disease, bilateral crepitations, leg oedema	Upper lobe diversion Pleural effusions Perihilar oedema Cardiomegaly	Signs of ischaemia or infarction	Type 1 or type 2 respiratory failure
Pulmonary embolism	Pleuritic chest pain, risk factors (immobility, hospitalisation), haemoptysis, signs of deep vein thrombosis	Usually normal Occasionally wedge-shaped infarcts or small effusion	Most commonly sinus tachycardia. Right heart strain (RBBB, S1 Q3 T3 sign) or atrial fibrillation	Type 1 respiratory failure

Some patients with COPD are at risk of developing acute acidotic CO_2 retention and this can be worsened by high inspired oxygen concentrations. Therefore, you should aim to use as low a concentration of (controlled) oxygen therapy as possible to get saturations between 88 and 92%. You should use a controlled oxygen device such as a Venturi mask to supply the oxygen (usually at 24, 28, 40 or 60% O_2). The patient should have regular blood gas measurement until stable (by arterial gas, arterial line or capillary blood gas sampling (Fig. 7.3.1)).

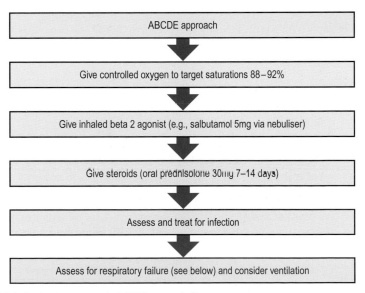

Figure 7.3.1 Acute management of COPD exacerbation

7

Respiratory failure

This is classified by the ABG result. Respiratory failure is defined as an arterial oxygen concentration (PaO_2) <8 kPA (60 mmHg). This can be difficult to interpret if the patient is receiving oxygen, but approximately the oxygen concentration in kPA should be inspired oxygen concentration minus 10 (e.g., if inspired oxygen is 40%, the kPA should be about 30 — if it is less than this, there is a ventilation-to-perfusion mismatch). To calculate the ventilation/perfusion mismatch accurately you can use a formula such as the alveolar:arterial oxygen gradient.

Respiratory failure is further classified into the following:

- *Type 1 respiratory failure* (example pH 7.42, $PaCO_2$ 3.5 kPA, PaO_2 7.5 kPA, HCO_3 24 mmol/l).
- A low PaO_2 but a normal (or low) $PaCO_2$ — indicates a ventilation/perfusion mismatch, for example, PE or pneumonia.
- *Type 2 respiratory failure* (example pH 7.20, $PaCO_2$ 8.5 kPA, PaO_2 7.5 kPA, HCO_3 24 mmol/l)
- A low PaO_2 and a high $PaCO_2$ — most commonly due to acute exacerbations of COPD but also occurs:
  - If patients are tiring due to prolonged periods of breathlessness (e.g., in pneumonia or asthma).
  - If there is a neuromuscular problem such as in motor neurone disease or if the patient is drowsy (e.g., from sedative drugs).
  - In COPD there can be some metabolic compensation to chronic hypercarbia — the pH can then be normal (example pH 7.39, $PaCO_2$ 8.5 kPA, PaO_2 7.5 kPA, HCO_3 30 mmol/l).
  - Patients with acute exacerbations of COPD with type 2 respiratory failure should be considered for non-invasive positive pressure ventilation (NIPPV). Prior to starting, a decision should be made about a ceiling of care; i.e., should there be escalation to invasive ventilation if NIPPV fails?
  - Patients without COPD who develop type 2 respiratory failure should be considered for invasive ventilation.

⚠ WARNING

- Not all patients with type 2 respiratory failure have COPD — in patients with asthma or pneumonia it indicates a patient is tiring and invasive ventilation should be considered urgently.

✓ How to excel in this station

Action	Reason	How
Oxygen prescription.	Patients with COPD can be oxygen sensitive and prescribing fixed oxygen therapy is good practice.	Write it on the prescription chart (some may have a specific place to prescribe); e.g., 'Oxygen 28% via Venturi mask at 4 l/min'.
Ask about allergies.	This is an essential part of safe prescribing.	Ask the patient prior to writing the prescription.
Know about oxygen masks.	You may be asked to apply one to a simulated patient.	Spend time on the ward or in the simulation lab getting to know the types of oxygen mask, how they are applied and the indications for each.
Assess baseline functional status.	This is important in guiding decisions about escalation of care.	Ask the patient or a relative about how limited they are by breathlessness—you could ask about how far can they walk, if they can climb a flight of stairs and whether they use oxygen at home.

Common error	Remedy	Reason
Uncontrolled oxygen therapy.	Use fixed-flow oxygen delivery titrated to the patient's oxygen saturations.	Uncontrolled oxygen therapy can be dangerous in a section of patients with COPD. You should aim to give the lowest concentration of oxygen that achieves target saturation levels.
Missing alternative diagnoses.	Assess CXR and ECG as well.	You could miss a pneumothorax or pneumonia, both of which are alternative reasons why a person with COPD could destabilise.

✗ Common errors in this station

STATION VARIATIONS

○ Basic

You could simply be given a set of blood gas results to discuss with an examiner.

○ Advanced

In an advanced station you could be asked to assess the patient for non-invasive ventilation and consider their escalation status (usually for postgraduates).

Further Reading

Station 3.3, Examining the breathless patient.

Macleod's Clinical Diagnosis, Chapter 12, 'Dyspnoea'.

Global initiative for Obstructive Lung Disease (GOLD) guidelines, http://www.goldcopd.org.

7

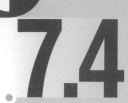

Acute management of abdominal pain

7.4

CANDIDATE INFORMATION

Background: You are a junior doctor and are asked to review a patient admitted to the Surgical Assessment Unit complaining of increasing abdominal pain over the past 48 hours. The pain was initially central but today became more localised to the right side, and in the past couple of hours has become very severe.

Task: Perform an initial assessment of the patient and initiate any necessary immediate management steps.

APPROACH TO THE STATION

Acute appendicitis is common in both adults and children. Most patients remain relatively well and often their observations are within normal limits once they have had pain relief. However, progression of acute appendicitis to perforation and peritonitis can occur and these patients can be very unwell and may develop shock. Ensure you are familiar with the main features of acute appendicitis, including symptoms and signs, necessary investigations, treatment and potential complications (Table 7.4.1).

This station may be conducted as a structured oral examination or as a clinical scenario with a manikin. When assessing acutely unwell patients, it is important to use the ABCDE approach and perform the necessary investigations or basic management at each stage, prior to moving on. This approach will always mean that you have treated the most important things first and don't miss anything out.

Table 7.4.1 Features of acute appendicitis	
Symptoms	Abdominal pain, classically starts centrally then localises to the right iliac fossa (RIF) Malaise Poor appetite Fever Diarrhoea (due to retroperitoneal irritation)
Signs	Tachycardia Tachypnoea Fever Abdominal pain with guarding—classically at McBurney's point in RIF (see Fig. 7.4.1), also Rovsing's sign may be positive (pressure in the LIF causes pain maximally in the RIF) Rigidity of the abdomen—suggests peritonitis and perforation

Table 7.4.1 Features of acute appendicitis—cont'd

Investigations	WCC + CRP may be increased USS—may show inflammation of the appendix, though this is normally only performed if there is diagnostic uncertainty Erect CXR if perforation is suspected
Complications	Perforation Appendix mass Appendix abscess
Treatment	Appendicitis—appendectomy (open or laparoscopic) Appendix mass or abscess—normally require IV antibiotics and the appendix is ideally removed a few weeks later when it is less inflamed, though they sometimes require removal or drainage acutely

Figure 7.4.1 McBurney's point

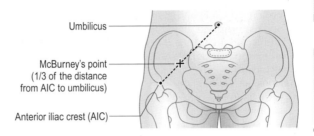

Umbilicus

McBurney's point
(1/3 of the distance
from AIC to umbilicus)

Anterior iliac crest (AIC)

7

PATIENT INFORMATION

Name: John Jones **Age:** 24 years **Sex:** Male

Clinical information (provided by the examiner):

Airway: Patent and patient is talking.

Breathing: Respiratory rate 28/min. O$_2$ saturations 98% on air. Chest clear on auscultation.

Circulation: Pulse 130/min. Temperature 38.5 °C. BP 90/65. CRT 3 s, peripherally feels warm.

Disability: GCS 15/15. A on AVPU score. BM 5.6.

Exposure: Looks sweaty and uncomfortable, complaining of severe pain. Palpation of the abdomen reveals rigidity.

CLINICAL KNOWLEDGE AND EXPERTISE

Airway
- Introduce yourself and explain what you are about to do.
- If they talk in response, the airway is patent.
- If not, consider opening the airway (head tilt, chin lift) and reassessing.

- Only move on to B when you are happy the airway is patent.
  - In this case, the patient is talking and responding, therefore the airway is clear and you may move on.

Breathing

- Take, or ask for, the respiratory rate and oxygen saturations.
- Auscultate the chest and percuss if relevant.
- Apply high flow oxygen if the patient has an increased respiratory rate or low saturation, or appears unwell.
- Ask for further investigations (CXR, blood gas) as appropriate:
  - In this case, the respiratory rate is high but there is no apparent chest cause; therefore, commence high flow oxygen, request a CXR and move on.

Circulation

- Take or request the pulse, blood pressure, CRT and urine output.
- Insert 1–2 cannulae if there are signs of circulatory shock (tachycardia, hypotension, prolonged CRT) and give an IV fluid bolus.
- Send appropriate blood tests—for example, a U+E, CRP, FBC, LFT, amylase and lactate to aid the diagnosis, a blood culture if the patient is febrile and a cross-match sample and clotting studies, if the patient might be going to theatre.
- Consider placing a urinary catheter and commencing a fluid balance chart.
- If the patient is febrile and the cause is unknown, start broad-spectrum antibiotics.
  - In this case, the patient has signs of shock; therefore, you should call for help if you had not already done so.
  - Reassess after the bolus for clinical improvement and consider repeating the bolus if there is no improvement.
  - Commence antibiotics in view of the fever—for example, cefuroxime and metronidazole.
  - State that you would like a urinary catheter inserted.
  - If you see clinical improvement after your interventions, you may move on.

Disability (+ glucose)

- Calculate their AVPU or GCS.
- Ask for a capillary glucose (BM).
  - In this case, the patient is alert and the glucose is satisfactory. You may move on.

Exposure

- Expose the patient looking for rashes, haemorrhage, or swellings.
- Inspect and palpate the abdomen for clinical signs.
- Ask for the temperature.
  - In this case, further assessment of the patient reveals a rigid and extremely painful abdomen. This is highly suggestive of a perforation leading to peritonitis.
  - Appropriate management is to request an erect CXR (looking for free air under the diaphragm), start antibiotics if not already given and urgently call the surgical senior trainee for assessment of the patient, who is likely to arrange urgent transfer to theatre.

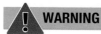 **WARNING**

- If a patient has signs of peritonitis, even without any signs of shock, the surgical team must urgently see them, as they require resuscitation and transfer to theatre for definitive management.

- Features of shock must be taken very seriously as patients can rapidly deteriorate. Initial management involves gaining intravenous access and giving fluid boluses, titrated to clinical response. If no clinical improvement, care needs to be escalated to senior staff and potentially to the intensive care team.

✓ How to excel in this station		
Action	**Reason**	**How**
Assess and treat as per ABCDE.	From the background you will be suspecting appendicitis and it may be tempting to examine the abdomen before completing the other sections of ABCD.	If you did this, you would miss the features of shock that need to be dealt with urgently and this could lead you to fail. Do not be distracted by the case background and assess the patient using ABCDE, investigating and initiating management at each stage before moving on.

✗ Common errors in this station		
Common error	**Remedy**	**Reason**
Missing signs of shock.	Recognise warning signs of shock—tachycardia, narrow pulse pressure, hypotension, prolonged CRT.	This is very important to show your knowledge of shock and that you can initiate resuscitative measures.
Missing signs of peritonitis.	Recognise signs of peritonitis—severe abdominal pain, often generalised and worse on moving and inspiration (shallow breathing) and a rigid abdomen on palpation.	Peritonitis can lead to septic shock if not recognised early and it is crucial you demonstrate your awareness of this. You should also show that you recognise the patient needs urgent review by the surgical team and resuscitation as required, and will likely need urgent transfer to theatre.

7

STATION VARIATIONS

⭘ Basic

Appendicitis

You may be informed that patient has clinical features of appendicitis, without signs of peritonitis. In this case you would still gain IV access and take bloods. However, you would probably not give antibiotics and while the patient needs to be referred for surgical assessment, this does not need to be immediate.

Further Reading

Macleod's Clinical Diagnosis, Chapter 4, 'Abdominal Pain', for further information on the acute abdomen.

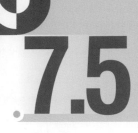

Acute management of a diabetic emergency 7.5

CANDIDATE INFORMATION

Background: You are a junior doctor and are called to review a patient admitted to the Medical Assessment Unit with abdominal pain and rapid breathing, who is normally fit and well. A capillary blood sugar is 28 mmol/l.

Task: Perform an initial assessment of the patient and state the immediate management.

APPROACH TO THE STATION

Diabetic ketoacidosis (DKA) can occur in adults and children, either as an initial presentation of new type 1 diabetes or in known patients. DKA is serious condition and is potentially fatal if not recognised promptly and managed. The diagnosis depends on the triad of a high blood sugar, acidosis and ketones present in the urine or blood (Table 7.5.1). There is national guidance for the management of DKA in adults and children, which is normally available locally (or local adaptation).

As in other stations within this chapter, this station may be conducted as a structured oral examination or as a clinical scenario with a manikin. Follow an ABCDE approach and request the necessary investigations or initiate basic management at each stage, prior to moving on. See Fig. 7.5.1 for a summary of the examination in DKA.

Table 7.5.1 Diagnostic criteria for DKA and 'severe' DKA

Hyperglycaemia	>11 mmol/l
Acidosis	pH <7.3 Bicarbonate <15 mmol/l
Ketonaemia	Blood ketones >3 mmol/l or significant urinary ketones (2+ or more on standard dipstick)
Markers of 'severe' DKA	Blood ketones >6 mmol/l, venous bicarbonate <5 mmol/l, venous pH <7.1, K <3.5 mmol/l GCS <12, systolic BP <90 mmHg, HR <60 or >100 bpm, saturations <92% If any of these features are present, seek senior support ± involve critical care

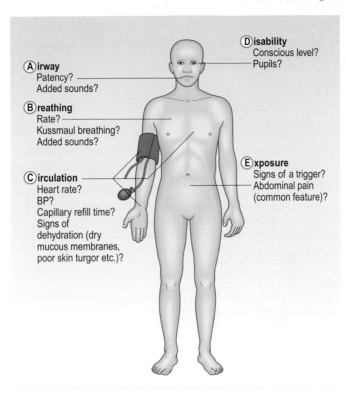

Figure 7.5.1 Examination summary in DKA

PATIENT INFORMATION

Name: Marie Wright **Age:** 26 years **Sex:** Female

Clinical information (from the examiner):

Airway: Patent and patient is talking.

Breathing: Respiratory rate 36/min, with rapid sighing breaths. O₂ saturations 98% on air. Chest clear on auscultation.

Circulation: Pulse 120/min. Temperature 36.7 °C. BP 100/70. CRT 3 s.

Disability: GCS 15/15. A on AVPU score. BM 28.5.

Exposure: Looks pale and tired. Lips and mucous membranes are dry.

CLINICAL KNOWLEDGE AND EXPERTISE

Airway
- Introduce yourself and explain what you are about to do; a patient who responds verbally has a patent airway. If there is no verbal response, consider opening the

7

airway (head tilt, chin lift) and reassessing. Only move on to B when you are happy the airway is patent.

- In this case, the patient is talking and responding to you; therefore, the airway is clear and you may move on.

Breathing

- Take, or ask for, the respiratory rate and oxygen saturations.
- Auscultate the chest and percuss if relevant.
- Apply high flow oxygen if the patient has an increased respiratory rate or low saturation, or appears unwell.
- Ask for further investigations of breathing as appropriate; for example, if the patient is unwell and the cause is unknown, it may be appropriate to perform a blood gas and chest X-ray (CXR).
  - In this case, the respiratory rate is high with shallow, sighing respirations, but there is no apparent chest cause; therefore, it would be appropriate to commence high flow oxygen, request a blood gas and move on.
  - You are informed that the venous blood gas (or capillary gas in children) demonstrates a pH 7.19 and a bicarbonate of 10 mmol/l (see Table 7.5.3 below for information on blood gas interpretation).

Circulation

- Take, or ask for the pulse, blood pressure and capillary refill time (CRT). Attach cardiac monitoring and pulse oximetry.
- Insert 1–2 cannulae if there are signs of circulatory shock (tachycardia, hypotension, prolonged CRT) and give an IV fluid bolus.
- Send appropriate blood tests — for example, a U + E, CRP, FBC, LFT, amylase, blood ketone and lactate to aid the diagnosis, and a blood culture if the patient is febrile.
- Consider placing a urinary catheter and commencing a fluid balance chart.
- If the patient is febrile and the cause is unknown, start broad-spectrum antibiotics.
  - In this case, the patient has signs of shock and has fulfilled two of the diagnostic criteria for DKA (high blood sugar and acidosis).
  - You should call for help if you have not already done so.
  - Request a blood ketone (bedside tests are available) or urine sample for ketones. You are informed ketones are positive and can therefore make the diagnosis of DKA.
  - Commence initial emergency fluid management (as in Table 7.5.2).
  - Reassess regularly.
  - A urinary catheter would be useful but is not an immediate priority.
  - If you see clinical improvement after your interventions, you may move on.

Disability

- Establish the AVPU or GCS.
- Check that the pupils are equal and responsive to light.
- Request the blood sugar if not already known.
  - In this case, the patient is alert, though they may be drowsy and lethargic in DKA.

Exposure

- Expose the patient, looking for rashes, haemorrhage or swellings. Inspect and palpate the abdomen for clinical signs.
  - In this case, further assessment of the patient is unremarkable.
  - State that the diagnosis is DKA as a first presentation of type 1 diabetes (as the patient was previously fit and well). Further history from the patient or family may reveal recent polydipsia and polyuria.

Table 7.5.2 Initial management of DKA*

Management	Initial	Ongoing
Intravenous fluid therapy	If BP <90 mmHg give 500 ml of 0.9% saline as a bolus over 10 min If BP >90 mmHg give 1000 ml of 0.9% saline over 60 min	Repeat if BP remains <90 mmHg Follow this with 1000 ml 0.9% saline over the next 2 h
Potassium	Add 40 mmol/l K to each bag of IV fluid once K <5.5	
Insulin therapy	Commence a fixed rate intravenous insulin infusion at 0.1 unit/kg/h, made up with 50 units soluble insulin in 50 ml 0.9% saline If on long-acting insulin, continue at the same dose and time as well	Add 125 ml/h 10% dextrose once blood glucose <14 mmol/l
Investigations	Blood glucose Blood ketones Blood gas (venous) Urea and electrolytes Full blood count Other investigations as indicated (blood culture, CXR etc.)	Repeat hourly Repeat hourly Repeat at 1 h and then 2 hourly Repeat at 1 h, and then 4 hourly
Monitoring	At least hourly observations (HR, saturations, BP, RR, temperature and GCS) initially; consider continuous cardiac and pulse oximetry monitoring if abnormal observations.	

*Follow local guidance for ongoing management.

7

WARNING

- Involve senior support and critical care teams early if there are any of the features of severe DKA, particularly if these persist following initial resuscitation measures.
- Cerebral oedema is a potentially fatal complication of DKA. Watch for any change in the conscious level and escalate concerns promptly. Fluid resuscitation must be given with caution in patients who are elderly or pregnant or have known cardiac or renal failure.

How to excel in this station

Action	Reason	How
Recognise DKA.	DKA can be fatal if not recognised early and managed. Remember it can occur in patients not known to have diabetes.	Learn the three diagnostic criteria. The symptoms of DKA may be vague—feeling generally unwell, abdominal pain, vomiting, confusion and sighing breathing. Have a high index of suspicion and check a blood sugar.

Common errors in this station

Common error	Remedy	Reason
Bypassing A and B in ABCDE.	Always follow an ABCDE approach. Don't be tempted to start with C, even if you feel that is where the main problem is.	Given the high blood sugar and features of DKA (abdominal pain and sighing respirations), clarifying a diagnosis of DKA with a gas and ketones testing is a priority, but still should not be requested before the airway and breathing are checked.

7

STATION VARIATION

⭕ Advanced

Blood gas interpretation

As part of this station you could be asked to interpret blood gas results. A guide to the common abnormalities is outlined in Table 7.5.3.

Follow this 3-step approach to aid the interpretation:
1. **Assess pH** — acidaemia pH <7.35 or alkalaemia pH >7.45.
2. **Assess bicarbonate and base excess** — if abnormal, this suggests a metabolic component.
3. **Asses the carbon dioxide** — if abnormal, this suggests a respiratory component.

There may be abnormalities suggesting both respiratory and metabolic components, which may be due to compensation mechanisms (for example, increased respiratory rate to 'blow off' CO_2 during a metabolic acidosis, as is seen in DKA), or may be due to a true mixed cause.

Table 7.5.3 Interpretation of blood gases	
pH <7.35	pH >7.45
Metabolic acidosis Low bicarbonate or −ve BE Normal CO_2 Causes—DKA, lactic acidosis, chronic renal failure **NB:** The CO_2 may be low due to respiratory compensation or high in a mixed respiratory and metabolic acidosis.	**Metabolic alkalosis** High bicarbonate or +ve BE Normal CO_2 Causes—excessive GI losses, drug ingestion, electrolyte disturbance **NB:** The CO_2 may be high due to respiratory compensation or low in a mixed respiratory and metabolic alkalosis.
Respiratory acidosis High CO_2 Normal bicarbonate Causes—severe acute ventilator failure, airway obstruction **NB:** The bicarbonate may be high due to renal compensation, for example in chronic respiratory disease.	**Respiratory alkalosis** Low CO_2 Normal bicarbonate Causes—anxiety or central causes, e.g., brain injury **NB:** The bicarbonate may be low due to renal compensation, for example due to chronic central causes.

Further Reading

Macleod's Clinical Diagnosis, Chapter 12, 'Dyspnoea', specifically the 'Interpretation of arterial blood gases' clinical tool.

Macleod's Clinical Examination, Chapter 5, 'The Endocrine System', section on diabetes mellitus; Chapter 7, 'The Respiratory System', section on arterial blood gas analysis.

NICE guidance, Clinical Guideline 15, 'Type 1 Diabetes: Diagnosis and Management of Type 1 Diabetes in Children, Young People and Adults', July 2004 (revised since).

Acute management of sepsis

7.6

CANDIDATE INFORMATION

Background: You are a junior doctor and are asked to review urgently a 38-year-old woman directly admitted to the Medical Assessment Unit with a high temperature and rigors. The patient's baseline observations were abnormal with a high Early Warning Score (EWS) and she thinks that she has not passed urine for over 8 hours; before that she had some burning when passing urine.

Task: Perform an initial assessment of the patient and initiate any necessary immediate management steps.

APPROACH TO THE STATION

Sepsis is a huge problem worldwide. In the UK, 37,000 deaths per year can be attributed to sepsis. Evidence shows that the clinical outcome is substantially improved by providing rapid assessment and treatment in the form of a 'care bundle'. A care bundle is a group of investigations and therapies that need to be performed together to provide a high standard of care. For acute sepsis, the bundle (Box 7.6.1) consists of some basic investigations and therapies that need to be instituted within 3 hours of the clinical suspicion of sepsis alongside an appropriate patient assessment.

This station may be conducted as a structured oral examination or as a clinical scenario with a simulation manikin. When assessing acutely unwell patients, it is important to use the ABCDE approach and perform the necessary investigations or initiate basic management at each stage, prior to moving on. This will always mean that you have treated the most important things first and don't miss anything out.

Box 7.6.1 The sepsis care bundle

The following elements must all be instituted **within 3 h** of clinical suspicion of sepsis:
- Assess **blood lactate** with an ABG or venous lactate.
- Assess urine output by inserting a **urinary catheter.**
- Take **blood cultures** before starting antibiotic therapy (unless this would result in delay to administration of antibiotics).
- Give **high flow oxygen**, providing there are no contraindications.
- Give a **fluid bolus** of 30 ml/kg crystalloid and assess response.
- Start **broad-spectrum antibiotic therapy** without delay.

7

PATIENT INFORMATION

Name: Sarah Robertson   **Age:** 38 years   **Sex:** Female

Clinical information (from the examiner):

Background:

The patient is normally well and works as a teacher. She started to notice burning and stinging on passing urine 2 days ago and has been feeling increasingly unwell since.

Airway: Patent and patient is talking.

Breathing: Respiratory rate 32/min. O_2 saturations 96% on air. Chest clear on auscultation.

Circulation: Pulse 130/min. Temperature 39 °C. BP 88/65. CRT 3 s, peripherally feels warm.

Disability: GCS 14/15. V on AVPU score. BM 5.6.

Exposure: Looks sweaty, flushed, and unwell. Slightly drowsy but easily rousable. Some mild flank tenderness in the left renal angle but the abdomen is soft and non-tender and bowel sounds are present.

CLINICAL KNOWLEDGE AND EXPERTISE

The elements from the **sepsis care bundle** are highlighted below in bold.
The ABCDE approach in this scenario would be as follows (see also Fig. 7.6.1):

Airway
- Introduce yourself and explain what you are about to do.
- If they talk in response to you, the airway is patent.
- If not, consider opening the airway (head tilt, chin lift) and reassessing.
- Only move on to B when you are happy the airway is patent.
  - In this case, the patient is talking and responding, the airway is clear, you may move on.

Breathing
- Take, or ask for, the respiratory rate and oxygen saturations.
- Auscultate the chest and percuss if relevant.
- Apply high flow oxygen if the patient has an increased respiratory rate, low saturation or appears unwell.
- Ask for further investigations (CXR, blood gas) as indicated.
  - In this case, the respiratory rate is high but chest is clear on auscultation; therefore, it would be appropriate to commence **high flow oxygen** and request a CXR and **ABG** (Box 7.6.2).

Circulation
- Take or request the pulse, blood pressure, CRT and urine output.
- Insert 1–2 cannulae if there are signs of shock (tachycardia, hypotension, prolonged CRT) and give an IV fluid bolus.

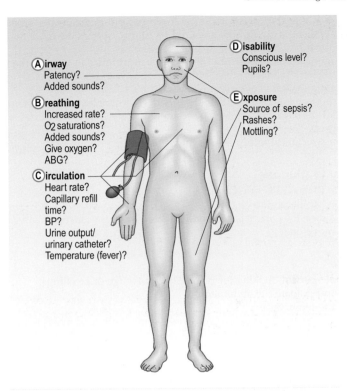

Figure 7.6.1 ABCDE assessment in sepsis

Box 7.6.2	ABG result on air (if requested)
pH	7.20
pCO_2	3.88
pO_2	10.4
HCO_3	16.2
Lactate	4.2
BE	−6.4

- Send appropriate blood tests—for example, a U + E, CRP, FBC, LFT, amylase and lactate to aid the diagnosis, a blood culture if the patient is febrile and a cross-match sample and clotting studies, if the patient might be going to theatre.
- Consider placing a urinary catheter and commencing a fluid balance chart.
- If the patient is febrile and the cause is unknown, start broad-spectrum antibiotics.
  - In this case, the patient has signs of shock; therefore, you should call for help if you had not already done so.
  - Place IV access (ideally two large-bore cannulae), take bloods (including U + Es) and **blood cultures** as the patient has a very high temperature.
  - Check a **venous lactate** or **ABG** if you have not already done so.
  - Give a **fluid bolus** of IV crystalloid.

7

- Reassess after the bolus for clinical improvement and consider repeating the bolus if there is no improvement, up to 30 ml/kg (may be more than 2 l of fluid for a 70-kg patient).
- **Commence broad-spectrum intravenous antibiotics** in view of the fever (ask to check the local prescribing policy but you must suggest an appropriate antibiotic such as piperacillin-tazobactam).
- Ask to place a **urinary catheter**, particularly important here as the patient has not passed urine for several hours and there may be a urinary source of sepsis.
- If you see clinical improvement after your interventions, you may move on.

Disability (+ glucose)

- Calculate their AVPU or GCS.
- Ask for a capillary glucose (BM).
  - In this case, the patient is responding to voice and the glucose is satisfactory. You may move on.

Exposure

- Expose the patient, looking for rashes, haemorrhage or swellings.
- Inspect and palpate the abdomen.
- Ask for the temperature.
  - In this case, further assessment reveals some flank tenderness but no clinical features suggestive of peritonitis or an acute abdomen. The history of dysuria suggests a urinary source but broad-spectrum antibiotics should be given initially until the results of more investigations are available.
  - The history of poor urine output could suggest an acute kidney injury caused by shock (most likely) or possibly urinary obstruction. In either case the insertion of a urinary catheter is crucial for further management.

⚠ WARNING

- You must remember to check the patient's allergies before administering antibiotic treatment.
- Features of shock must be taken very seriously as patients can rapidly deteriorate. Involve senior clinicians with any patient displaying signs of severe sepsis and shock. If there is no response to the initial care bundle, then care needs to be escalated and the patient will need to be managed in critical care.

 How to excel in this station

Action	Reason	How
Assess and treat as per ABCDE.	This allows a rapid and systematic assessment and initial treatment and management for severe sepsis.	Instituting thorough and appropriate systems-based treatment is more important initially than more complex investigations. Doing the basic things well is more likely to result in a good outcome.
Recognise severe sepsis and shock.	Septic shock is associated with a high mortality even in young patients.	Tell the examiner that the clinical signs are in keeping with septic shock. Outline your initial management and involve seniors at an early stage.

Common errors in this station		
Common error	**Remedy**	**Reason**
Poor knowledge of broad-spectrum antibiotics.	Have a good working knowledge of some antimicrobial agents that you could use to treat serious or life-threatening sepsis.	Complex and detailed knowledge of antibiotic pharmacology is not necessary, but it is important to be able to select appropriate initial antibiotic therapy and that it is given without delay.
Poor knowledge of the sepsis care bundle.	Demonstrate to the examiner that you would incorporate the sepsis care bundle into your management.	Guidance from the Surviving Sepsis campaign is widely used across Europe and this recommends the use of a sepsis care bundle to improve outcomes in sepsis.

STATION VARIATION

○ Advanced

Data interpretation and antibiotic prescribing

You may be provided with some clinical information and results from a microbiology report and be asked to select appropriate antibiotic therapy based on the clinical picture, then asked to prescribe it on a drug chart. You will be provided with a BNF to check drug doses. Refer to station 6.1 for how to approach such a station.

Further Reading

Macleod's Clinical Diagnosis, Chapter 28, 'Shock'.

Surviving Sepsis Campaign, in particular the use of sepsis care bundles and the research that led to their introduction, at http://www.survivingsepsis.org.

7

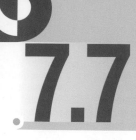

Acute management of postpartum bleeding

7.7

CANDIDATE INFORMATION

Background: You are a junior doctor in the Emergency Department and a 33-year-old woman has been brought in 2 weeks postpartum with brisk vaginal bleeding.

Task: Please assess her and start appropriate treatment.

APPROACH TO THE STATION

This station may be conducted as a structured oral examination, asking you to describe your management (and possibly explain to a simulated patient) or, where facilities are available, you may act out your management in a simulated environment with a manikin (see the chapter introduction, 7.0, for more details). In a simulated station you may also have a 'helper' (usually acting as a nurse to whom you can issue instructions), or your examiner may perform this role.

The key to the management of acutely unwell patients is to be systematic with an ABCDE approach and to call for help from your seniors. The structured, systems-based ABCDE will help ensure that you don't miss anything and that you deal with adverse signs in order of urgency. It is helpful to give a running commentary.

PATIENT INFORMATION

Age: 33 years   **Sex:** Female

You have given birth to your first baby (a boy) 2 weeks ago, who is well and thriving. You are using a mixture of breast and bottle feeds. You have been having ongoing abdominal cramps and quite heavy blood loss from the vagina since giving birth. This evening you started bleeding very heavily and the blood was soaking through your clothes. You are unsure of the volume—it looked like loads. Your partner panicked and called an ambulance when he saw all the blood. You have now started to feel dizzy.

Other information: You are a non-smoker and have no significant medical history. You have had one previous pregnancy but miscarried at 11 weeks.

Patient observations/clinical findings (given by examiner):

Airway: Patent, talking but feeling anxious and unwell.

Breathing: Respiratory rate 30/min. O_2 saturations 97% on air. Chest clear bilaterally with good air entry.

Circulation: Pulse 124/min. Temperature 35.9 °C. BP 88/66. CRT 4 s, peripherally feels cool. No catheter or IV access.

Disability: GCS 14/15. E3, M6, V5. V on AVPU score. Anxious. BM 6.1.

Exposure: Looks pale. Feels light-headed and breathless. Large volume blood loss PV.

CLINICAL KNOWLEDGE AND EXPERTISE

Major postpartum haemorrhage can occur immediately after the birth (primary) or be delayed and occur days or weeks after delivery (secondary). Immediate haemorrhage can be due to a number of causes but by far the commonest is uterine atony, whereas delayed haemorrhage is usually related to retained products. Although major postpartum haemorrhage requires specialist obstetric management, the immediate management of any major blood loss is the same (see also Fig. 7.7.1):
- IV access (2 × large-bore cannulae) and send blood urgently for full blood count, clotting and cross-match.

7

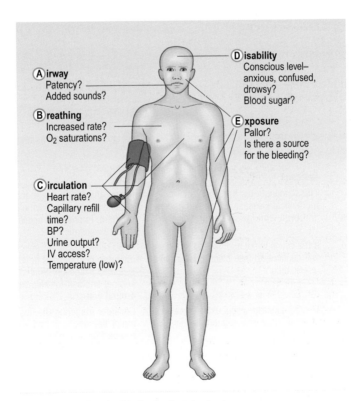

Figure 7.7.1 Examination of patient in hypovolaemic shock

7

- Call for immediate help—you will need other staff available to check blood, put up fluids and resuscitate.
- Call for specialist help—the cause of the bleeding needs to be dealt with, so alert the obstetric team urgently.
- Replace circulating volume with IV fluid (colloid is often used in preference, but crystalloid is acceptable) but only until blood is available.
- Replace blood, using un-cross-matched O negative blood until cross-matched blood is available.
- All bleeding patients should have urgent blood tests including cross-match, clotting and full blood count. An arterial blood gas can be helpful in assessing for signs of shock (high lactate) and may also give an estimated haemoglobin.
- A urinary catheter is very helpful for assessing response to fluid resuscitation.

  A particularly strong candidate may also exhibit knowledge of the following:
- Trigger the hospital's major haemorrhage pathway—this is usually done by calling the switchboard on the emergency number and saying 'major haemorrhage' and giving the patient's location. This allows the blood bank to allocate further O negative blood, and to allocate a 'blood runner' to quickly transport the blood and blood products from the lab.
- Ask advice regarding other appropriate treatments and transfusions—you can ask to speak to the haematologist on call, who will advise you what other blood products and treatments are indicated.
- Hypothermia causes clotting derangement and further bleeding—for massive transfusion it is good to get a blood warmer and a warming blanket™ for the patient (such as a Bair Hugger™).

⚠ WARNING

- Do not underestimate the situation—postpartum haemorrhage is a leading cause of perinatal maternal death in developed countries and world-wide.

✓ How to excel in this station

Action	Reason	How
Clear, systematic management.	This demonstrates that you can methodically assess a bleeding patient and begin emergency treatment.	Follow the ABCDE approach, establishing that circulation is the problem. Prioritise IV access and start fluid resuscitation.
Call for help.	If the cause is not addressed the patient will continue to lose blood despite fluid resuscitation.	It is crucial to call for specialist obstetric help to treat definitively. It is also necessary to alert your seniors and ask for help from those around you.
Consider further management.	This demonstrates your extra knowledge of emergency management to the examiner.	Consider triggering the hospital's major haemorrhage pathway, asking advice from haematology and keeping the patient warm.

Common error	Remedy	Reason
Unstructured approach.	Become familiar with the ABCDE approach by talking through cases, practising in simulation suites or observing in acute clinical areas.	If your ABCDE approach becomes second nature you can deal with cases of increasing complexity without overlooking things or getting flustered.
Getting too tied up in obstetric details.	Concentrate on the immediate management of the bleeding—you do not need to have obstetric knowledge.	A bleeding patient needs the same emergency treatment whatever the cause.

Common errors in this station

STATION VARIATIONS

○ ○ Intermediate/Advanced

This station could be bleeding due to any cause—gastrointestinal bleeding and trauma are other examples.

Further Reading

Royal College of Obstetricians and Gynaecologists, Green-top guideline 52, Prevention and Management of Postpartum Haemorrhage (2009). Available from http://www.rcog.org.uk.

7

Acute management of an unwell child

7.8

CANDIDATE INFORMATION

Background: You are a junior doctor on your Paediatric placement. You have been asked to see a child who has presented with a fever, irritability and lethargy.

Task: Perform an initial assessment of the child and initiate any necessary immediate management steps.

APPROACH TO THE STATION

Bacterial meningitis is a life-threatening condition that requires urgent medical attention. It can occur at any age, but it is common in childhood and adolescence and 20% of bacterial meningitis occurs in the first year of life. Symptoms and signs are often vague and non-specific, so it is important to have a high index of suspicion in children (Table 7.8.1). An overview of the examination findings structured as an A to E approach is included in Fig. 7.8.1. There is national guidance available for the

Table 7.8.1 Features of bacterial meningitis in children and infants	
Symptoms	Fever Vomiting or refusing food and drink Lethargy Irritability Headache
Signs	Shock—tachycardia, hypotension, prolonged capillary refill time, poor perfusion Rash—blanching or non-blanching Decreased conscious level or confusion Respiratory distress Focal neurological deficit or seizures Signs of meningism—bulging fontanelle, stiff neck, photophobia, Kernig's sign positive
Investigations	WCC + CRP may be increased, though they may be normal initially Blood cultures should be sent CT scan may be required prior to LP if there are signs of raised intracranial pressure, or if there is any neurological deficit CSF classically demonstrates a high white cell count (>5), low glucose and high protein

Table 7.8.1 Features of bacterial meningitis in children and infants—cont'd

Treatment	IV antibiotics—protocols depend on age of the infant or child and any specific clinical suspicion of a cause (such as tuberculosis). However, in infants over 3 months, the empirical antibiotic normally commenced is ceftriaxone (80 mg/kg once daily). Steroids—Dexamethasone (0.15 mg/kg qds for 4 days) should be commenced in those children >3 months of age, if there are any of the features below and it is within 12 h of commencing antibiotics. • CSF high WCC (>1000 per microlitre) • Frankly purulent CSF • Bacteria on Gram stain • CSF raised WCC, with protein >1 g/l

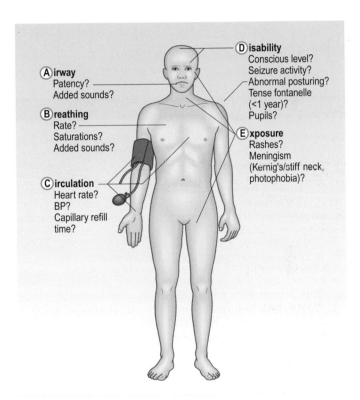

Figure 7.8.1 Possible examination findings in meningitis

assessment and management of children with suspected bacterial meningitis, and most hospitals have a copy of this or similar guidance locally. Comment that you would consult this guidance regarding ongoing management or for further information, for example, regarding specific antibiotic choices.

As in other stations within this chapter, this station may be conducted as a structured oral examination or as a clinical scenario with a simulation manikin. Remember to follow an ABCDE approach and request the necessary investigations or initiate basic management at each stage, prior to moving on.

PATIENT INFORMATION

Name: Connor Grove   **Age:** 2 years   **Sex:** Male

Clinical information (from examiner):

Airway: Patent and patient is crying.

Breathing: Respiratory rate 36/min. O_2 saturations 98% on air. Chest clear on auscultation.

Circulation: Pulse 130/min. Temperature 39.3 °C. BP not reading. CRT 2 s, centrally feels warm with cool peripheries.

Disability: V on AVPU score initially. BM 4.1.

Exposure: Blanching rash on trunk.

CLINICAL KNOWLEDGE AND EXPERTISE

Airway

- Introduce yourself to the child and parents and explain what you are about to do.
- If they are talking or crying, the airway is patent. Listen for added sounds (such as snoring, gurgling).
- If not, consider opening the airway (head tilt, chin lift) and reassessing.
- Only move on to B when you are happy the airway is patent.
  - In this case, the child is crying, therefore the airway is clear and you may move on.

Breathing

- Take, or ask for, the respiratory rate and oxygen saturations.
- Auscultate the chest and percuss if relevant.
- Apply high flow oxygen if the patient has an increased respiratory rate or low saturation, or appears unwell.
- Ask for further investigations (CXR, blood gas) as appropriate.
  - In this case, the respiratory rate is high but there is no apparent chest cause; therefore, it would be appropriate to commence high flow oxygen, request a CXR and a capillary gas and then move on.

Circulation

- Take or request the pulse, blood pressure, capillary refill time and urine output.
- Insert an intravenous cannula if there are signs of circulatory shock (tachycardia, hypotension, prolonged CRT) and give an IV fluid bolus.
- Send appropriate blood tests — for example, a U+E, CRP, FBC and LFT to aid the diagnosis, and a blood culture and meningococcal PCR if the patient is febrile.
- Consider placing a urinary catheter and commencing a fluid balance chart.
- If the patient is febrile and the cause is unknown, start broad-spectrum antibiotics.
  - In this case, although the child is tachycardic, you are informed they are crying and febrile, so they are not necessarily in shock. The normal capillary refill is reassuring. It is often hard to get a BP reading on an unsettled child. In this situation, it would be reasonable to suggest an antipyretic such as paracetamol, recheck the BP and monitor the child carefully, rather than giving a fluid bolus at this stage; however, giving a fluid bolus (10 ml/kg of 0.9% saline would also be a reasonable option).

- Place IV access and take bloods as above, including a blood culture.
- Reassess after the bolus for clinical improvement.
- Commence antibiotics (ceftriaxone 80 mg/kg) in view of the fever and irritability.
- If you see clinical improvement after your interventions, you may move on.

Disability (+ Glucose)

- Calculate their AVPU or GCS.
- Ask for a capillary glucose (BM).
  - In this case, the patient is responding to verbal stimuli initially, though you are told this improves after the fluid bolus. Bedside blood sugar is 4.1. You may move on.

Exposure

- Expose the child, looking for rashes, injuries or signs of meningism.
- Inspect and palpate the abdomen for clinical signs.
- Ask for the temperature.
  - In this case, further assessment of the child reveals a blanching rash and stiff neck, suggesting a diagnosis of bacterial meningitis.
  - Appropriate management is to continue IV antibiotics and transfer the patient to an area of high dependency to carefully monitor them systemically and neurologically. This child will probably require a CT scan prior to a lumbar puncture, once they are clinically stable. Steroids may need to be given if the above criteria are met (see Table 7.8.1).

⚠ WARNING

- If parents report a high-pitched or abnormal cry or that their child is irritable and 'not themselves', take these concerns seriously, as they are often very reliable.
- Lumbar puncture is contraindicated in children who have signs of raised intracranial pressure, as there is a potential it could lead to brain herniation, and in children who are clinically unstable. In these cases, the LP should be delayed until the child is stable or a CT scan of the head has been performed.

✓ How to excel in this station

Action	Reason	How
Recognise meningitis.	This allows for early antibiotics and observation of the child in an appropriate setting.	Although signs and symptoms are often vague, the combination of a temperature and irritability must be taken seriously, especially if there are other features of meningism or shock.

✗ Common errors in this station

Common error	Remedy	Reason
Missing signs of shock.	Recognise warning signs of shock—tachycardia, low blood pressure, prolonged CRT.	This is clinically very important to demonstrate you have knowledge of the features of shock and that you can initiate resuscitative measures if they are present. Tachycardia alone in infants and children may have multiple causes, and does not necessarily signify shock.

7 | STATION VARIATION

⭕ Advanced

Shock and meningococcal septicaemia

If there are features suggesting that the child is in shock, especially if there is also a non-blanching rash, the diagnosis of meningococcal septicaemia should be considered. In these cases it is useful to send a meningococcal PCR sample from the blood tests and a clotting sample as this may be deranged. Management involves IV antibiotics as in bacterial meningitis, but these children may also require extensive fluid resuscitation, and potentially inotropic support. Call for help from seniors early as the child may need transfer to an intensive care setting.

Further Reading

Macleod's Clinical Diagnosis, Chapter 18 'Headache', specifically the section 'Any Features of Meningitis?'.

NICE Clinical Guidance, NICE CG102, 'The Management of Bacterial Meningitis and Meningococcal Septicaemia in Children and Young People Younger than 16 years in Primary and Secondary Care' (June 2010). Available at http://www.nice.org.uk.

Index

Note: Page numbers followed by *b* indicate boxes, *f* indicate figures and *t* indicate tables